Handbook of Orthopaedic Trauma

Surgical Management from Admission to Rehabilitation

Edited by

Paul V Fearon FRCS(Tr&Orth) MD
Consultant Orthopaedic Trauma Surgeon
Department of Trauma and Orthopaedic Surgery
Great North Trauma and Emergency Centre
Royal Victoria Infirmary
Newcastle upon Tyne, UK

Andrew Gray MD FRCS
Consultant Trauma and Orthopaedic Surgeon
Department of Trauma and Orthopaedics
James Cook University Hospital
Middlesbrough, UK

Paul Duffy MD FRCS(C)
Division Chief of Orthopaedic Trauma
Foothills Medical Centre
Calgary, Canada

JP medical publishers

London • New Delhi • Panama City

Published by JP Medical Ltd,
83 Victoria Street, London, SW1H 0HW, UK
Tel: +44 (0)20 3170 8910 Fax: +44 (0)20 3008 6180
Email: info@jpmedpub.com Web: www.jpmedpub.com

ISBN: 978-1-909836-15-0

British Library Cataloguing in Publication Data
A catalogue record for this book is available from the British Library

Library of Congress Cataloging in Publication Data
A catalog record for this book is available from the Library of Congress

Publisher:	Richard Furn
Development Editor:	Gavin Smith
Editorial Assistant:	Katie Pattullo
Design:	Designers Collective Ltd

Preface

Handbook of Orthopaedic Trauma has been written to provide practicing trauma and orthopaedic surgeons, at all levels, with a clinically oriented guide to fracture management, setting out practical and reproducible patient management pathways from admission to treatment and rehabilitation.

The format of the chapters will enable the reader to:

- evaluate injury patterns correctly
- identify those fractures that require surgical intervention
- position patients correctly for surgery
- utilize appropriate surgical equipment
- approach and reduce fractures safely
- reduce intraoperative and postoperative complications
- improve patient outcomes

All the chapters are similarly structured in support of the book's goal of focusing on the patient's journey, from admission, evaluation and surgical intervention through to discharge planning and rehabilitation. A unique feature is the inclusion of specially commissioned cadaveric photographs which illustrate the surgical approach to the patient.

Each chapter includes clinical cases depicting real-life scenarios. Corresponding X-rays and CT scans relating to each clinical case are included to demonstrate management options that are reproducible in clinical practice. Throughout the book we have emphasized safe surgical approaches and highlighted common pitfalls to help the reader limit clinical complications, maximize function in the patient and improve overall outcomes.

We have compiled *Handbook of Orthopaedic Trauma* with the assistance of a dedicated team of practicing surgeons from North America and the UK. Whilst it is not all encompassing, we nonetheless hope the book will enable the reader to treat the majority of clinical presentations encountered in fracture management.

Surgical education is continually developing with enhanced knowledge, improvements in equipment and simulated learning for improved practical skills. If this book can be used to improve the clinical outcome for your patients then it will have achieved what it was intended to do.

Paul V Fearon
Andrew Gray
Paul Duffy
August 2017

Acknowledgements

I would like to thank the medical photography department at The Newcastle upon Tyne Hospitals NHS Foundation Trusts, and staff at the Newcastle Surgical Training Centre. And to Kelly, Conall, Isla and Caitlin, for all the times I was too busy. PVF

To my family and friends for their support and to Paul Fearon for involving me in this project. AG

Special thanks to Paul Fearon for leading the charge on this venture and as always to my family, Suzanne, Liam and Robyn for their everlasting support. PD

Contents

Contributors

Stephen E Aldridge MD FRCS(Tr&Orth)
Consultant Trauma and Orthopaedic Surgeon
Department of Trauma and Orthopaedic Surgery
Great North Trauma and Emergency Centre
Royal Victoria Infirmary
Newcastle upon Tyne
UK

Rebecka Asp FRCS(Tr&Orth)
Specialty Trainee, Trauma and Orthopaedics
Wessex Deanery
South Central Strategic Health Authority
Winchester
UK

Richard E Buckley MD FRCS
Professor of Orthopedic Trauma Surgery
Department of Surgery
Foothills Medical Centre
University of Calgary
Calgary, Alberta
Canada

David J Deehan MD DSc FRCS(Tr&Orth)
Professor of Orthopaedic Surgery
Department of Orthopaedic Surgery
Freeman Hospital
Newcastle upon Tyne
UK

Antoine GC de Gheldere MD
Department of Trauma and Orthopaedic Surgery
Great North Children's Hospital
Royal Victoria Infirmary
Newcastle upon Tyne
UK

Nicholas M Desy MD FRCS
Attending Orthopaedic and Trauma Surgeon
Division of Orthopaedic Trauma
Rockyview General Hospital
Calgary, Alberta
Canada

Paul Duffy MD FRCS(C)
Division Chief of Orthopaedic Trauma
Foothills Medical Centre
Calgary, Alberta
Canada

Clive Duncan MB MSc FRCSC
Professor and Emeritus Chair
Department of Orthopaedic Surgery
University of British Columbia
Vancouver, British Columbia
Canada

Paul V Fearon FRCS(Tr&Orth) MD
Consultant Orthopaedic Trauma Surgeon and
Head of Orthopaedic Trauma
Great North Trauma and Emergency Centre
Royal Victoria Infirmary
Newcastle upon Tyne
UK

David Fender FRCS(Tr&Orth)
Consultant Spinal Surgeon
Department of Trauma and Orthopaedic Surgery
Great North Trauma and Emergency Centre
Royal Victoria Infirmary
Newcastle Upon Tyne
UK

Daren P Forward MA FRCS DM
Consultant Orthopaedic Surgeon
Department of Trauma and Orthopaedics
Queen's Medical Centre
Nottingham
UK

Kanishka Milton Ghosh MD FRCS(Tr&Orth)
Consultant Trauma and Orthopaedic Surgeon
Department of Trauma and Orthopaedic Surgery
Great North Trauma and Emergency Centre
Royal Victoria Infirmary
Newcastle Upon Tyne
UK

Andrew Gray MD FRCS
Consultant Trauma and Orthopaedic Surgeon
James Cook University Hospital
Middlesbrough
UK

Nicholas Hancock FRCS(Tr&Orth)
Consultant Trauma and Orthopaedic Surgeon
Department of Trauma and Orthopaedics
University Hospital Southampton
Southampton
UK

Philip Henman FRCS (Tr&Orth)
Consultant Orthopaedic Surgeon
Orthopaedic Department
Royal Victoria Infirmary
Newcastle upon Tyne
UK

James Holland MB ChB FRCS (Orth)
Consultant in Trauma and Orthopaedics
Freeman Hospital, Royal Victoria Infirmary,
Newcastle upon Tyne
UK

Peter Hull FRCS (Tr&Orth) MBChB
Trauma and Orthopaedic Consultant
Division of Trauma and Orthopaedic Surgery
Cambridge University Hospitals NHS Foundation Trust
Cambridge
UK

Phillip Johnston MD FRCS (Tr&Orth)
Consultant Orthopaedic Surgeon, Associate Lecturer
Department of Orthopaedics
Cambridge University Hospitals NHS Trust
Cambridge
UK

Alan Johnstone FRCSEd(Orth)
Professor and Consultant Trauma and Orthopaedic Surgeon
Orthopaedic Trauma Unit
Aberdeen Royal Infirmary
Aberdeen
UK

Mike Kelly MBBS MD FRCS (Tr&Orth)
Consultant Orthopaedic Surgeon
Orthopaedic Department
North Bristol NHS Trust
Bristol
UK

Charlotte P Lewis MBBS MRCS FRCS(Tr&Orth)
Consultant Orthopaedic Trauma Surgeon
Queen Alexandra Hospital
Portsmouth
UK

George Mataliotakis MD
Senior Spinal Fellow
Spinal Surgery Department
Salford Royal – NHS Foundation Trust
Salford
UK

Ben J Ollivere
Clinical Associate Professor
University of Nottingham
Honorary Consultant Orthopaedic and Major Trauma Surgeon
Queens Medical Centre
Nottingham
UK

Nigel D Rossiter FRCSEd(Tr&Orth) FFSTEd
Consultant Trauma and Orthopaedic Surgeon
Basingstoke & North Hampshire Hospital
Basingstoke
UK

Omar Sabri FRCS(Tr&Orth)
Consultant Trauma and Orthopaedic Surgeon
Department of Orthopaedics and Trauma
St George's University Hospitals
London
UK

Faiz Shivji BMBS BMedSci MRCS (Eng)
Specialist Registrar, Trauma and Orthopaedics
Department of Trauma and Orthopaedics
Queen's Medical Centre
Nottingham
UK

Iain Stevenson MbCHb FRCS (TR & Orth)
Consultant Trauma and Orthopaedic Surgeon
Department of Trauma and Orthopaedic Surgery
Aberdeen Royal Infirmary and Woodend Hospital
Aberdeen
UK

Neil White MD FRCS
Clinical Lecturer
University of Calgary
South Health Campus
Calgary, Alberta
Canada

John Williams MA(Oxon) DM(Oxon) FRCS(Orth)
Consultant Orthopaedic Trauma Surgeon
Great North Trauma and Emergency Centre
Royal Victoria Infirmary
Newcastle upon Tyne
UK

Grace CK Yip MA MB/BChir MRCS
Trauma and Orthopaedic Specialty Registrar
Cambridge University Hospitals NHS Foundation Trust
Cambridge
UK

1 Clavicle fractures

Faiz Shivji, Ben J Ollivere

Introduction

Clavicle fractures are sustained usually as the results of high energy trauma and may be associated with severe injury to the chest wall or shoulder. At one end of the spectrum fixation of the clavicle may be part of the management of other complex injuries (such as scapula-thoracic disassociation, floating shoulders or chest wall trauma), while at the other end isolated sporting injuries may require fixation to maximize postoperative function.

Incidence

The clavicle is the most commonly injured bone in the shoulder girdle accounting for nearly half of these injuries, but representing just 2.5% of fractures seen in clinical practice. Most commonly seen as middle third fractures (accounting for around 80% of fractures) the anatomical position of the fracture lines in relation to the stabilizing acromioclavicular, sternoclavicular and coracoclavicular ligaments is essential in determining optimum treatment.

High energy clavicle fractures have a propensity for nonunion, and secondary migration and displacement. Patients sustaining high energy clavicle fractures should be followed up with interval radiographs if the decision is made to treat them nonoperatively. In the vast majority of cases clavicle fractures will heal with conservative management although rates of nonunion are appreciable and higher in those with high energy injuries.

Mechanism of injury

The vast majority of clavicle fractures are the result of a direct blow to the shoulder, usually on the super-lateral aspect. Commonly sustained during contact sports or higher energy falls (such as from a horse) these are usually isolated injuries and can be treated in the outpatient setting. Higher energy fracture patterns are associated with seat belt injuries in road traffic accidents and traction injuries to the arm. These injuries may be associated with other injuries including neurovascular, and concomitant chest wall or shoulder fractures. Although originally described as occurring as the result of a fall to an outstretched hand, this is a less common mechanism of injury but is commonly associated with clavicle fractures in the elderly.

Initial management/ prioritization

The patient is reviewed in accordance with Advanced Trauma Life Support (ATLS) protocol if the injury is a result of a high-energy mechanism of injury. Evaluation of patients for surgery should include exclusion of neurovascular injury to the shoulder girdle, exclusion of other fractures and a weight bearing anteroposterior (AP) radiograph. Many patients managed in the resuscitation room are imaged supine, which can give a false impression of an undisplaced fracture.

Considerations for surgery

Midshaft fractures

The majority of midshaft clavicular fractures can be treated either operatively or nonoperatively. There have been a number of recent large multicenter randomized controlled trials that favor operative intervention in certain groups. Patients with displaced higher energy midshaft clavicular fractures have been shown to have improved functional outcomes and fewer complications when treated nonoperatively. Indications for surgical intervention can include significant displacement, associated requisite vascular or neurological repair, penetration of the deltoprapezial fascia or can be associated with floating shoulder or chest wall injuries (e.g. rib fractures, flail chest). Although surgery carries with it risks including brachial plexus and vascular injuries, it should be considered in patients with risk factors for nonunion.

Lateral fractures

Lateral clavicle fractures have higher rates of nonunion due to the deforming forces of the shoulder girdle and gravity. Patients with displaced fractures in which the coracoclavicular ligaments are not functioning to reduce the fracture should be considered for plate fixation ideally with augmentation of the coracoclavicular ligaments or with a hook plate.

Medial fractures

Medial fractures or fracture dislocations of the medial clavicular physis should be treated with a sling if anteriorly displaced. However, if driven posteriorly into the chest cavity they should be stabilized after open reduction to avoid injury to or compression of the mediastinal structures.

Case example: Diaphyseal clavicle fracture

A fit and well male cyclist came off his bike while racing, sustaining a closed displaced clavicle fracture (**Figure 1.1**). This was an isolated injury. Following discussion of the treatment options he elected for surgical fixation, hoping to limit his absence from sport. Postoperative X-rays (**Figure 1.2**) show the results, using the principles of absolute stability.

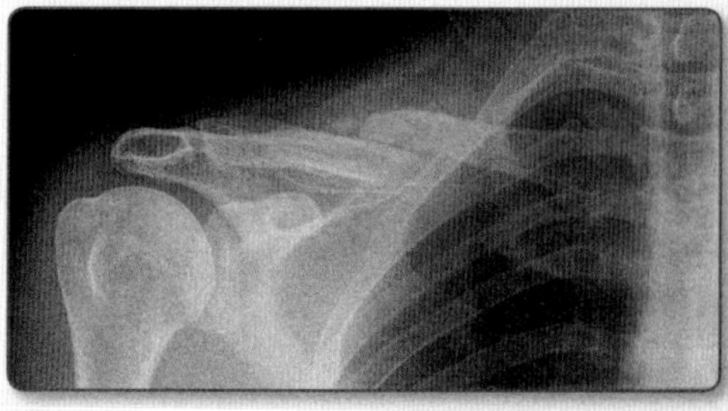

Figure 1.1 Anteroposterior X-ray of the patient's displaced right diaphyseal clavicle fracture.

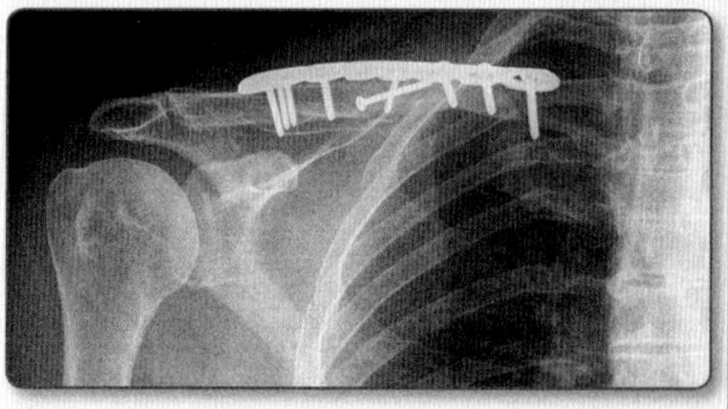

Figure 1.2 Postoperative X-ray of the fracture reduced and fixed with interfragmentary lag screws before an anterior plate is applied.

Theater layout and patient positioning

Optimal access is achieved to the majority of clavicle fractures with the patient positioned supine on a carbon fiber table with a small sandbag between the shoulders. Although many surgeons perform surgery in the beach chair position this tends to displace the fracture, whilst positioning supine will tend to reduce the fracture. The patients head should be turned away and positioned on a headring (positioning the endotracheal tube away from the operated side). This allows for unrestricted access of the whole length of the clavicle (**Figure 1.3**).

For posteriorly displaced sternoclavicular joint dislocations or medial physeal fractures the use of the carbon fiber table also allows vascular access and the positioning of an endoluminal balloon prior to reduction, in case of significant bleeding.

Review of surgical approaches

The anterior approach is the workhorse approach for clavicle fixation (**Figure 1.4a**).

Anterior approach

The skin incision should not be undermined and the clavicle exposed directly under the claviopectoral fascia (**Figure 1.4b**). The small supraclavicular sensory nerves innervate the upper-outer quadrant of the breast and should be preserved if possible.

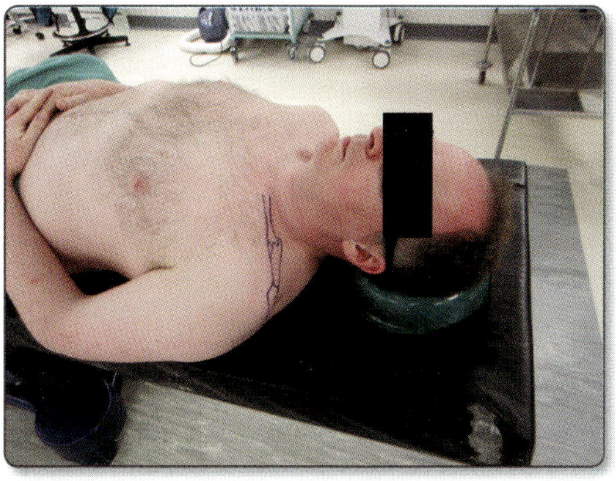

Figure 1.3 Clinical setup. Patient supine with head on head ring, allowing the image intensifier to come from the contralateral side or from the top end.

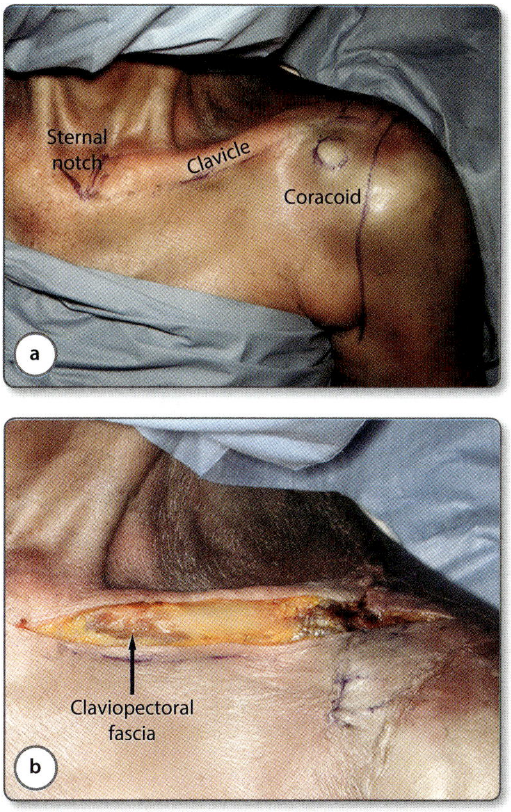

Figure 1.4 (a) Surgical surface anatomy of clavicular area. (b) Surgical exposure of clavicle.

Equipment requirements

- Radiolucent table and small sandbag
- Pre-contoured clavicle plates
- Separate lag screws (either 3.5 mm or 2.7 mm screws)
- Small fracture reduction clamps
- Large see through hip/DHS fracture drape (so the head and eyes can be visualized and protected throughout the surgery)

Reduction and stabilization methods

Diaphyseal fractures are easiest to reduce with the patient supine on a carbon fiber table.

A simple fracture pattern such as this can be approached directly, and anatomically reduced. Reduction is best achieved with small Tulloch brown reduction forceps.

If fixation is delayed by even a few days release of the periosteum on the under surface of the clavicle is recommended and can be easily achieved under direct vision with a periosteal elevator. This reduces the risk of traction injury to the nerves or vessels.

Placement of one or two 3.5 mm or 2.7 mm lag screws will secure the fixation and allow neutralization with a plate.

The clavicle is subject to significant torsional and bending forces. The use of thicker dynamic compressive plate (DCP) or pre-contoured plates is preferred to reconstruction or other plate types to reduce the rates and incidence of metalwork failure. Care should be taken with shortened or older fractures to free the under-surface of the clavicle prior to fracture reduction to avoid traction on the brachial plexus.

Lateral fractures can often be better approached with a bra-strap incision as these are often driven posteriorly and access for either a suture anchor or tape around the coracoid is best effected with an anterior-posterior bra-strap incision.

The use of 2.7 mm lag screws for simple fracture patterns with small butterfly or other fragments can often improve fixation and improve the application of plates.

The 'S' bend on the clavicle varies in arc of curvature from patient to patient and on occasion the reversal of the contralateral pre-contoured plate can give a better fit than the 'intended' side.

Plates can be contoured to the anterior clavicle and resist the deforming forces better in this orientation, however, care should be taken to avoid too much soft tissue stripping and medial screws are heading directly toward the subclavian vein.

Case example: Medial fracture

A man playing rugby sustained a direct blow to the medial end of his clavicle (**Figure 1.5a**). A CT scan was organized which shows the clavicle to be abutting and indenting the great vessels (**Figure 1.5b**).

Surgery in this case was undertaken in conjunction with interventional radiologists and vascular surgeons who can place a balloon in the aortic arch in case of significant hemorrhage when the clavicle is reduced. Facilities and instruments are available for an emergency thoracotomy should this be required.

The patient is placed supine on a carbon fiber table and accessed gained through the groin to the aortic arch and an uninflated balloon placed under fluoroscopic guidance endovascularly adjacent to the fractured ends.

A direct approach to the medial clavicle is undertaken and the mediastinum entered under direct vision. The clavicle is carefully mobilized and reduced under direct vision.

Application of two 2.7 plates to the superior and anterior surface of the medial clavicle with lateral screws applied first as buttress plates (**Figure 1.5c**). Care should be taken not to penetrate the medial surface of the manubrium when inserting the medial screws.

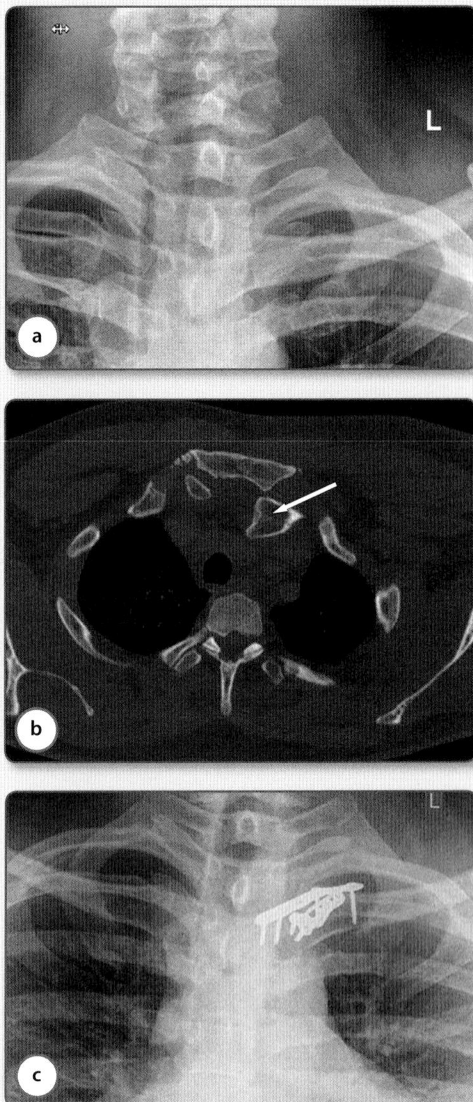

Figure 1.5 (a) Anteroposterior X-ray following rugby injury to medial end of left clavicle. (b) Axial CT image of displaced posterior medial end of clavicle with compression of great vessels. (c) Postoperative X-ray of reduced and plated medial clavicle dislocation.

Rehabilitation

Rehabilitation should be active early mobilization, with little time in a sling. Patients should avoid contact sports until sound union has occurred (usually 3 months). Initial range of motion exercises and active assisted shoulder rehabilitation should be undertaken from day 1 postoperatively but weight bearing should be avoided for 3 weeks.

Avoiding postoperative complications

Care should be taken with drilling as injury to the subclavian vein, artery and brachial plexus are well-described complications. When performing fixation sub-acutely (after 7 days) the complication rates from traction injuries are higher and careful mobilization of the clavicle prior to reduction can reduce these rates.

When addressing lateral clavicle fractures the fixation should be augmented with either a hook plate or a coracoclavicular ligament reconstruction (with either a suture anchor or Surgilig).

Summary of learning points

- Tailor patient management to clinical situation and fracture pattern
- In the poly trauma patient, surgical fixation may be necessary for progression of mobility and rehabilitation
- Careful surgical dissection with limited soft tissue stripping of bony fragments

Further reading

Canadian Orthopaedic Trauma Society. Non-operative treatment compared with plate fixation of displaced mid-shaft clavicular fractures. A multicenter randomized clinical trial. Bone Joint Surg Am 2007; 89:1–10.

Robinson CM. Fractures of the clavicle in the adult. Epidemiology and classification. J Bone Joint Surg Br 1998; 80:476–484.

Robinson CM, Goudie EB, Murray IR, et al. Open reduction and plate fixation versus nonoperative treatment for displaced midshaft clavicular fractures: a multicenter, randomized, controlled trial. J Bone Joint Surg Am 2013; 95:1576–1584.

Sambandam B, Gupta R, Kumar S, Maini L. Fracture of distal end clavicle: A review. J Clin Orthop Trauma 2014; 5:65–73.

Sidhu VS, Hermans D, Duckworth DG. The operative outcomes of displaced medial-end clavicle fractures. J Shoulder Elbow Surg 2015; 24:1728–1734.

2 Scapula fractures

Stephen E Aldridge, Paul V Fearon

Introduction

Extra-articular scapular fractures can be managed nonoperatively with sling support, analgesia and early active assisted physiotherapy to maintain movement.

Incidence

Scapula fractures account for 3–5% of all shoulder girdle fractures. When scapular fractures are secondary to major trauma, associated injuries can include the following: chest injuries (rib fractures, flail chest, pneumothorax, pulmonary contusion etc.), clavicle fractures (floating shoulder), spine fractures, intra-abdominal injuries (spleen, liver, etc.), and lower limb fractures. Scapula fractures affect different parts of the bone (**Figure 2.1**).

Mechanism of injury

The majority of younger patients have a history of a high-energy injury, such as motor vehicle crashes, fall from height, etc. Although less common, intra-articular fractures in isolation can occur in the elderly following a fall from standing height.

Initial management/ prioritization

Advanced Trauma Life Support (ATLS) assessment takes priority, including the assessment of pulmonary function, followed by careful assessment of soft tissue status and upper limb neurology (brachial plexus examination). The vast majority of extra-articular fractures can be managed nonoperatively with splintage, analgesia and rehabilitation.

Considerations for surgery

The main indications include intra-articular involvement of the glenoid in functionally active patients. Glenoid fracture displacement can result in secondary glenohumeral subluxation-dislocation. Fractures affecting 25% of the anterior glenoid fossa or 33% of the posterior fossa may result in instability with resultant pain and instability. Younger patients with rim fractures may also develop instability. Other

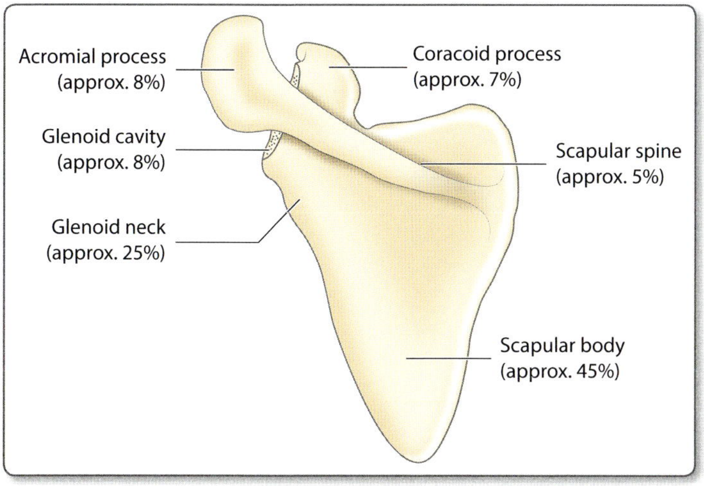

Figure 2.1 Scapula fracture locations.

considerations for operative intervention involve scapula fractures with double displacement of the superior suspensory complex of the shoulder (such as with clavicle fracture or AC joint disruption 'floating shoulder pattern').

X-rays and supplementary CT scans are used for fracture evaluation and pattern description.

Theater layout and patient positioning

A proposed theater set up and lay out is illustrated in **Figure 2.6a**. Positioning the patient in such a manner allows free movement of the ipsilateral arm to aid in fracture reduction, and if necessary

Case example: Scapula fracture with intra-articular gleaned involvement

A 28-year-old man sustained direct shoulder blade trauma, by running into a wall while playing indoor five-a-side football (**Figure 2.2**). He underwent ATLS assessment before being referred to the receiving orthopaedic team. To better assess the fractured pattern a CT scan was undertaken (**Figure 2.3**). This shows the displaced posteriorly located interarticular glenoid fracture. This was approached via a classical Judet approach. The medial border of the scapular was reduced initially, before 3 mm Schanz pins were inserted into separate articular fragments and reduced and held with the application of a mini-external fixture (**Figure 2.4**). Supplementary stabilizing k-wires can then be inserted as necessary, before definitive stabilization with appropriately sized plates, i.e. 3.5 mm reconstructive plate on medial border and 2.7 mm plates on posterior articular gleaned surface (**Figure 2.5**).

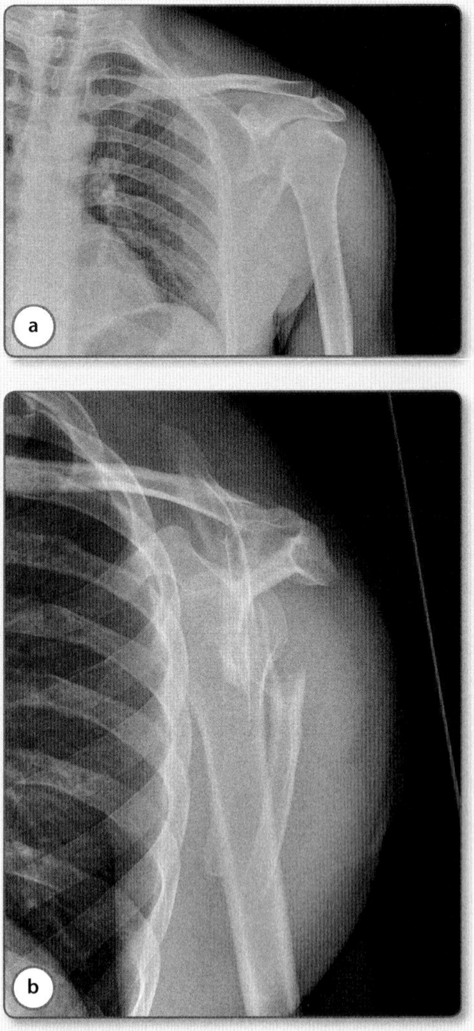

Figure 2.2 (a, b) Anteroposterior and scapula Y view X-rays of left shoulder region, showing intra-articular left scapula fracture.

Case example: *continued.*

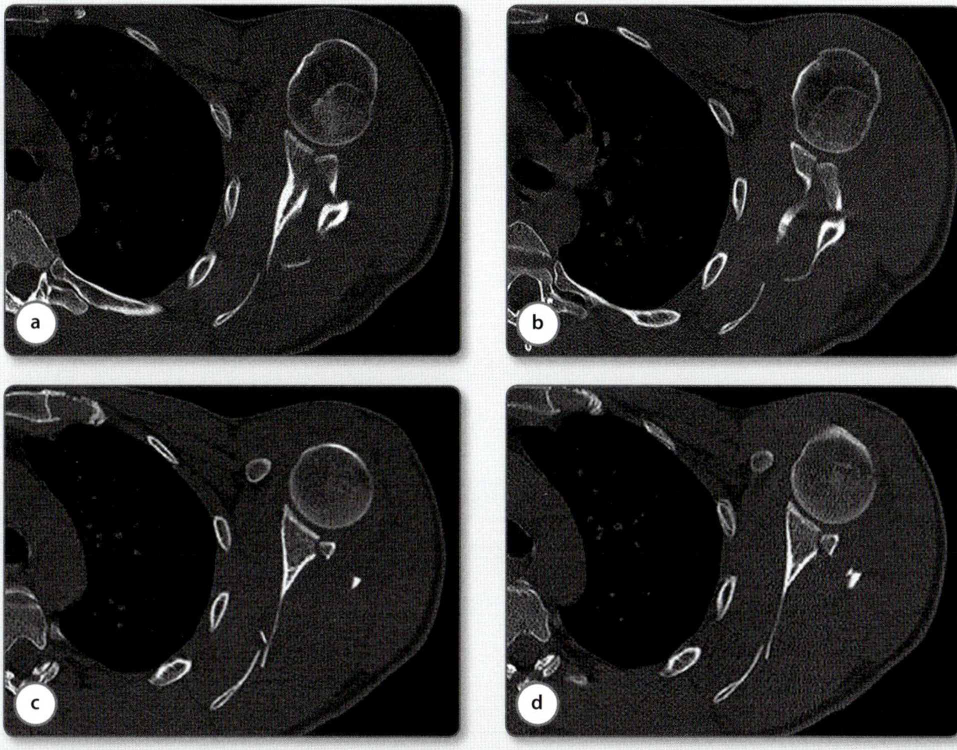

Figure 2.3 (a–d) Axial CT scan images from proximal to distal showing a displaced posterior glenoid fracture fragment with extra-articular blade component.

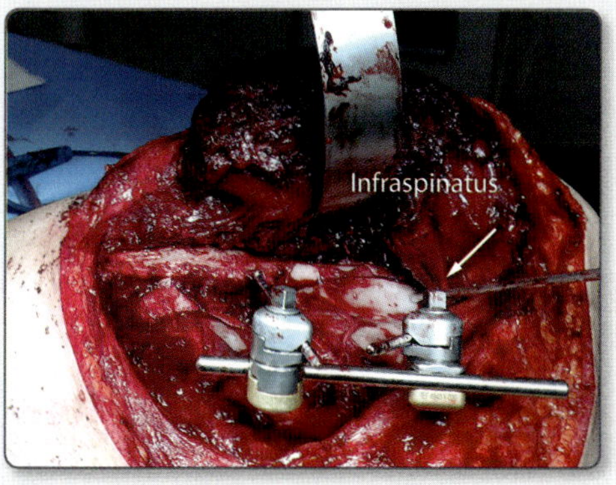

Figure 2.4 Temporary reduction with mini-external fixator. 3 mm Schanz screws are inserted with T-handles and joy-sticked into position before temporary K-wire fixation and construction of the external fixator. The Deaver retractor holds the infraspinatus and the suprascapular neurovascular bundle is identified and protected (white arrow).

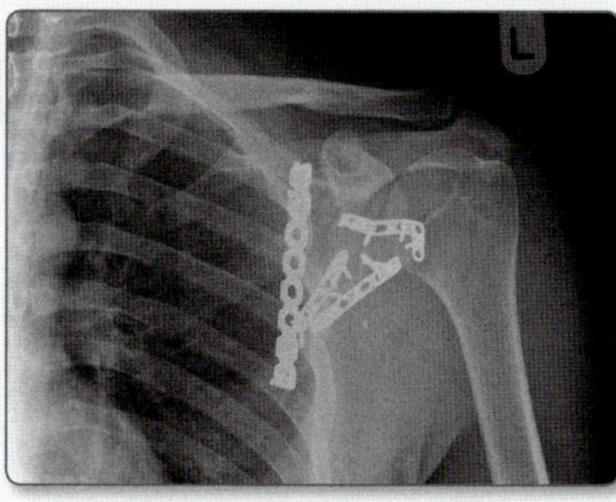

Figure 2.5 Postoperative check X-ray. Medial border 3.5 mm reconstruction plate, with laterally placed 2.7 mm wrist plates.

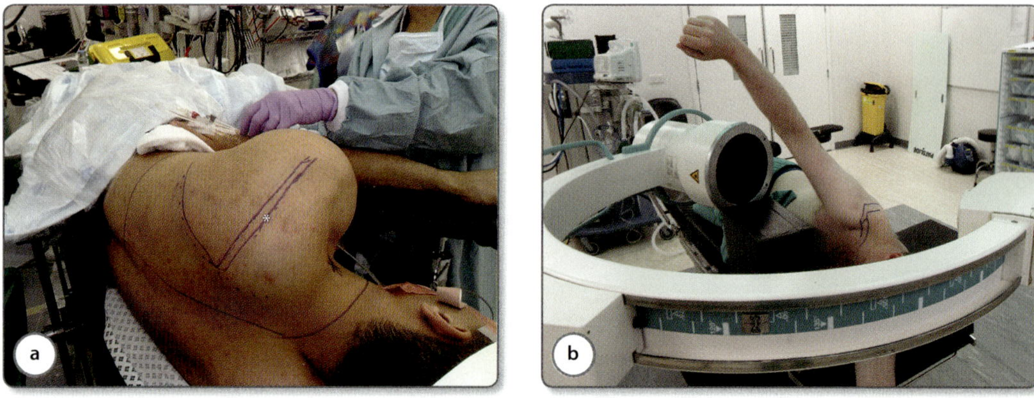

Figure 2.6 (a) Lateral positioning of patient with free draping of injured arm, supported on arm gutter or foam block to allow movement of the glenohumeral joint during surgery. This patient set up is for posterior approaches to the scapula, but it also allows anterior clavicle access if necessary (* scapula spine). (b) Set up with image intensifier to obtain intra-operative X-ray views.

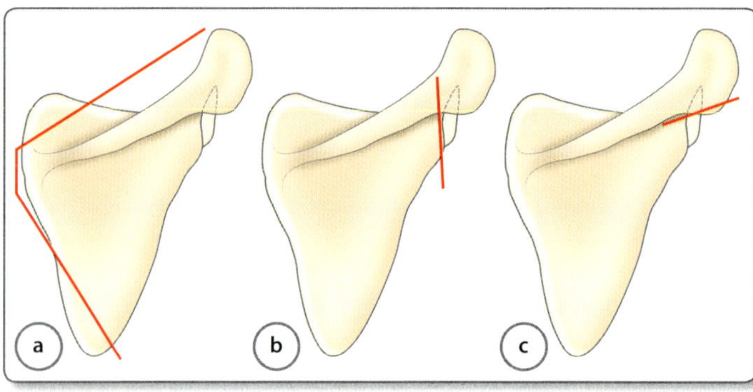

Figure 2.7 (a–c) Possible skin incisions for classical Judet approach and limited exposures (unless dealing with an isolated posterior glenoid fracture it is recommended to undertake the L-shaped approach as this is the only extensile approach).

allows anterior access to the clavicle for fixation, while still allowing X-rays to be obtained intraoperatively.

Review of surgical approaches

Options will depend upon fracture configuration:

Classical Judet approach

- This is a good approach for body and neck fractures, particularly if there has been a delay to surgery as can debride all callous that has developed. Not as good for intra-articular viewing as the suprascapular nerve (SSN) limits the extent of lateral extension
- Lateral or prone position, with free arm drape and support
- Check X-rays prior to prepping pre-preparation and draping of patient to ensure intraoperative X-rays can be obtained [requiring anteroposterior (AP) and axillary views]
- Make skin incision along scapula spine and curved inferiorly along medial aspect (boomerang type incision; **Figure 2.7a**)
- Elevate medial aspect of deltoid off the scapula spine and reflect superolaterally as necessary (**Figure 2.8a**)
- Mobilize infraspinatus from the medial scapula border and reflect it on its neurovascular bundle passing from the

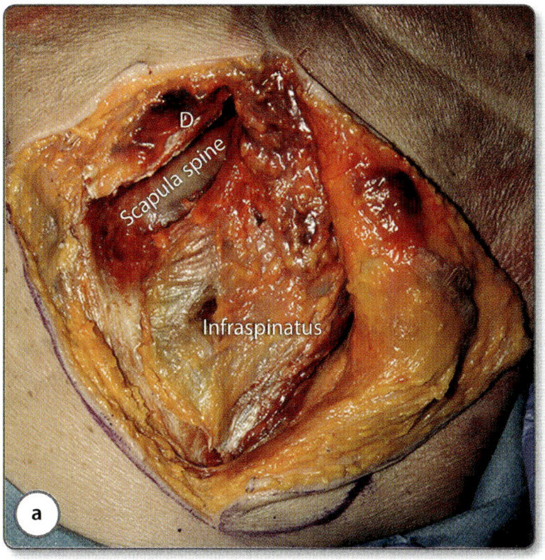

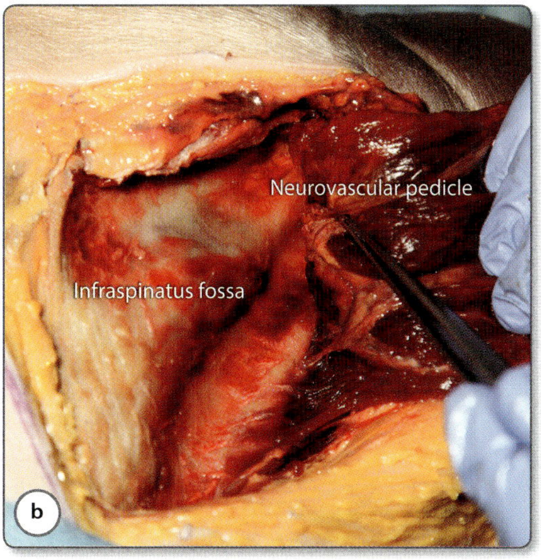

Figure 2.8 (a) Elevation of deltoid (D) from the scapular spine giving access to the infraspinatus muscle belly. (b) Infraspinatus elevated from posteromedial scapular border, maintaining neurovascular pedicle, giving access to posterior glenoid.

spinoglenoid notch. Elevation off the posterior scapular surface, gives access to the infraspinous fossa and posterior aspect of the glenoid (**Figure 2.8b**). Care and attention is required when handling the neurovascular pedicle and muscle mass

Infraspinatus splitting approach

- The skin incision for the classical Judet approach can be utilized, again with release of the deltoid off the scapular spine as necessary. Otherwise a more limited vertical or horizontal incision centered on the posterior glenoid neck can be utilized (**Figure 2.10b** and **2.10c**). The approach is between the two heads of infraspinatus (**Figure 2.9**)
- Good for posterior glenoid fractures (less good for body or neck fractures)
- Exposure greater than 1.5 cm medially to the glenoid is to be avoided due to the increased risk of damage to the SSN

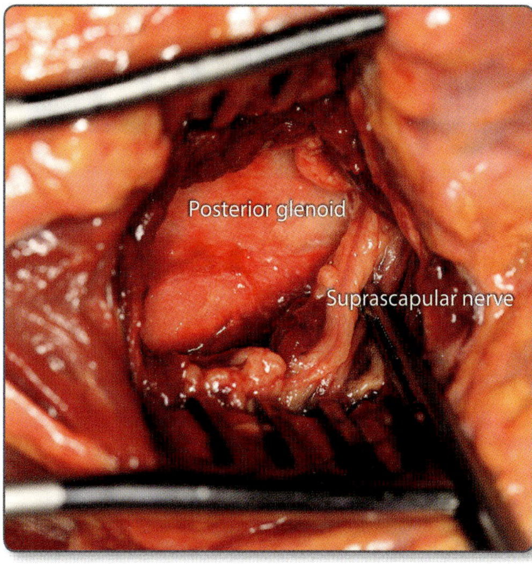

Figure 2.9 Infraspinatus splitting approach; suprascapular nerve identified.

Interval infraspinatus and teres minor approach

- Similarly to the infraspinatus splitting approach, variable skin incisions can be utilised (**Figure 2.7 a-c**)
- Good for posterior glenoid and scapular neck fractures, and can use windows to get to the body if necessary
- Develop laterally the interval between infraspinatus superiorly and teres minor inferiorly

- Ligate the ascending branch of the circumflex scapular artery. This approach gives access to the lateral scapular border and can be used for indirect reduction of glenoid fractures

Deltopectoral approach

- Position patient supine or in beach chair
- Good for anterior glenoid fractures
- Ensure intraoperative X-rays obtainable before standard preparation and draping
- Identify coracoid and make skin incision in interval over deltopectoral region (**Figure 2.10a**)
- Identify cephalic vein and retract either medially or laterally depending on vascular tributaries. This will allow access to subscapularis (**Figure 2.10b**) following division of the clavipectoral fascia
- Carefully dissect subscapularis off the underlying joint capsule, using stay sutures for later repair. Do not dissect inferiorly to subscapularis due to axillary nerve being at risk
- Make a separate vertical capsulotomy, allowing visualization of the anterior glenoid region for reduction and fixation (**Figure 2.10c**).

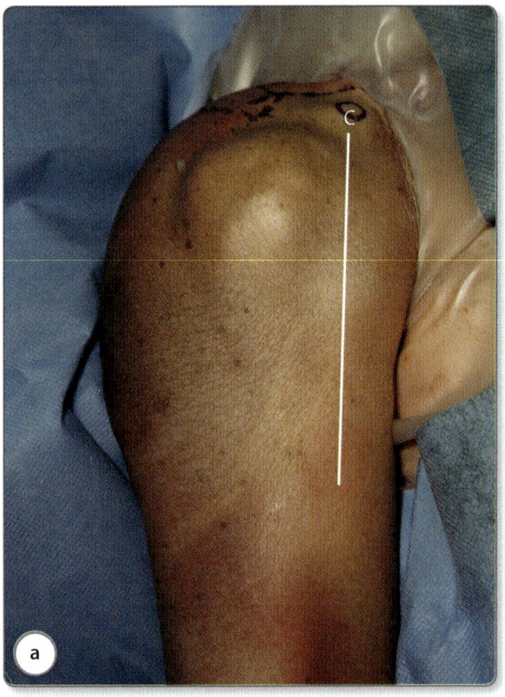

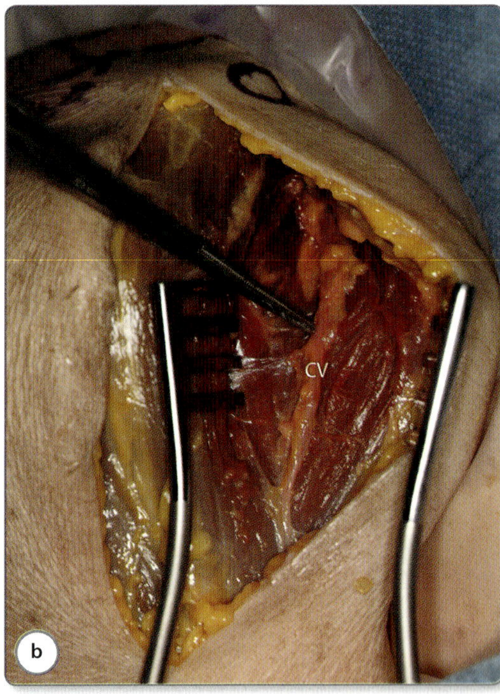

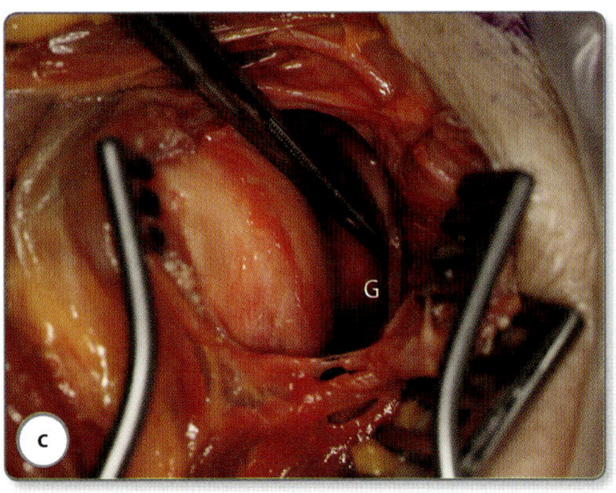

Figure 2.10 (a) Skin incision marked (C, coracoid process). (b) Deltopectoral interval opened with protection and lateral retraction of cephalic vein, giving access to subscapularis. Use of self-retaining retractors necessary to aid exposure. (c) Stay sutures can be placed in subscapularis and capsule to aid retraction-access and for later repair. Glenoid (G) visualized in depth of approach.

Separating the subscapularis from the capsule allows the fracture fragment to be mobilized and fixed extra-articularly, whereas if the capsule and subscapularis are divided as one layer the reduction and fixation must be made within the joint, which might lead to difficulty positioning screws. Visualization of the glenoid is aided by the use of Fukuda retractor.

An alternative approach to the glenoid is to split the subscapularis muscle medial to the tendon at the junction between the upper two-thirds and lower one-third. The muscle is elevated off the glenoid neck with a swab, and the tendon incised laterally if the glenoid rim is not visible. This gives a direct view onto the fracture, and a capsulotomy is made in line of the fibers at the level of the fracture to allow visualizition of the joint surface for anatomical fixation. This is a useful approach if there is concerns about tenotomizing the subscapularis (e.g. in the presence of associated proximal humeral fracture). Gelpey retractors are useful for this approach as are short K-wires into the neck to hold the subscapularis fibers apart.

Equipment requirements

This depends on institution availability and the surgeon's preference. In the majority of cases, the following are utilized:

- Small fragment and minifragment sets
- Anatomical plates/locking options
- K-wires
- Reduction clamps
- Retractors: Gelpi self retainers/Deaver
- Mini-external fixator as reduction aid
- Cannulated screw set

Reduction and stabilization methods

Often reduction of the medial and lateral scapular borders initially aids in the reduction of the posterior glenoid fracture. A combination of clamps, K-wires or a mini external fixator can be used initially (**Figure 2.4**), before definitive fixation, with appropriately sized plates.

In a case of anterior glenoid fracture the fragment is often smaller than that in the posterior glenoid fractures, and can also be fragmented. It is useful in these situations to use screws placed on the medial border of the fragments with washers buttressing against the fragments. As the capsular attachment is usually still attached to the fragment the rotation stability of the fragment is re-gained gained once the capsule is reattached. The use of a Dewar's or Bristow instrument can lever the fragment into its fracture bed utilizing the intact periosteum/capsule to hold it stable whilst wires are inserted.

Rehabilitation

Request physiotherapy review and input when surgical wounds are satisfactory.

- Rest in poly sling device initially
- No heavy lifting until fracture union
- Passive range of motion exercises building up to active assisted and active as symptoms and serial X-rays allow

Avoiding postoperative complications

The most common postoperative complications are listed below, along with techniques to reduce their incidence.

- Infection/wound healing complications:
  - Careful soft tissue handling
  - Prescription of antibiotics
  - Attention to hemostasis intraoperatively
  - Avoidance of hematoma formation in infraspinatus fossa if using classical Judet approach (consider suction drain for 24 hours postoperatively)
- Infraspinatus and deltoid detachment from bony attachment. Reattachment of infraspinatus/deltoid via nonabsorbable transosseous sutures
- Neurovascular damage:
  - Careful soft tissue handling when mobilizing infraspinatus on its pedicle
  - The SSN may be trapped in the fracture, and needs to be identified before fracture reduction
  - Careful retraction of conjoint tendon medially to avoid musculocutaneous nerve damage

- Care when dissecting along inferior border of subscapularis to avoid damage to the axillary nerve
- Loss of reduction:
  - Thorough review of CT scans with accurate surgical planning and approach
  - Stable fixation of fracture components
- Post-traumatic stiffness:
  - Accurate joint reconstruction with stable fixation allowing early protected physiotherapy

Summary of learning points

- It may be necessary to initially reduce the medial border in order to attend to the lateral and intra-articular components, when using posterior approaches
- Radiolucent table with radiolucent blocks allowing support of ipsilateral arm and clear image intensifier images
- Appropriate equipment selection to aid surgery
- The SSN may be trapped in fracture components

Further reading

Cole PA, Gauger EM, Schroder LK. Management of scapular fractures. J Am Acad Orthop Surg March 2012; 20:130–141.

Cole PA, Gauger EM, Herrera DA, Anavian J, Tarkin IS. Radiographic follow-up of 84 operatively treated scapula neck and body fractures. Injury 2012; 43:327–333.

Edwards SG, Whittle AP, Wood GW. Nonoperative treatment of ipsilateral fractures of the scapula and clavicle. J Bone Joint Surg Am 2000; 82:774–780.

Ideberg R, Grevsten S, Larsson S. Epidemiology of scapular fractures Incidence and classification of 338 fractures. Acta Orthop Scand 1995; 66:395–397.

Jeray KJ, Cole PA. Clavicle and scapula fracture problems: functional assessment and current treatment strategies. Instr Course Lect 2011; 60:51–71.

Nordqvist A, Petersson C. Fracture of the body, neck, or spine of the scapula. A long-term follow-up study. Clin Orthop Relat Res 1992; 283:139–144.

3 Proximal humerus fractures

Stephen E Aldridge

Introduction

Proximal humeral fractures are common injuries, which are often difficult to manage and frequently cause long-term dysfunction of the arm due to stiffness and pain. Treatment aims are to enable early movement and to reduce the stiffness.

Incidence

Proximal humerus fractures account for 5% of all fractures. When these fractures are secondary to major trauma, associated injuries can include the following: chest injuries, ipsilateral upper limb injuries, spine fractures, intra-abdominal injuries and lower limb fractures. However, the vast majority of these fractures are the result of simple falls in older osteoporotic patients.

Mechanism of injury

The majority of younger patients have a history of a high-energy injury, or shoulder dislocation. Common associated injuries in this situation are of dislocation of the shoulder, glenoid fracture, and neurovascular injury, particularly of the axillary nerve and artery.

Initial management

Advance Trauma Life Support (ATLS) assessment takes priority, including the assessment of pulmonary function, followed by careful assessment of soft tissue status and upper limb neurology with particular attention to the axillary nerve and vascular supply.

Preoperative workup

- General assessment for surgery
- Neurovascular assessment
- Radiological review [anteroposterior (AP) of glenohumeral joint, scapula-Y and modified trauma axial, if tolerated]
- CT scan if necessary (assessment of fracture configuration, glenoid involvement and metaphyseal extension)

Considerations for surgery

The general health and functional expectations of the patient are the primary consideration for surgery. There are very few absolute indications for surgery, such as open fractures or vascular compromise, both of which are rare. That being the case there is no significant emergency for surgery, and the treatment can be considered and discussed with and if necessary referred to a specialist upper limb surgeon, whilst the patient is immobilized in a sling. Delay for a significant period, however, may lead to more difficult surgery and worse outcomes, as the tuberosities start to heal in situ, and the cuff muscles become less compliant, and the subdeltoid space hematoma starts to organize quickly. It is my experience that leaving these fractures for more than 2 weeks affects the long-term outcome.

Indications for surgery in patients who are fit for surgery and have the functional requirement for independent living are based on the displacement of the fragments and the stability of the fracture. Undisplaced fractures can be treated nonoperatively. Isolated, displaced tuberosity fractures, which are essentially avulsion fractures as part of a dislocation episode, need to be fixed surgically (undisplaced tuberosity fractures require close observation with regular X-rays as they can displace due to the pull of the cuff insertion). In the absence of a dislocation, be aware that an 'isolated' tuberosity fracture is unusual and is likely to have an associated surgical neck fracture and/or lesser tuberosity fracture. Surgical neck fractures tolerate significant displacement well, such that they are likely to heal if bony contact between the two fragments is maintained. These can frequently be managed in a collar and cuff sling, with physiotherapy to start early passive movement. Three and four part fractures are combinations of the above fracture patterns. Three-part fractures typically involve the surgical neck and greater tuberosity and treatment is based on the

Case example: Four-part humeral fracture

A 39-year-old man fell from 100 feet, landing in mud. He was assessed in the emergency department under the ATLS principles and on secondary survey, which included a whole-body CT scan, was found to have stable thoracic spine fractures, rib fractures and a multi-fragmentary proximal four-part humeral fracture (**Figure 3.1**). Further assessment of the shoulder revealed a closed neurologically normal limb with no vascular compromise. The shoulder was contused but the soft tissues were healthy. He was immobilized in a sling for comfort, and his other injuries were assessed before considering the treatment options. Postoperative radiographs in **Figure 3.2** show the result of treatment by humeral nail fixation.

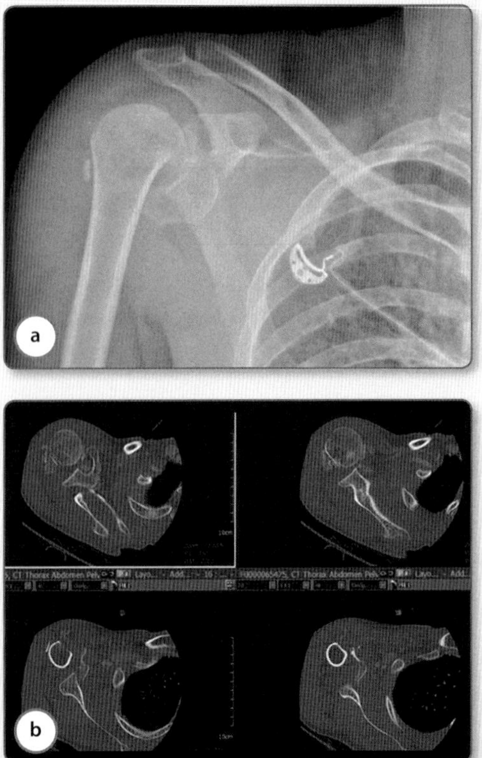

Figure 3.1 (a) Anteroposterior view of right shoulder region. (b) Axial CT scans of four-part proximal humerus fracture.

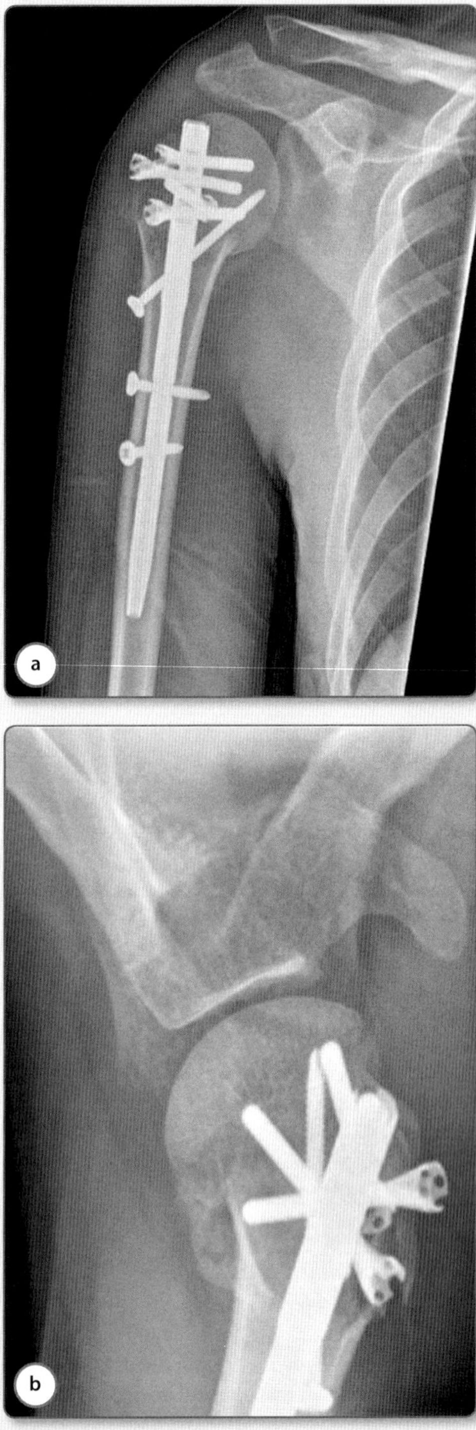

Figure 3.2 Humeral nail fixation of four-part proximal humerus fracture.

displacement of the tuberosity or humeral head. Three-part fractures should have a blood supply maintained to the humeral head through the soft tissue attachment of the associated nonfractured tuberosity, and so should be amenable to fixation. Four-part fractures by definition have displacement of the tuberosities such that the blood supply to the humeral head may be compromised. The exception to this is the valgus impacted fracture, where the capsular attachment of the medial 'hinge' inferiorly is intact between the humeral head and shaft, with the periosteal vessels able to maintain the blood supply. Thus, valgus impacted fractures may be fixable if at the time of surgery this soft tissue attachment is intact. For other four-part fractures consideration between fixation versus replacement should be entertained. In younger patients maintaining the native humeral head even with a chance of avascular necrosis is better than replacement, in the long term.

Review of treatment options

Nonoperative

Radiological review of the injury looking for displacement of the constituent parts is undertaken. Assessment of the patients' functional demands and fitness for surgery is also considered. Depending upon the above two components a treatment option is then undertaken.

Frequently deciding between the benefits of surgical treatment and conservative treatment are difficult. The PROximal Fracture of the Humerus: Evaluation by Randomisation (ProFHER) trial has shown that if there is no clear indication for surgery then conservative treatment is best.

Open reduction and internal fixation

Suture fixation or screw fixation

Isolated tuberosity fractures are avulsion fractures and often have a shell of bone attached to the rotator cuff tendon, these are usually simple to reduce, and 'key-in' to the bed of the fracture on the humerus. Fixing them can be difficult as the bone can fracture with screw fixation. Alternatives include tension band fixation. My preferred method is to suture the tuberosity with trans tendinous sutures passed through drill holes in a cruciform arrangement (**Figure 3.3**).

Plate fixation

Over the last 10 years the advent of locking plates has led to an increase interest in fixing these fractures as the angular stable screws give greater stability to the construct. This hasn't been without its problems; with the risk of osteoporotic bone collapsing over the screws leading to a significant risk of screw penetration into the joint. Thus, what was thought to be the answer to this complex injury still leaves problems. Using a plate to fix the fracture, is able to control the humeral head and shaft fragments well, but the tuberosity fragments may not be captured fully by the array of screws. Thus it is important to reattach the tuberosities to each other and also to the plate. Using a plate to fix the fracture requires the fracture to be reduced prior to fixation, which can be difficult to maintain during application of the plate.

Intramedullary nail

These have recently started to come back into favor with nails specifically designed to lock screws into the nail to give angular stability and designed to incorporate the tuberosity fractures. Although the fixation is with a nail, it is important not to think that this means it is a minimally

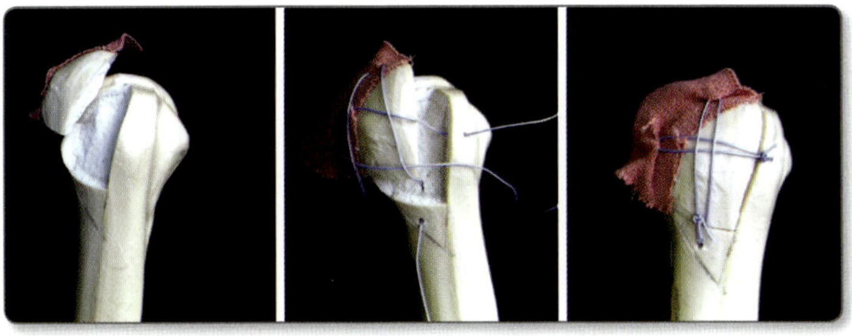

Figure 3.3 Placement of sutures for greater tuberosity fixation. This relies on the pull of the rotator cuff to maintain compression of the fragment.

invasive technique. The approach and reduction is the same as for plate fixation, so that the tuberosities are identified and reduced around the head and shaft. The two main advantages of the nail are that after preparing the fracture. The nail can be inserted and the composite parts of the fracture reduced around the nail, before locking the screws into place, allowing small adjustments with the implant in place. The other advantage is that the nail fills the bony defect left by the fracture, so that the void that the head might collapse back into is eliminated by the presence of the nail. The cuff tendons may still need to be sutured to each other and also around the nail/screws to neutralize the muscle pull.

Arthroplasty

In fractures with no soft tissue attachment to the humeral head in older patients, replacement is the best option for pain relief, but the functional outcomes are variable. Hemiarthroplasty has been the mainstay of replacement surgery, but is reliant on the healing of the tuberosities onto the implant for function. The alternative is to eliminate the need for supraspinatus function, by changing the biomechanics of the implant using a reverse anatomy replacement. This then uses the deltoid as an abductor by medializing the center of rotation of the shoulder. Recently evidence in favor of reverse shoulder arthroplasty has become available from randomized controlled trials, but these currently only have short-term follow-up in an older patient population. The long-term outcome of reverse shoulder replacement in younger patients for trauma is still not clear. It is beyond the scope of this chapter to describe the full decision making and technique for arthroplasty of the shoulder, but if fixation is being attempted in older patients with three or four part fractures, it should be performed by a surgeon with the skills and experience to undertake the appropriate replacement at the time, with the appropriate implants available.

Theater layout and patient positioning

In general terms, the patient's head should be 180° from the anesthetic machine. Generally beach chair position is employed, with the table toward the side of the laminar flow area, to give as much space for surgeon, assistant, scrub nurse and trolleys. The patient is positioned with their injured side at the edge of the table, and the arm overhanging the edge, to allow full extension and access for the image intensifier C-arm (**Figure 3.4**). A mobile Mayo table is useful to rest the arm at the appropriate height during the surgery. The II C-arm is positioned at the head end of the table, to allow imaging of the shoulder, anteroposterior (AP) and axillary views. The screen should be on the opposite side of the table from the operative side.

Review of surgical approaches

Deltopectoral

- Position patient supine or in the beach chair position. The arm should be able to move freely into extension (by having the shoulder over the edge of the bed)
- Ensure intraoperative X-rays are obtainable before standard preparation and draping. It is

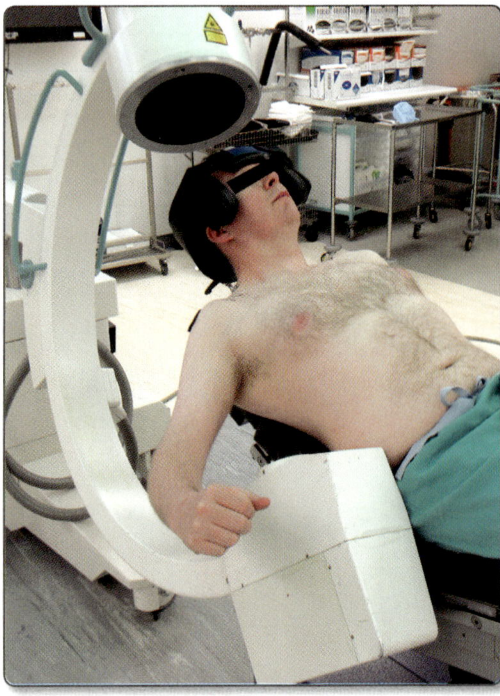

Figure 3.4 Proposed clinical set up for surgical procedures.

important to be able to get AP and axillary views intraoperatively to avoid screw penetration and to assess the lesser tuberosity reduction
- Identify the coracoid and make skin incision in the interval between the deltoid and pectoralis major (**Figure 2.8a**), which can extend distally along the lateral border of the biceps
- Identify the cephalic vein and retract either medially or laterally depending on vascular tributaries, this will allow access to subacromial and subdeltoid space (**Figure 2.8b**) following division of the clavipectoral fascia lateral to the conjoint tendon. Once the subacromial space is entered, Hohmann retractors can be inserted over the rotator cuff and around the shaft to lever the deltoid posteriorly, exposing the cuff, tuberosities and the fracture

Deltoid splitting

- Patient positioning and image intensifier setup are identical. The acromion and clavicle are marked, and the skin incised over the anterior edge of the acromion, and distally along the lateral border of the deltoid (**Figure 3.5a**)
- Skin flaps are raised and the anterior raphe of the deltoid exposed. The deltoid is released as subperiosteal dissection from the anterior acromion, and the raphe split in line with its fibers. This exposes the underlying subdeltiod and subacromial space (often filled with hematoma)
- Holman retractors allow exposure of the posterior and anterior subdeltoid space to allow control of the tuberosities. Care is taken not to divide the deltoid further than 5 cm from the acromial edge, to avoid injury to the axillary nerve. If this approach is used for plate fixation, then the nerve should either be identified and dissected and protected, or a window either side of the nerve used to pass the plate deep to the nerve (**Figure 3.5b**)

Combined deltopectoral and deltoid split

- The advantage of using this approach is that it allows access through both approaches getting the benefit of each approach
- Saber incision is made from the deltopectoral groove, over the lateral border of the acromion, and posteriorly over the posterior border of the acromial spine (**Figure 3.6a**)
- Full thickness skin flaps raised reflecting the lateral fasciocutaneous flap laterally to expose both the deltopectoral groove and cephalic vein anteriorly and the anterior raphe and the anterior acromion laterally (**Figure 3.6b**). This allows the approach through each window as described above

Equipment requirements

This will depend on institution availability and surgeon preference. In the majority of cases the following are utilized:

- Small fragment and minifragment sets
- Anatomical plates/locking options
- K-wires
- Retractors: Gelpie, Hohmann's and Atlantech self-retaining instruments

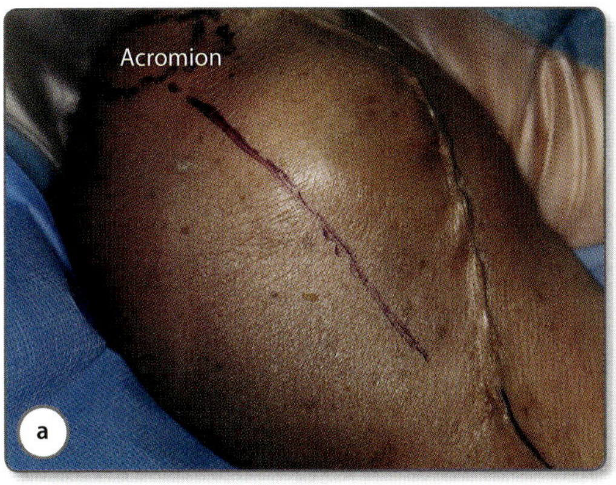

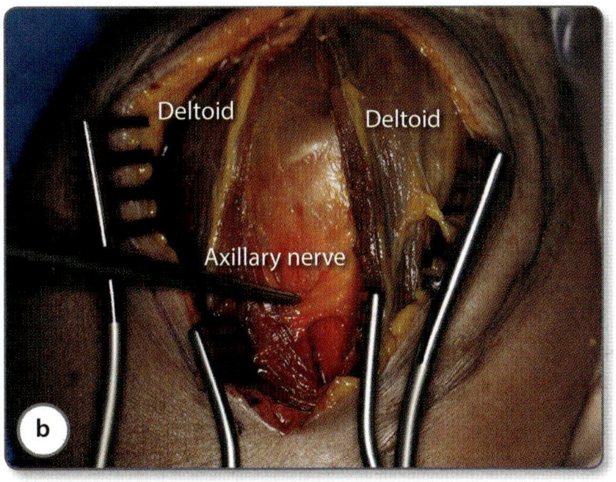

Figure 3.5 (a) Cadaveric image of skin incision. (b) Cadaveric image showing approach and axillary nerve.

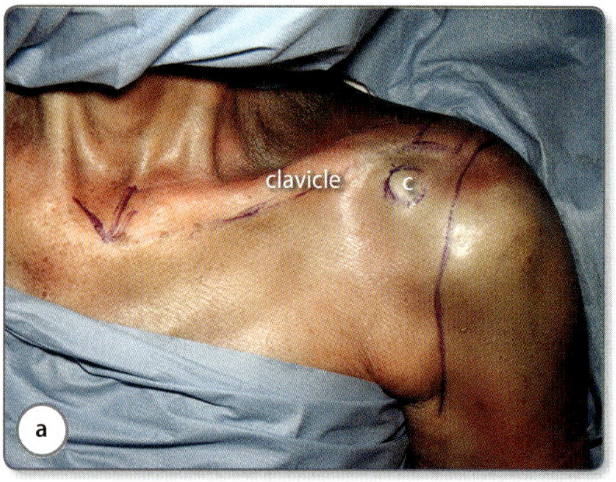

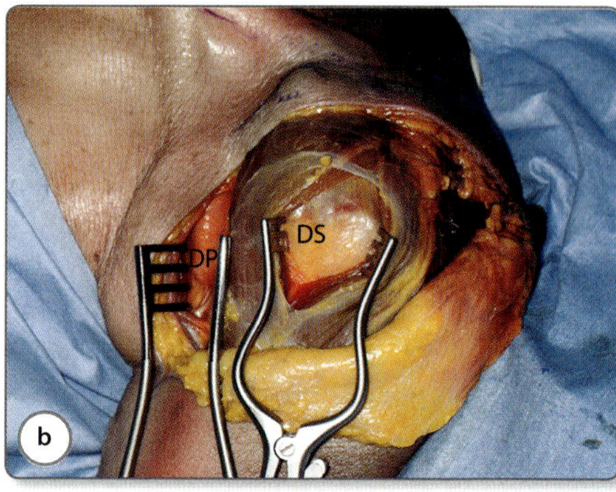

Figure 3.6 (a) Cadaveric image of skin incisions. (b) Cadaveric image of two-window approach.

- Sutures for cuff (large needle) heavy braid
- Cannulated screw set
- Mayo table to position the arm during surgery

Reduction and stabilization methods

Fracture lines are identified (this is sometimes difficult as overlying contused bursa can obscure the fractures). The fracture between the tuberosities is normally posterior to the bicipital groove, and to expose this, the supraspinatus fibers should be split in line with the fracture line, to reveal the humeral head. If the tuberosities are grossly displaced, the greater tuberosity is often pulled posteriorly by the cuff insertion, and needs to be retrieved, by holding the arm in abduction and internal rotation.

The tendons of the rotator cuff are identified and tagged with sutures to allow the tuberosities to be controlled once they are released (the tuberosities should not be handled with grasping instruments as they are liable to fragment). Soft tissue attachments should not be released from the tuberosities.

The fractures can be cleaned and then reduced. The head is pushed against the glenoid, and the tuberosities reduced around the head by pulling on the suture around the tuberosities.

Temporary stabilization may be necessary with stout K-wires, and if the construct is grossly unstable the wires traversing the head into the glenoid may be required to build the humeral shaft and tuberosities around the head, which is no longer mobile.

If using a plate, the fracture should be held reduced with whatever temporary measures are required before placing the plate over the greater tuberosity just posterior to the bicipital groove. Care is taken to keep the plate distal enough so that the proximal edge will not impinge against the acromion in abduction. Once the plate is held in place the screws are filled into the head, taking care not to perforate the articular surface, with either the drill or the screws. Following bony fixation the cuff sutures are passed through suture holes in the plate and tied off to neutralize the deforming forces on the tuberosities (**Figures 3.7**).

If using a nail, the fracture can be reduced and temporarily held prior to insertion, or alternatively the nail can be inserted into the shaft and the fracture fragments reduced around the nail. The reduction is undertaken in the same way as for a plate, and the tuberosity sutures are passed around the nail and tied to hold the tuberosities around the nail and against each other laterally. The proximal screws can then be passed into the head through the jig, and the distal locking screws through distal stab incisions. The cuff sutures can then also be tied around the screw heads (some systems have holes in the screw heads allowing suture passage) to neutralize the pull of the cuff (**Figure 3.2**).

Rehabilitation

Request physiotherapy review and input when surgical wounds are satisfactory.

- Rest in poly sling device initially, but there should be early passive movement

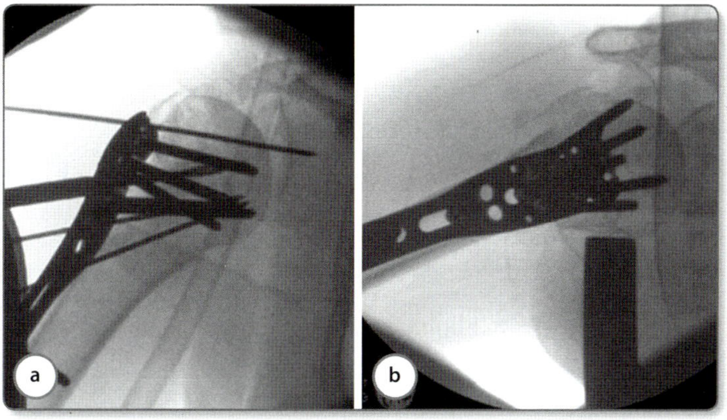

Figure 3.7 (a, b) Intraoperative fluoroscopy of anatomical contoured locking plate fixation.

- No heavy lifting until fracture union
- Passive range of motion exercises building up to active assisted and active as symptoms and serial X-rays allow

Avoiding postoperative complications

Infection/wound healing complications

- Careful soft tissue handling
- Prophylactic antibiotics
- Attention to hemostasis intraoperatively

Deltoid detachment from acromion

- Reattachment of deltoid via nonabsorbable transosseous sutures

Neurovascular damage

- Limitation of deltoid split distally to avoid axillary nerve
- Identification and protection of the axillary nerve when using calcar screws into the nail/plate
- Careful retraction of conjoint tendon medially to avoid musculocutaneous nerve damage
- Care when dissecting along inferior border of subscapularis to avoid damage to the axillary nerve

Loss of reduction

- Thorough review of CT scans with accurate surgical planning and approach
- Stable fixation of fracture components
- Use of neutralizing sutures from cuff to implant

Post-traumatic stiffness

- Accurate fracture reconstruction with stable fixation allowing early protected physiotherapy
- Appropriate positioning of the implant to avoid any impingement against the acromion or irritation of the subdeltoid bursa
- No penetration of the joint with screws confirmed with appropriate imaging at operation

Summary of learning points

- Careful review of radiographs and CT scans to understand fracture configurations and to plan fixation
- Positioning of the patient and C-arm prior to surgery, to get acceptable intraoperative images (imaging never gets better during the procedure)
- Exposure and control with careful handling of the tuberosities to allow reduction and stable fixation is key to long-term function
- Appropriate equipment selection to aid surgery
- Avoid prominent metalwork and screw penetration to reduce subdeltoid adhesions
- Avoid axillary nerve injury during surgical dissection, fracture reduction and implant insertion

Further reading

AO Foundation: AO Surgery Reference. www2.aofoundation.org/wps/portal/surgery (accessed 28 March 2017).

Jordan RW, Modi CS. A review of management options for proximal humeral fractures. Open Orthop J 2014; 8:148–156.

Neer CS 2nd. Displaced proximal humeral fractures. I. Classification and evaluation. J Bone Joint Surg Am 1970; 52:1077–1089.

Rangan A, Handoll H, Brealey S, et al. Surgical vs nonsurgical treatment of adults with displaced fractures of the proximal humerus: the ProFHER randomized clinical trial. JAMA 2015; 313:1037–1047.

Stanbury SJ, Voloshin I. Reverse shoulder arthroplasty for acute proximal humeral fractures in the geriatric patient: a review of the literature. Geriatr Orthop Surg Rehabil 2011; 2:181–186.

4 Diaphyseal humeral fractures

Nigel Rossiter, Paul V Fearon

Introduction

Most nonpathological diaphyseal humeral fractures in adults and children will heal without surgery and nonoperative management remains the mainstay of management of these injuries. Healing time will vary with age, patient comorbidities, body habitus, compliance, drug/nicotine/alcohol consumption amongst other variables. The patient, not the picture, needs to be treated.

Pathological fractures in adults are often secondary to malignant causes, the most common being multiple myeloma, followed by metastatic lesions from other primary tumors: breast, lung, thyroid, kidney and prostate, being the 'big five' but others will include bowel, ovary and, rarely, primary bone tumors.

Incidence

Overall fractures of the diaphysis of the humerus make up 1–3% of all acute fractures. In trauma registries – which include patients with major trauma but exclude isolated fractures not requiring admission, pediatric fractures, nor pathological injuries – the rate is 1%. This rate is said not to vary with age, but recent data suggest an increasing incidence in the aging population due to frailty, falling, osteoporosis and the increasing incidence of pathological lesions.

Mechanism of injury

The mechanism of a diaphyseal humeral fracture may be due to:

- A fall onto an outstretched hand
- A direct blow: often as a result of a motor vehicle collision
- Rotational forces (e.g. 'arm wrestling')
- Throwing injuries: fractures have reported after baseball pitching, javelin throwing, etc.
- Penetrating trauma (e.g. gunshot/ballistic trauma)
- Pathological lesions causing weakening of the bone

Initial management/ prioritization

As with any fracture, a fracture of the humeral diaphysis is painful and like any other fracture the same principles apply. The patient as a whole must be assessed addressing life-threatening issues first. Careful assessment of the integument/skin is performed noting any penetrating injury, any obvious open fracture, distal neurovascular function (in particular radial nerve motor function: looking especially for the ability to extend the wrist, not the fingers, as this function can be performed by the intrinsic muscles supplied by the median nerve) and/or vascular injury.

Once assessment has been completed and fully documented and any open wound cleaned of any gross contamination, photographed and dressed, a splint can be applied. Splintage will aid in analgesia and protect the soft tissues from further injury. The easiest and most comfortable split is a 'U-slab'. This is also known as a 'sugar tong splint' or 'coaptation splint'. Barring indications for surgery, below, the U-slab is usually left in place for approximately 10 days. There is no reason to X-ray the injury in this time. Appropriate analgesia is administered. Nonsteroidal anti-inflammatory drugs (NSAIDs) should be avoided if at all possible, as the bone is healing utilizing relative stability, which relies on the formation of callus. The formation of callus requires an inflammatory response, and therefore any drug that diminishes this response may delay or stop bone healing. There is much debate and evidence both for and against this hypothesis. In the author's opinion, it makes sense to avoid NSAIDs unless the pain cannot be controlled by any other means.

After approximately 10 days, as the swelling diminishes and the patient becomes more comfortable, the U-slab can then be exchanged for a functional brace. These were popularized by Sarmiento, who in his original series of over 660 cases reported a 98% union rate (although few other studies have managed to repeat this very high union rate, most authors quote rates in excess of 90%). They can be made from a variety of materials but all should comply with Sarmiento's original principles:

- They should be made of a material that allows some compression and moulding
- They should have a minimal layer of padding beneath them
- They should be in two sections or allow overlap to enable tightening
- They should have the ability for a patient or carer to tighten them on an almost daily basis
- They should allow movement of the elbow and ideally shoulder (and usually do not require extension over the top of the shoulder)

These function using tissue turgor as the brace is tightened to splint the fracture and using that tissue turgor to effect a reduction. The patient is encouraged to move the arm, in particular the elbow and shoulder. Once comfort of the fracture allows the brace may be removed for hygiene. The brace will be required usually for a minimum of 8 weeks in an adult but rarely longer than 24 weeks. This is the mainstay of management for the vast majority of patients with an isolated, closed injury.

Malunion with nonoperative management is common, but well tolerated. Klenerman's seminal paper in 1966 suggested that 3 cm of shortening, 20° of apex anterior or posterior angulation, and 30° of varus is tolerated. Valgus is rare. Rotational deformity is also not common, but possibly up to 15–20° of rotation is also well tolerated as long as there is normal shoulder and elbow function.

Considerations for surgery

These can be listed as 'hard' and 'relative'. Hard indications include:

- Open fractures
- Vascular injury requiring surgery
- Ipsilateral forearm fracture(s) – the 'floating elbow'
- Bilateral humeral fractures
- As part of polytrauma, in particular in combination with a lower limb and/or pelvic/acetabular injury when the upper limbs will be required to mobilize
- Neurological injury in combination with a penetrating injury
- Significant intra-articular extension with displacement
- 'Unacceptable' position
- Pathological fracture in an adult

Most clinicians would agree that the majority of these are good indications for surgery. Few require emergent surgery other than vascular injury with vascular compromise and severe open injury with gross contamination.

Relative indications for surgery include:

- Radial nerve injury postmanipulation of fracture/application of U-slab or splint, when function was normal prior (see below)
- Segmental fracture (due to the relatively higher incidence of delayed/nonunion of one of the fracture segments)
- Radial nerve palsy that fails to recover (see below)
- Transverse fractures at level of deltoid tuberosity – due to difficulty in controlling deforming forces of deltoid and pectoralis with a splint causing significant deformity and high rates of nonunion
- Obesity
- Large breasts
- Delayed/nonunion

Obesity and patients with large breasts are relative indications for operative fracture stabilization. The large chest tissue acts as a fulcrum over which the fracture tends to deform meaning that controlling the fracture with a splint is difficult and uncomfortable for the patient and tends to delayed/nonunion.

Radial nerve injury

The radial nerve is the most commonly injured neuro-vascular structure in association with a diaphyseal humeral fracture. The rate is quoted as up to 18% of all injuries. The 'Holstein-Lewis' fracture pattern – an oblique fracture of the distal one-third of the humerus – is the injury most associate with radial nerve injury. However, it is more commonly seen in mid diaphyseal/junction of middle and distal diaphyseal injury where the

Case example: Bilateral open humeral diaphyseal fractures

A young adult male pedestrian was hit by a car, sustaining bilateral open upper anterior arm fractures (**Figure 4.1**), a head injury and a segmental closed right tibia fracture. He was positioned supine on a radiolucent table and underwent temporary external fixation of his tibial fracture before, debridement, lavage and stabilization of both humeral fractures using compression plating (**Figure 4.2**) via anterolateral approaches (absolute stability). He did not require any plastic surgery intervention in terms of skin closure/coverage.

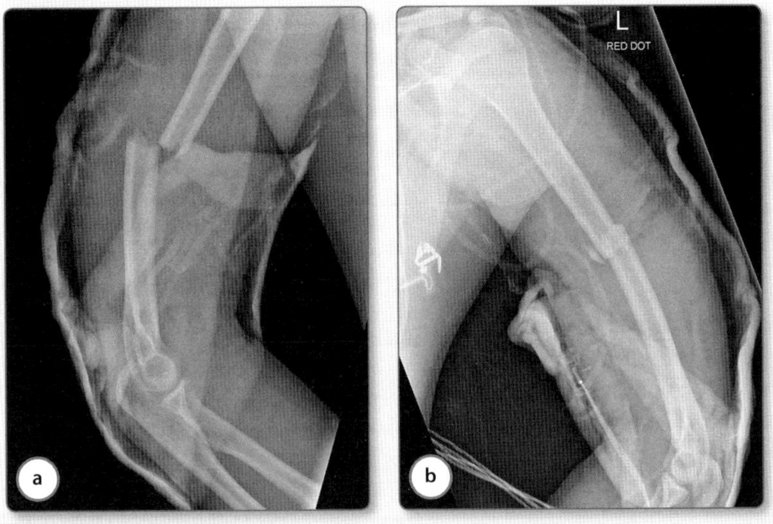

Figure 4.1 (a) Anteroposterior radiograph right upper arm, showing diaphyseal fracture. (b) AP radiograph left upper arm similar to contralateral side.

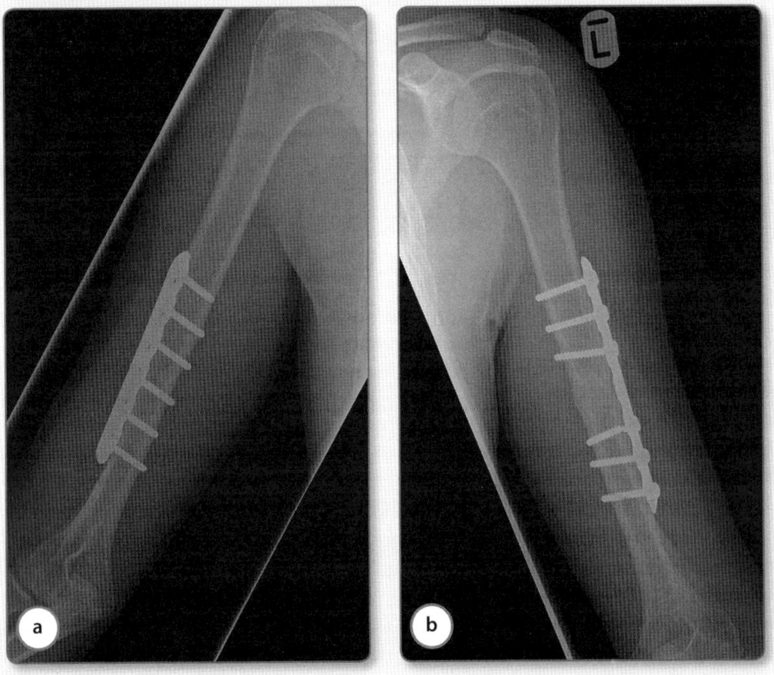

Figures 4.2 (a) Postoperative X-ray of case. Bilateral humeral plating with large fragment plates in compression mode, via anterolateral approaches. (b) Note breakage of screw prior to union on left side.

nerve is injured as it crosses behind the humerus obliquely from supero-medial to inferolateral around the 'spiral/radial groove' on the back of the humerus. The vast majority of these injuries are neuropraxias and will recover: 90% are said to recover by 3–4 months. The advice in most texts is to manage the patient expectantly, unless there is a hard indication for surgery. This actually also includes those patients who develop Radial nerve symptoms after manipulation or application of a U-slab or splint. If there is no evidence of recovery at 4 months then the nerve should be explored.

The problems are:

- Identification of the patient who is unlikely to/will not recover
- That at 4 months, almost all nerves that are explored are injured and only 50% of these subsequently recover function after another year
- Exploration of the fracture and nerve beyond 3–4 months is technically demanding, the nerve becoming encased in scarring and callus

For these reasons, it is the author's practice to:

1. Explore all radial nerve injuries early in patients where the radial nerve was functionally normal prior to manipulation or application of a U-slab or splint and to surgically stabilize the fracture
2. In a patient with a closed humeral diaphyseal fracture who presents with a radial nerve injury and no other indication for surgery, to splint the fracture for 10–14 days and if there is no clinical sign of obvious radial nerve recovery within those first 2 weeks, to advise open surgical exploration of the nerve and stabilization of the fracture as soon as possible

This is purely personal opinion without any hard evidence, but seems to makes surgical sense to the author and certainly makes the exploration of the nerve and stabilization of the fracture technically easier. The patient has to be informed that the operation may be unnecessary, as the evidence is that they have a 90% chance of recovery with no surgical intervention. However, if they are one of the 10% of patients who do not recover by 4 months, they then have a 50% chance of permanent damage, face an operation that is much more technically challenging and therefore has greater associated risks of infection and iatrogenic nerve injury, not to mention having waited a further 4 months with an uncertain outcome.

Using classification to guide operative management

Understanding the fracture pattern will guide management. Once the AO/OTA classification of the fracture pattern has been made this will guide the surgeon.

- Type A fractures: these generally do best with absolute stability techniques ('compression plating')
- Type B fractures: these may have absolute or relative stability techniques
  - B1 fractures in general may be best managed using absolute stability
  - B2 fractures in general can have either technique though surgeons tend towards to absolute stability
  - B3 fractures in general tend to be managed with relative stability techniques [this can be achieved with plates, nails (or external fixation)]
- Type C fractures: usually managed using relative stability techniques
  - Plates
  - Open or MIPO/MIPPO (minimally invasive plate osteosynthesis/minimally invasive percutaneous plate osteosynthesis)
  - Intra-medullary nails
  - Ante- or retro-grade
  - Interlocking (elastic stable)
  - External fixation

Theater layout and patient positioning

Separate theater setups and layouts are proposed in **Figure 4.5** for anterolateral and posterior approaches. As with all setups, careful positioning is mandatory to avoid pressure damage to the patient, especially in the lateral decubitus or prone position. It is also important to confirm radiological access prior to draping the patient.

Review of surgical approaches

Anterolateral approach

- With the patient supine on a radiolucent table, ensure adequate radiological access prior to draping

Case example: Complex extra-articular distal humeral fracture

Isolated closed upper arm fracture in a young man (**Figure 4.3**) sustained following a fall from a bicycle. Following temporary splintage and repeat neuromuscular examination he was admitted for surgical stabilization. This was undertaken by positioning the patient prone on a radiolucent table and arm board. Open reduction was undertaken utilising the posterior approach with identification and protection of the radial nerve. Fixation was undertaken with the application of a plate in spanning mode to achieve relative fracture stability and healing by callus (**Figure 4.4**). The intraoperative notes record the position of the radial nerve in relation to the screw holes in the underlying plate.

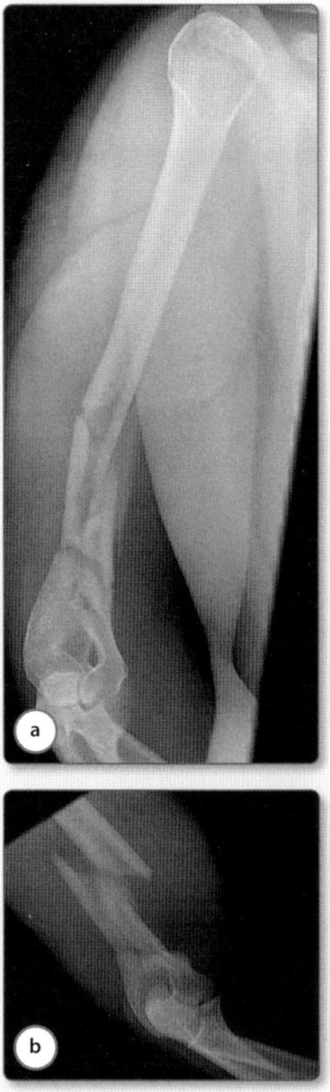

Figure 4.3 (a) Anteroposterior radiograph showing communicated distal humeral fracture. (b) Lateral radiograph of communicated distal humeral fracture.

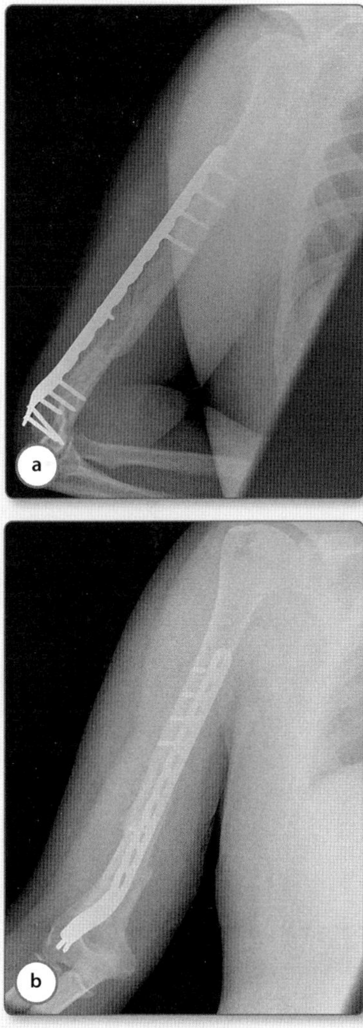

Figure 4.4 Postoperative X-rays of case shown in Figure 4.3 via posterior approach with plate applied in spanning mode (relative stability) to posterior surface of humerus. Intraoperative notes clearly record the position of the nerve in relation to numbered plate holes

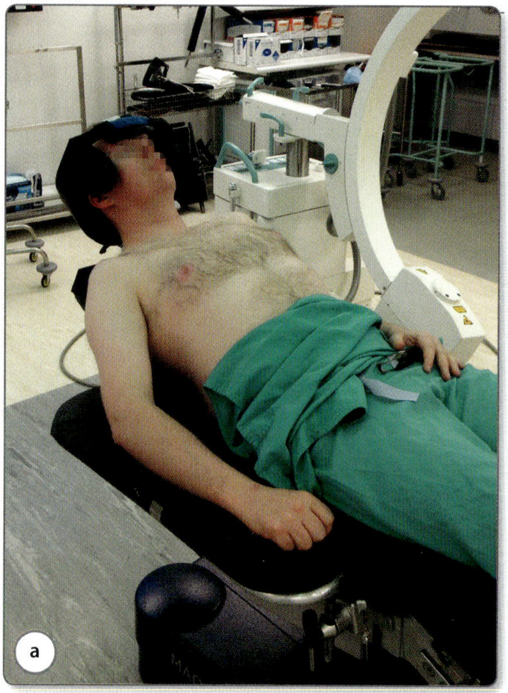

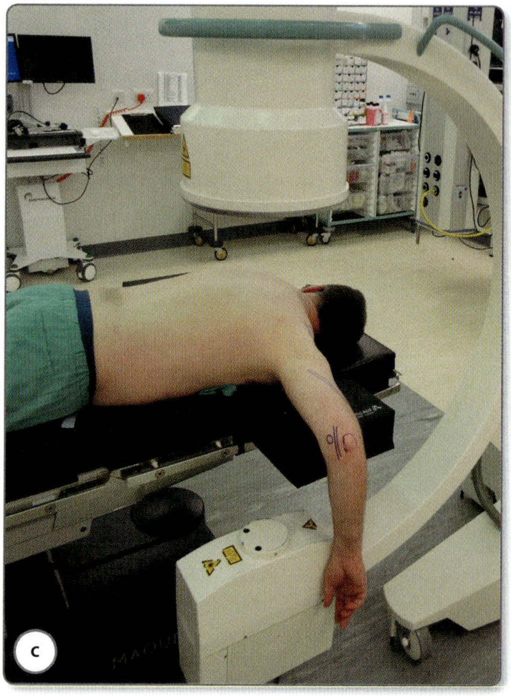

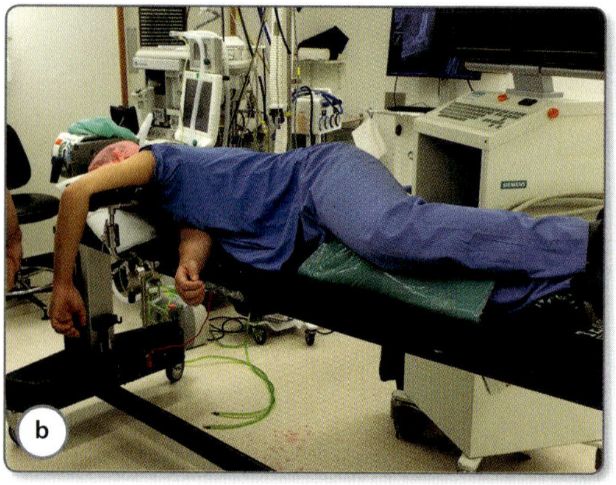

Figure 4.5 (a) Supine position for anterolateral approach. Often, a modified beach chair position can be employed for humeral nailing with the arm parallel to the torso, but care needs to be taken to ensure radiological access. (b) Lateral decubitus positioning with padding of all pressure areas and dependant arm moved away from under torso to avoid undue compression. (c) Prone positioning of patient with padded mattress allowing abdomen to hang free. The humerus can be screened in orthogonal views by just moving the image intensifier arm.

- Make a skin incision over anterolateral border of biceps (**Figure 4.6a**), which is then exposed and retracted medially
- Split the brachialis to access the anterior border of the humerus (**Figure 4.6b**)
- Identify the radial nerve distally as it pierces the intramuscular septum (**Figure 4.6c**)

Posterior approach

- The patient should be placed in the lateral decubitus or prone position with an image intensifier coming in parallel to head end of table
- Make a posterior skin incision from the acromial tip to the olecranon (**Figure 4.7a**)
- Identify the nerve proximally in the interval just inferior to teres major and trace it distally, splitting the triceps (**Figure 4.7b**)
- The fracture can then be exposed and reduced. In the operative notes, always record position of nerve in relation to the plate holes in case later exploration is ever required

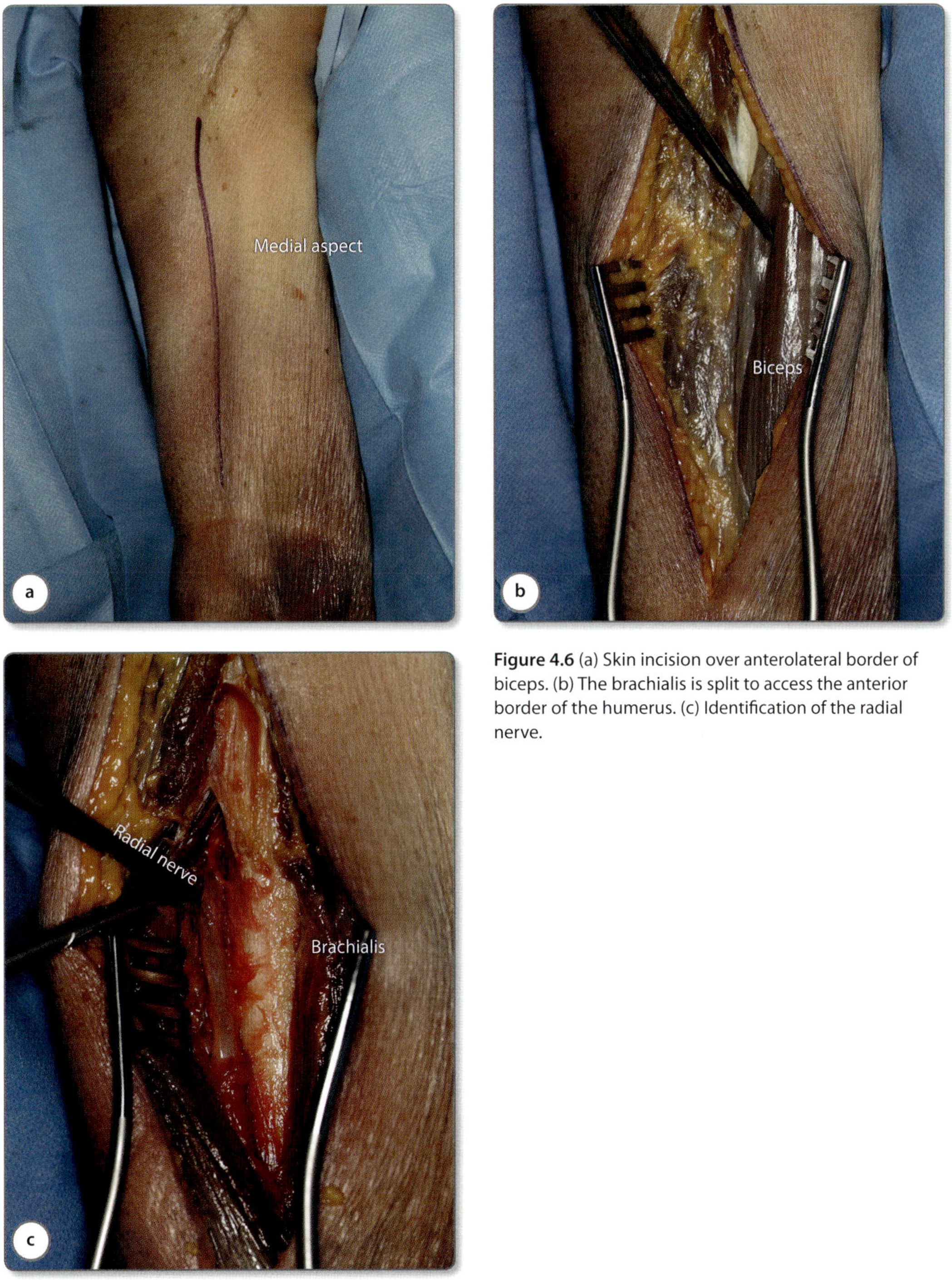

Figure 4.6 (a) Skin incision over anterolateral border of biceps. (b) The brachialis is split to access the anterior border of the humerus. (c) Identification of the radial nerve.

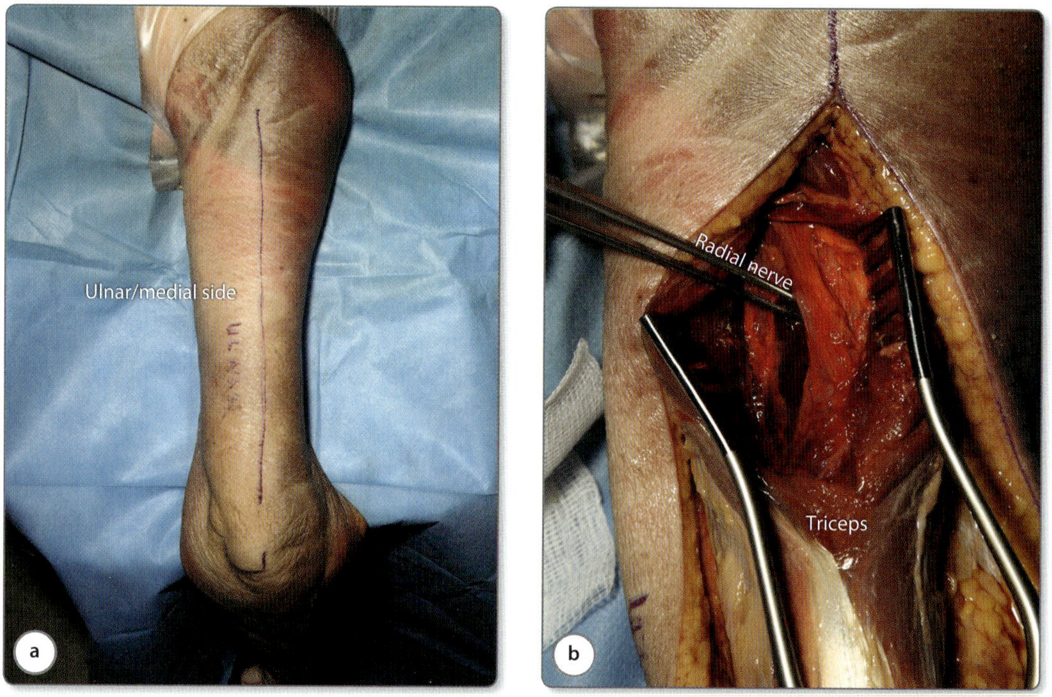

Figure 4.7 (a) Posterior skin incision from acromial tip to olecranon. (b) Identification of the nerve proximally.

Equipment requirements

- Radio-lucent arm table
- Positioning aids (e.g. gutter if patient lateral)
- Gel pads for pressure areas
- Standard orthopaedic surgical instruments, suction and light handles
- Image intensifier cover
- Self-retaining retractors: Norfolk & Norwich, Travers, Gelpi vascular sloop to go around radial nerve. The 'F tool' from the Elastic nailing set is very useful to aid with closed fracture reduction
- Ball tipped pusher (Kugelspitze) reduction device (from pelvic/acetabular sets)

Reduction and stabilization methods

If operative intervention and stabilization of a humeral shaft fracture is chosen the author in general choses to plate the vast majority of fractures, utilizing a formal open approach and reduction, using the plate in a mode appropriate to the fracture pattern, plus achieving fracture reduction as close as possible with as little soft tissue disruption to the fracture fragments as possible. If the fracture is pathological in an adult, an antegrade interlocked intramedullary nail is chosen instrumenting as much of the length of the intramedullary canal as possible, and, ensuring that meticulous surgical technique is employed at the shoulder with any implant well below the articular surface and proximal interlocking screws carefully positioned.

Grafting

The author has not needed nor used a bone graft, nor any form of bone growth 'stimulant' (e.g. ultrasound, pulsed electromagnetic fields, bone morphogenic proteins, etc.) for humeral fractures either acutely or for non-unions where there is no bone loss for over 10 years. The author has yet to find an indication for any of these.

Rehabilitation

Usually full active use of the arm, shoulder and elbow is allowed immediately with no lifting of anything heavier than one pint for approximately 1 month. NSAIDs are avoided if possible. A formal postoperative X-ray is taken before discharge. Once the wound is dry the author advises exposure of the wound to the air and normal washing is allowed 2–3 days postoperatively. Appropriate clinic and radiological follow-up is arranged until bony union is confirmed.

Avoiding postoperative complications

- Appropriate preoperative planning combined with team communication
- Access to appropriate equipment and knowledge of biomechanics and strain required for fracture healing
- Avoidance of unnecessary surgical dissection
- Identification and protection of structures at risk
- Appropriate fracture reduction and correct usage of fixation devices
- Early mobility of shoulder and elbow

Summary of learning points

- The majority of humeral fractures can be treated nonoperatively
- Careful planning with approaches, patient positioning and radiological access allows easier progression of the procedure
- Meticulous dissection and identification of structures at risk is essential
- Use implants in appropriate modes for relative or absolute stability

Further reading

AO Foundation: AO Surgery Reference (humeral shaft). www2. aofoundation.org/wps/portal/surgery (accessed 28 March 2017).

Castellá FB, Garcia FB, Berry EM, et al. Nonunion of the humeral shaft: long lateral butterfly fracture – a non-union predictive pattern? Clin Orth Relat Res 2004; 424:227–230.

Garcia A Jr, Maeck BH, Perelló EB, et al. Radial nerve injuries in fractures of the shaft of the humerus. Am J Surg 1960; 79:625–627.

Gosler MW, Testroote M, Morrenhof J, Janzing HMJ. Surgical versus non-surgical interventions for treating humeral shaft fractures in adults. Cochrane Database Syst Rev 2012; 1:CD008832.

Kettlekamp D, Alexander H. Clinical review of radial nerve injury. J Trauma 1967; 7:424–432.

Klenerman L. Fractures of the shaft of the humerus. J Bone Joint Surg Br 1966; 48:105–111.

Kurup H, Hossain M, Andrew JG. Dynamic compression plating versus locked intramedullary nailing for humeral shaft fractures in adults. Cochrane Database Syst Rev 2011; 6:CD005959.

Postacchinni F, Morace GB. Fractures of the humerus associated with paralysis of the radial nerve. Ital J Orthop Traumatol 1988; 14:455–464.

Sarmiento A, Zagorski JB, Zych GA, et al. Functional bracing for the treatment of fractures of the humeral diaphysis. J Bone Joint Surg Am 2000; 82:478–486.

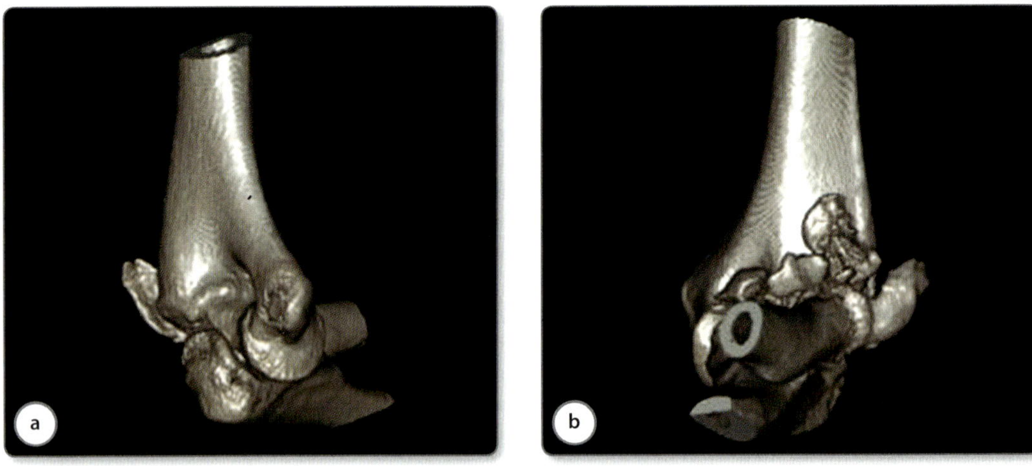

Figure 5.4 (a, b) Preoperative surface rendered CT scans of case shown in Figure 5.1.

arm and to reduce the tendency of the distal segment to fall, with gravity, into flexion.

Review of surgical approaches

The olecranon osteotomy is the work horse approach for surgical exposure of intra-articular fractures and will only be discussed below.

Olecranon osteotomy

- Position prone or lateral decubitus position
- Ensure adequate radiological access prior to draping
- Tourniquet optional
- Make posterior skin incision curved away from subcutaneous olecranon point (**Figure 5.6a**)
- Can create pilot hole in ulnar border now and pass wire for later tension band repair of osteotomy
- Identify and protect/isolate ulnar nerve (**Figure 5.6b**)
- Perform chevron olecranon osteotomy (**Figure 5.6c**) at mid-level of joint with oscillating saw, and complete osteotomy with osteotome, to give access to distal humeral articulation The proximal ulna and triceps is then reflected off the inter-muscular septum in a proximal direction (**Figure 5.6d**). This then allows fracture reduction and fixation to proceed

Careful repair of the osteotomy must be carried out using a tension-band-wire. Plating the osteotomy is expensive and unnecessary. Experienced surgeons may favor varieties of 'triceps-on' approaches but whatever approach is used the fracture must be adequately visualized to ensure anatomical reduction and nonpenetration of the metal-ware into the joint.

Equipment requirements

This will depend upon surgeon and institution preference, but in the majority small fragment (3.5 mm/2.7 mm) sets are utilized:

- 1.6 mm and 1.25 mm K-wires
- Battery drill and fine saw
- Osteotomes
- Tension band set
- Anatomical/locking plates
- Reduction clamps
- Headless screws

Reduction and stabilization methods

With C-type fractures there are two main strategies: first to reconstruct the articular block to produce an A-type fracture and then fix this block in the correct length, alignment and rotation to the shaft. This works best

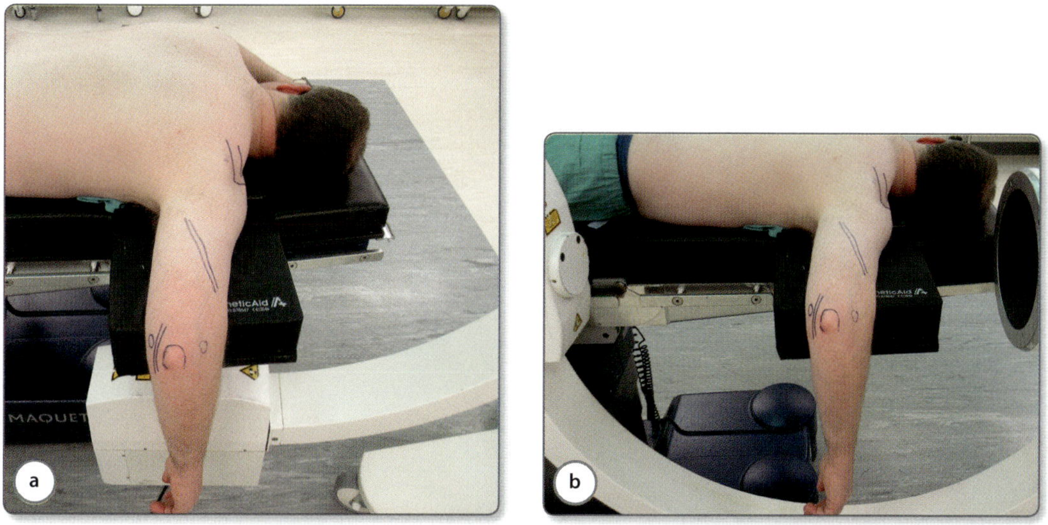

Figure 5.5 (a, b) Prone setup with image intensifier allowing AP and lateral images without moving the arm, the arm is resting on a padded wooden vein board.

with relatively simple articular fractures. The second method is to form a B-type fracture by provisionally stabilizing the largest of the articular fragments to the shaft and then progressively working across the joint, reducing and stabilizing the other fragments until the reconstruction is complete. Both methods require attention to detail and to avoid getting the overall alignment wrong; it is not uncommon to require several attempts at provisional fixation with K-wires before anatomical reconstruction is achieved. It is fair to say that no one technique will work for all configurations of fracture and a certain flexibility of approach is needed.

It is important to be able to obtain a good AP and lateral image of the elbow joint without having to move the limb; temporary fixation is often precarious and movement of the limb can lead to loss of implants and position.

Definitive fixation is usually obtained by placing appropriate plates along the medial and lateral columns as needed (**Figure 5.3:** case example). For C-type fractures two plates are needed; for B-type usually only one plate; if the column is intact, such as with a simple capitellar shear fracture, then only screws (conventional or headless) can be utilized. The plates can be put a 90° to each other where the lateral plate runs down the back of the lateral column to the level of the capitellar articular surface and the medial plate is around the medial column and thus the screws and plates are perpendicular to each other.

Precontoured anatomically specific plates when correctly positioned can be perfect but care needs to be taken of metalwork clashes and joint penetration. O'Driscoll has popularized the parallel plating method with plates down the edges of the medial and lateral columns. Although there is no doubt this is a very stable construct it does require additional dissection laterally and the plates need to be right around on the columns so screws passing through one plate engage with a fragment on the opposite side. Too often plates are placed relatively posterior to the required position and then the screws do not pass right across to the other side of the bone or come out of the front of the joint. Additionally, the lengths of the plates should be staggered to reduce the stress riser in the humeral shaft.

In elderly osteoporotic patients, highly comminuted fractures are often better served by total arthroplasty or resurfacing of the distal humerus, allowing early functional mobility (**Figure 5.7**).

For total arthroplasty olecranon osteotomy is contraindicated and either a triceps-on or triceps turn-down approach is favored. Thus, a decision needs to be made early on based on imaging

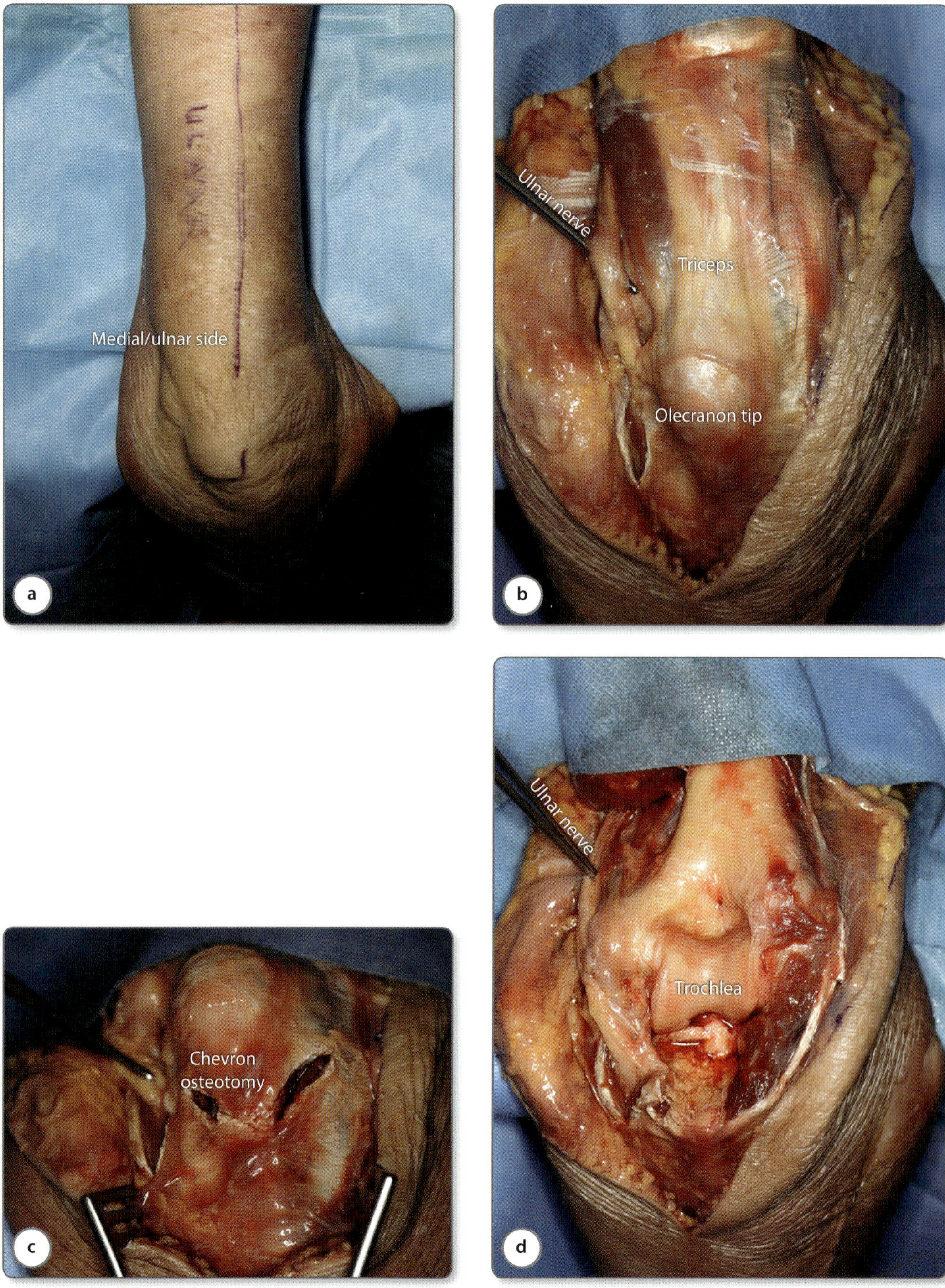

Figure 5.6 (a) The posterior skin incision is marked. (b) The ulnar nerve is identified and isolated to protect it during the procedure. (c) Cuts for a chevron osteotomy are marked. (d) Visualization of the intra-articular distal humeral surface.

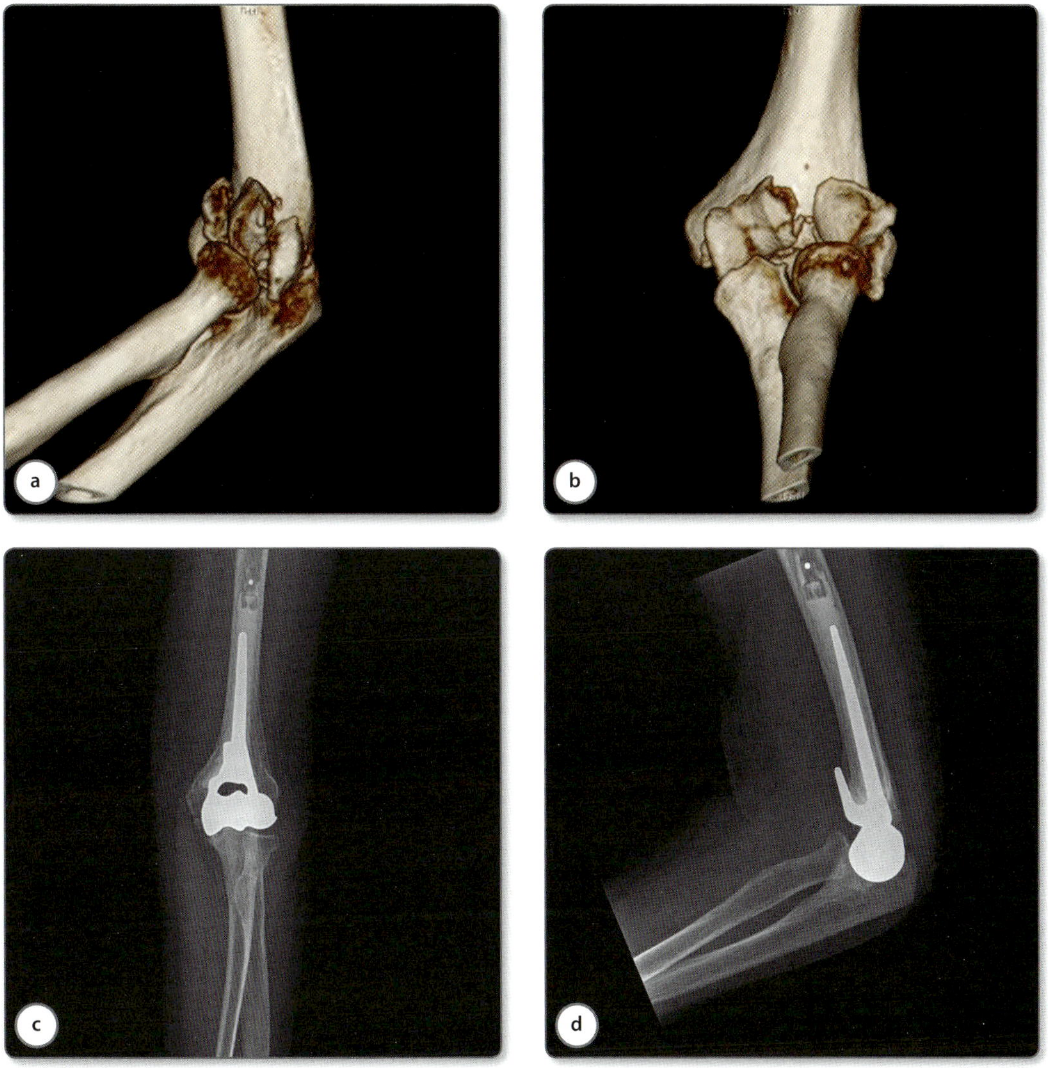

Figures 5.7 (a, b) Preoperative rendered 3-D CT scans of elderly osteoporotic comminuted articular elbow fracture. (c, d) Postoperative X-rays of distal humeral replacement to treat comminuted distal articular fracture.

or initial operative finding as to whether an arthroplasty is the best choice prior to committing to an osteotomy. With distal humeral replacement the implant can be inserted if an osteotomy has been performed but it is not ideal.

Rehabilitation

The adult elbow is intolerant of any prolonged immobilization. Loss of extension is the most common problem although losses of up to 20° are well tolerated. Once the wounds have healed, early physiotherapy is recommended: in this acute setting passive stretches do not lead to heterotopic bone formation. Continuous passive movement devices are available but cumbersome and disliked by patients. In some situations, thermoplastic extension braces can help with reducing flexion contractures. Movement, in the absence of bone or metal blocking it, will continue to improve for at least 9 months.

Avoiding postoperative complications

Infection

- Appropriate perioperative prophylactic antibiotics

Iatrogenic mal-reductions and metal-ware mal-positioning

- Meticulous surgical technique and intraoperative imaging

Stiffness

- Discussed above in rehabilitation section
- Early range of movement
- Sometimes planned soft tissue releases after at least 9 months are needed, along with metalwork removal

Damage to the nerves crossing the elbow

- Careful dissection and handling of ulna nerve
- On occasion, the ulna nerve may sit better in relation to any medial plate by being transposed anteriorly; documenting its final position in the operative record is mandatory. The operation often takes several hours so the tourniquet should be released after 90 minutes if utilized

Salvage options after failed fracture fixation

- Failed ORIF is a difficult problem and may require re-fixation or arthroplasty depending on the circumstances
- Infection should always be considered a possible cause of a nonunion

Summary of learning points

- Good imaging is essential for understanding the fracture and planning: surface-rendered CT scans and perioperative traction views are both helpful
- It is the author's view that a good AP and lateral traction radiograph taken at the beginning of the case prior to definitive patient positioning (with time for contemplation of the images) is one of the most valuable imaging maneuvers (**Figure 5.8**)
- The olecranon osteotomy approach is still the most versatile work-horse of approaches; reattaching it with a tension-band wire construction
- Varied reduction clamps and K-wires for temporary fixation
- There are increasing numbers of B-type fractures which are challenging to manage
- Careful staged reduction and building of fragments to stable diaphysis, or articular block reconstruction as appropriate
- Document position of ulnar nerve at the end of the procedure as metalware may need removing at a later date
- Distal humeral replacement may have advantages compared with total elbow replacement
- Trauma networks need to have referral pathways for appropriate patients to receive arthroplasty in specialist centers

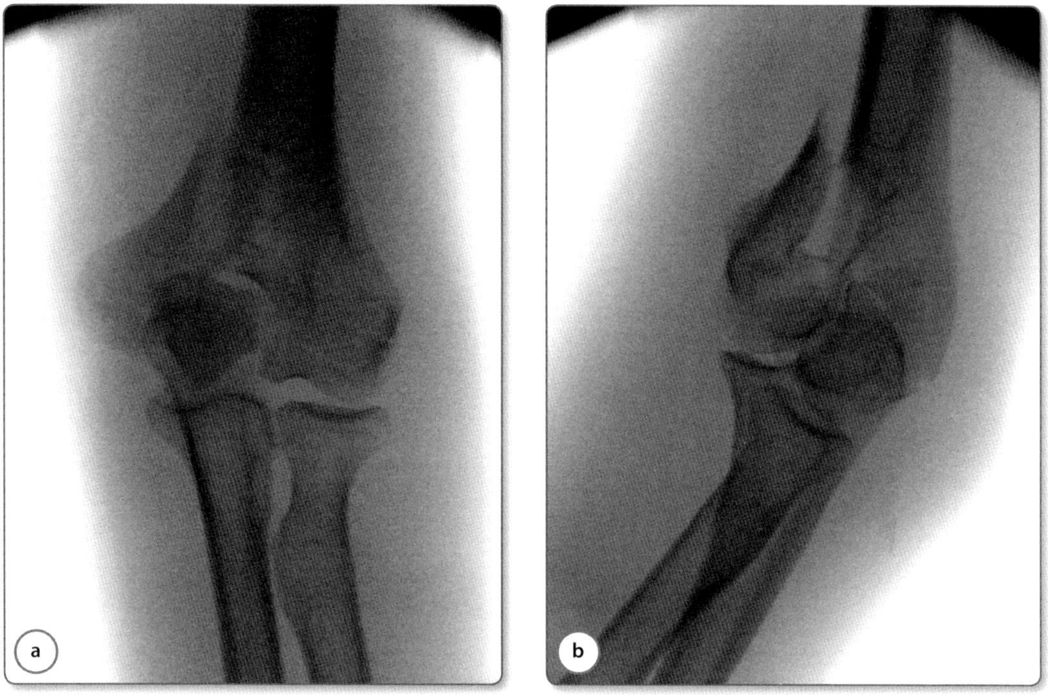

Figure 5.8 (a) AP and (b) lateral traction views of the case example discussed in this chapter.

Further reading

Athwal GS, Hoxie SC, Rispoli DM, Steinmann SP. Precontoured parallel plate fixation of AO/OTA type C distal humerus fractures. J Orthop Trauma 2009; 23:575–580.

Caravaggi P, Laratta JL, Yoon RS, et al. Internal fixation of the distal humerus: a comprehensive biomechanical study evaluating current fixation techniques. J Orthop Trauma 2014; 28:222–226.

Jupiter JB. The management of nonunion and malunion of the distal humerus – a 30-year experience. J Orthop Trauma 2008; 22:742–750.

Ring D, Gulotta L, Chin K, Jupiter JB. Olecranon osteotomy for exposure of fractures and nonunions of the distal humerus. J Orthop Trauma 2004; 18:446–449.

Ring D, Jupiter JB, Gulotta L. Articular fractures of the distal part of the humerus. J Bone Joint Surg Am 2003; 85:232–238.

6 Elbow fracture dislocations

Neil White

Introduction

Elbow dislocations can result from minor falls to high energy trauma, with or without associated fractures of the surrounding bones. As such they can be technically demanding fractures to manage.

Incidence

The elbow joint is among the most commonly dislocated major joint, second only to the shoulder. Elbow dislocations are classified as simple dislocations if they are not associated with concomitant periarticular fractures or complex when they are.

Elbow dislocations are named for the direction of the displacement of the distal fragment, with posterior dislocation by far being the most common. The anterior dislocation and divergent dislocation (the humerus goes in between the radius and ulna) are rare and associated with higher energy trauma. The elbow joint can also dislocate through a widely displaced olecranon fracture, referred to as a transolecranon dislocation.

Mechanism of injury

Elbow dislocations and fracture dislocations are usually the result of a fall on an outstretched hand or arm. A posteriorly directed force transmits up the forearm on an extended elbow and levers the ulna out of the trochlea yielding dislocation. Depending on the angle, rotation and force this may additionally cause a fracture of the coronoid as it impacts the trochlea and/or of the radial head as it impacts the capitellum. When all three components are present (dislocation, coronoid fracture, radial head fracture) this has been labelled a terrible triad injury.

Alternately elbow fracture dislocations may be caused from high-energy mechanisms such as motor vehicle crashes or falls from height. These injuries are not surprisingly more complex and challenging to treat.

Initial management/ prioritization

As with other orthopaedic injuries the patient must be seen as a whole. It is key to identify ipsilateral wrist injuries and to obtain quality wrist X-rays. Although rare, longitudinal injury between the radius and ulna can occur further complicating the elbow fracture dislocation.

All elbow fracture dislocations should undergo an attempted reduction in the emergency room. Generally traction and manual pressure on the olecranon will reduce the ulnotrochlear joint. The limb should be immobilized in a well-fitting splint. Neurovascular examination should be documented before and after reduction, and postreduction X-rays should be obtained.

The goal of closed reduction is usually not definitive treatment but rather to protect the soft-tissues while the definitive procedure is planned.

If a reduction cannot be obtained the definitive surgery should be expedited. In some cases, the surgeon on call will not have the skill set to deal with these complex injuries. In this case, the patient should go to theater for repeat attempted closed reduction and possible temporizing spanning external fixator.

Postreduction the patient needs to be made aware of the possibility and importance of changing neurovascular status. If admitted to hospital this should be regularly monitored.

Considerations for surgery

The optimal management for fracture dislocations of the elbow is early definitive reduction and reconstitution of a stable elbow to allow for early motion. It is important to take a thorough history including patient's medical profile, level of function, employment and social history. Not only will this help to avoid unwanted complications, it will also help to set realistic goals from a functional outcomes point of view.

Definitive surgery should be carefully planned. The surgeon needs to be prepared to follow a stepwise intraoperative algorithm, as the stability of the elbow cannot be predicted until the operation is underway (**Figure 6.1**).

All of the major nerves crossing the elbow are at risk during surgery. Regardless of the situation, protection of intact and functioning nerves should be at the forefront of the surgeon's mind throughout planning and execution of these often complex and lengthy procedures.

Theater layout and patient positioning

The patient is placed supine with the arm on a radiolucent hand table. A few pillows are taped to the patient's chest allowing the surgeon to change positions and access the entire elbow (**Figure 6.4**). If using a global posterior approach, the surgeon can start with the arm over the patient. Once a skin flap is carried laterally and the Kocher interval opened the arm can stay over the patient or be placed on the hand table. This positioning is versatile and allows for easy imaging by moving the C-arm and not the elbow, avoiding undue stress on the ligamental complexes.

The usual (or common) technique of getting a lateral X-ray is to keep the fluoro machine in the AP position and internally or externally rotate the shoulder around to a lateral. Internal rotation puts a huge stress on the lateral collateral ligament (often just repaired). External rotation puts stress on the medial collateral (usually not repaired). Both views usually open the elbow in varus or valgus and result in poor image quality with a perfect lateral of the humerus and an oblique joint. A true neutral rotation lateral must be obtained to assess reduction. By moving the fluoro machine close to the patient and

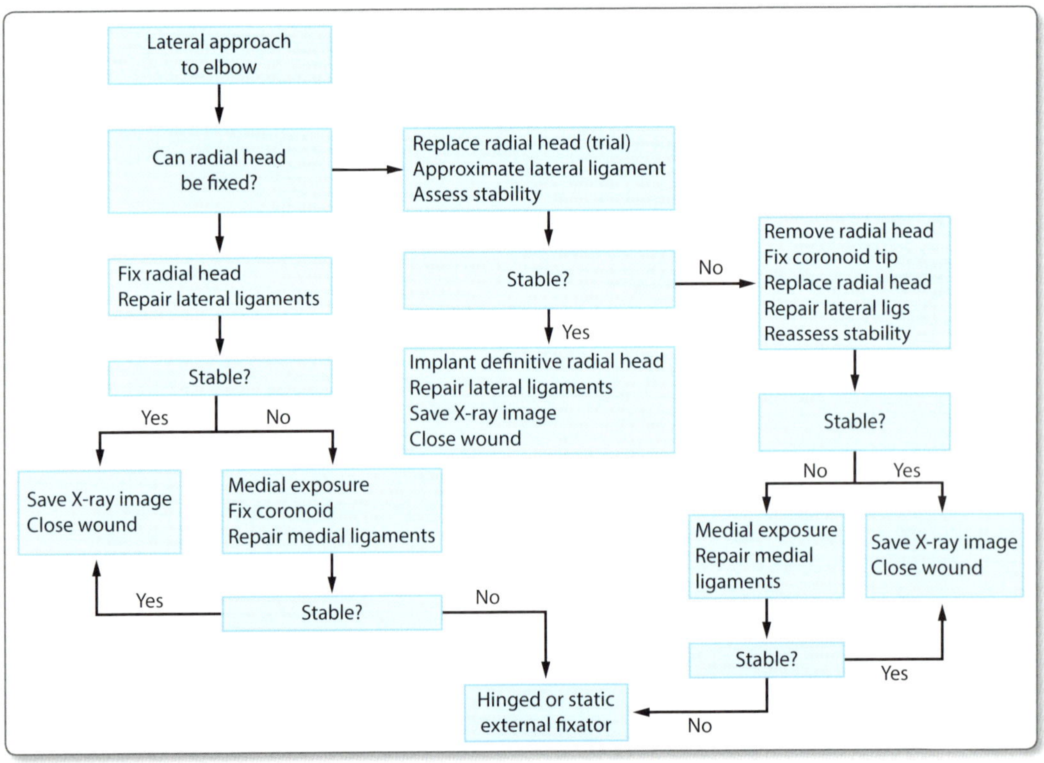

Figure 6.1 Proposed management algorithm for the treatment of fracture dislocations of the elbow.

Case example: Fracture dislocation of the elbow

A middle-aged woman lost her footing while boarding a train, sustaining a closed fracture dislocation of her elbow. The joint was reduced in the emergency department and splinted but redislocated (**Figure 6.2**). She was taken to theater and, using a lateral approach to the elbow, underwent radial head replacement and lateral ligament repair to stabilise the joint (**Figure 6.3**).

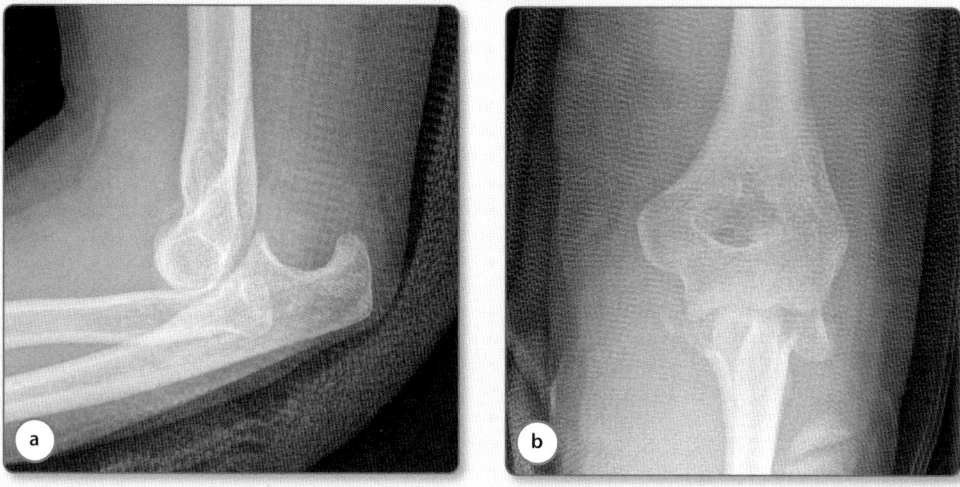

Figure 6.2 (a) AP and (b) lateral X-rays of posterior fracture dislocation with comminuted radial head fracture and suggestion of type 1 coronoid fracture.

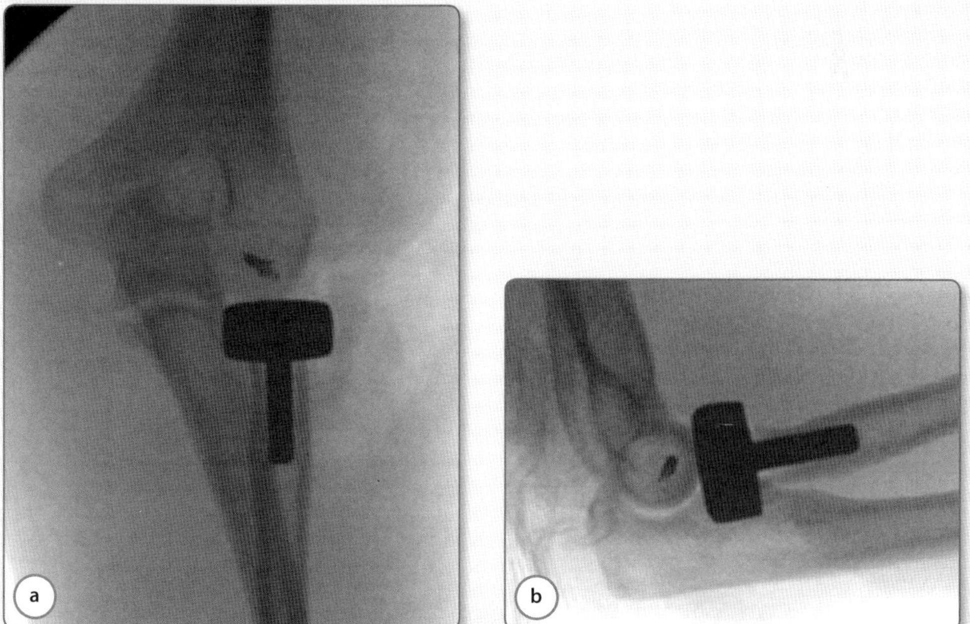

Figure 6.3 Intraoperative images from the patient depicted in Figure 6.2. Note the symmetry between the trochlea and ulna suggesting appropriate radial head sizing.

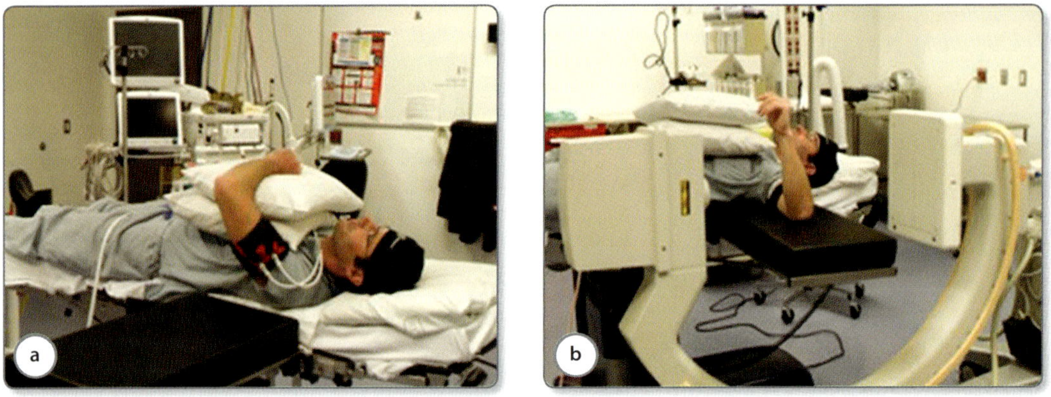

Figure 6.4 (a, b) Patient positioning for elbow surgery. Note moving of C-arm to obtain AP and lateral elbow images without stressing the medial and lateral soft tissues of the elbow.

coming through the arc to a true lateral, a neutral rotation film can be acquired (**Figure 6.5c**). The bed usually needs to be raised and it is a bit of a production but very worth it.

Review of surgical approaches

Kocher

- The skin incision can be made along the lateral border of the humerus over the lateral epicondyle across the joint and toward the subcutaneous palpable border of the ulna. Alternatively, a posterior universal skin incision can be utilized (**Figure 6.5a**)
- The interval between extensor carpi ulnaris (ECU) and anconeus is identified distally (**Figure 6.5b**). Look for a fat stripe and the characteristic fibers of anconeus that fan from horizontally orientated proximally to vertically orientated distally. Dissection then allows access to the joint (**Figure 6.5c**)
- Staying posterior to the ECU muscle ensures protection of the lateral collateral ligament (LCL). Keep the arm pronated to move the posterior interosseous nerve (PIN) anterior and away from surgical field. Dissection cannot be safely carried distal to the annular ligament without putting the posterior interosseous nerve at undue risk
- Most often the LCL is avulsed off of the humerus and this plane can be used to carry dissection proximally between triceps and brachioradialis

Medial approach to coronoid process

- After skin incision and identification/protection of the ulnar nerve, the nerve is followed into the natural split between heads of flexor carpi ulnaris (FCU). This plane is carried down to capsule and proximally up the flexor pronator mass (**Figure 6.6a**)
- The FCU splitting approach offers more exposure to the anteromedial facet of the coronoid (**Figure 6.6b**). The anterior portion of FCU and the flexor-pronator mass can be safely elevated off of the coronoid

Equipment requirements

- Small headless compression screws
- Radial head specific plates
- Radial head replacement set
- Suture anchors for ligament repair
- Suture passer for tip of coronoid avulsions
- Small buttress plates for larger coronoid fractures
- External fixator set

Reduction and stabilization methods

When fixing a 'typical' terrible triad, usually fixing or replacing the radial head and repairing the lateral ligaments is sufficient. Occasionally, the surgeon will need to fix a tip of coronoid fracture and, or the medial ligaments.

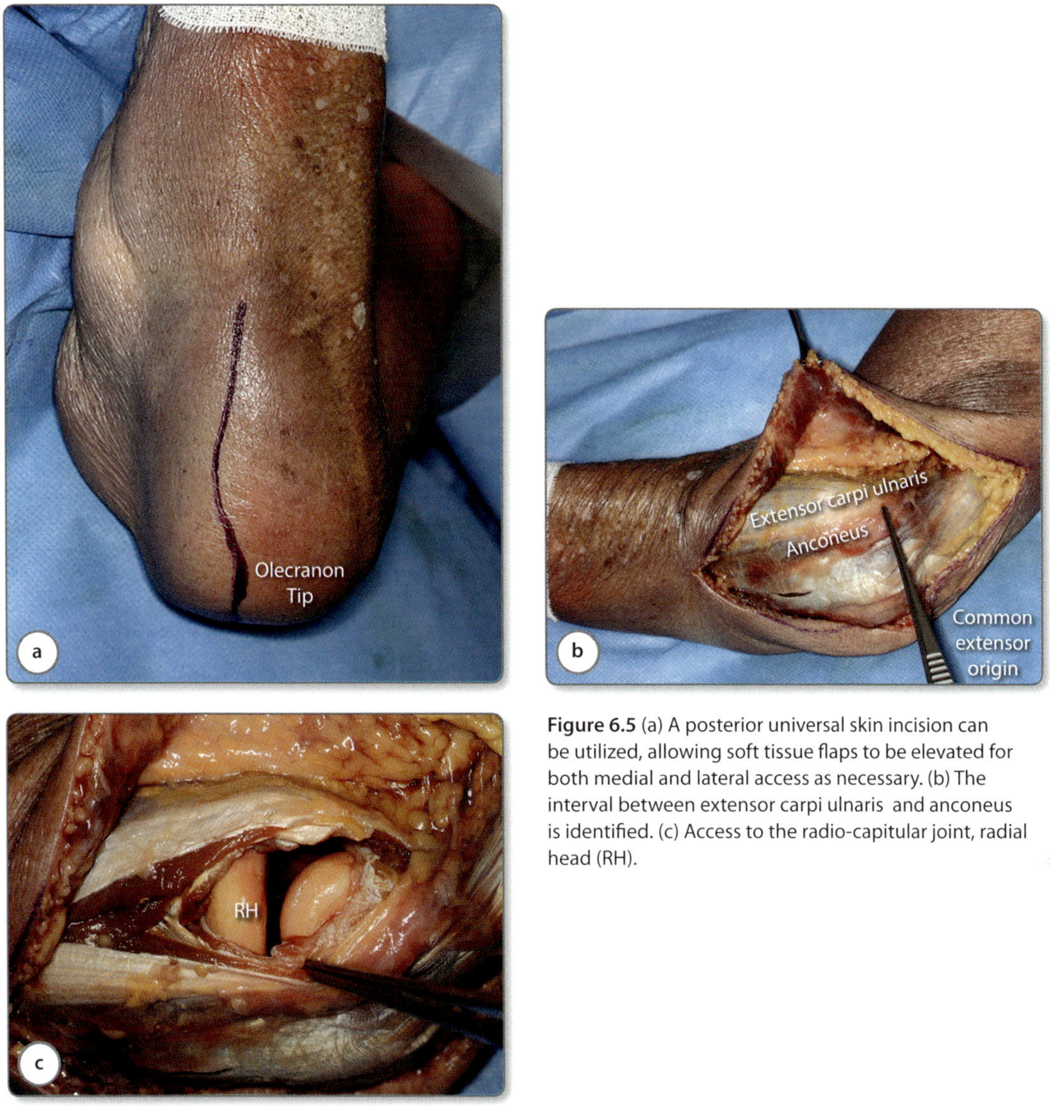

Figure 6.5 (a) A posterior universal skin incision can be utilized, allowing soft tissue flaps to be elevated for both medial and lateral access as necessary. (b) The interval between extensor carpi ulnaris and anconeus is identified. (c) Access to the radio-capitular joint, radial head (RH).

Radial head

Once exposed a decision needs to be made regarding the radial head. If the surgeon decides to fix the radial head they should set a time limit of about 30 minutes. A well done radial head replacement will perform better than a poorly fixed radial head. If using buried headless compression screws try to start in the small fragment with multiple wires. When inserting screw use the tip of thumb or finger to act as compression and counter-rotation (often in small fragments counter-rotation wire will cut out due to limited real estate). If using a plate or prominent hardware then be mindful of the non-articulating arc of the radial head.

If replacing the radial head use the native head as a sizer by putting it back together on the back table. If unsure, always downsize. Overstuffing the radial head is a common mistake, and will lead to a stiff elbow. There are several clues available to assess head size. Note, It always looks big on X-ray. This is because the thick articular cartilage of the native head does not show up on X-ray. The following tips can be helpful.

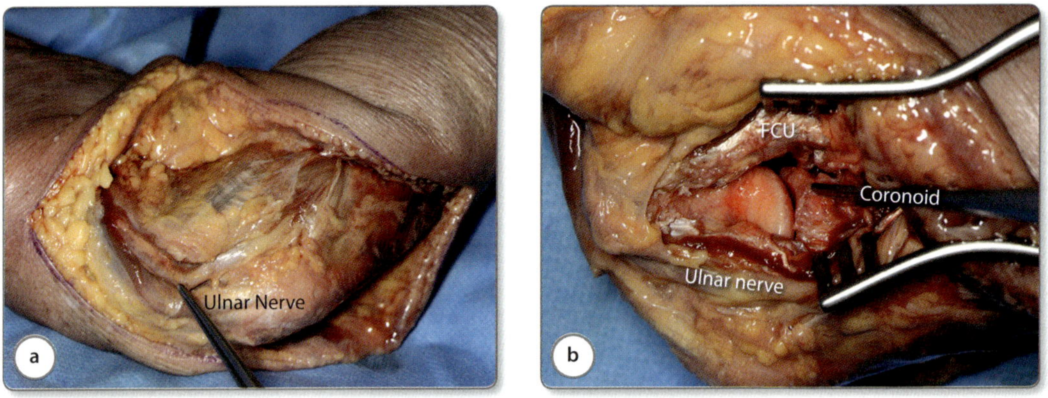

Figure 6.6 (a) The ulnar nerve is followed into the natural split between heads of flexor carpi ulnaris (FCU). (b) The anterior portion of FCU and the flexor-pronator mass can be safely elevated off of the coronoid for exposure . Care needs to be taken with self retainers on and around the ulnar nerve, as in Figure 6.6b, to avoid possible damage.

- Size the native radial head on the back table
- Use a planer to smooth out the neck
- When trialling, view the radial notch of the ulna and articular coronoid. The metal should be flush with this surface (**Figure 6.3a**)
- The radiocapitellar joint line needs to be symmetrical on anterioposterior X-ray (**Figure 6.3a**)

Coronoid fracture

If the radial head is being replaced, then radial head removal provides an excellent view of the tip of the coronoid. This can be secured with a suture and pulled back down. After grabbing the anterior capsule/coronoid with stitch, two divergent drill holes can be directed from the subcutaneous ulna to the base of the coronoid. The suture can then be passed and tied over a bony bridge. An ACL guide can be used to help with drill hole placement.

For the most part, fixation is unnecessary for small tip of the coronoid fractures. Although repair does confirm stability, it also can create stiffness. The minimum surgery required to create a stable elbow is all that should be done. Generally, with the radial head trial in place, the lateral ligaments can be approximated and stability assessed. If still unstable, the coronoid tip can be addressed after trial radial head is removed.

If the coronoid fracture is more than just the tip or the radial head amenable to fixation (not replaced) a medial approach is required. Care needs to be taken to protect the medial collateral ligaments of the elbow by working over the top of the anterior band. The apex of the coronoid fracture anteriorly on the ulna needs to be visualized and buttressed. Sometimes this can be done indirectly with posterior to anterior lag screws.

Lateral ligaments

A lateral suture anchor is placed at the isometric centre of rotation. An 18-gauge needle can be use with fluoroscopy to confirm the true centre. Generally, this is a few milimeters distal and anterior to the prominence of the lateral epicondyle.

The ligaments are almost always stripped from lateral epicondyle leaving it bare. They are usually easy to identify. Grabbing the lateral ligament with a separate stitch (heavy braided coated suture) allows several passes and a secure Mason-Allen type repair. This stich can then be approximated to the anchor with a slip knot or a bow. Stability can be assessed prior to committing to the repair.

Method of applying a static external fixator

The patient should be positioned supine with the arm on a radiolucent hand table. Pillows are placed on the patient's chest to allow the arm to periodically be positioned over the patient's chest if required (as above).

With the arm supine, two half pins are established in the distal third of the humerus.

Care needs to be taken to protect both the radial and ulnar nerves, and the pins should be inserted using an open approach. The radial nerve exits the intramuscular septum about 10–14 cm proximal to the lateral epicondyle travelling from posterior to anterior (**Figure 6.7**). The ulnar nerve is sitting in line with the direction of the pins on the medial side and is at risk with drill plunging or over insertion of the half-pins.

The incision should be about 4 cm proximal to the lateral epicondyle and extended 5–7 cm proximally along the lateral ridge. Spreading and blunt dissection to the bone is used, being sure to visualize everything that is being cut (radial nerve injury is an avoidable complication). Once on bone, drill guides can be used to protect the soft tissues. Drilling should take place laterally or slightly anterolaterally to avoid plunging. Pins should be placed by hand using fluoroscopic guidance. Blunt tipped pins are preferable because the threads are closer to the tip and they only need to be advanced about 2 mm beyond the medial cortex (thus protecting the ulnar nerve from injury). The arm can now be placed over the chest of the patient and the subcutaneous approach to the ulna is used to insert pins in a posterolateral to anteromedial direction. The elbow is then held reduced while the frame is constructed.

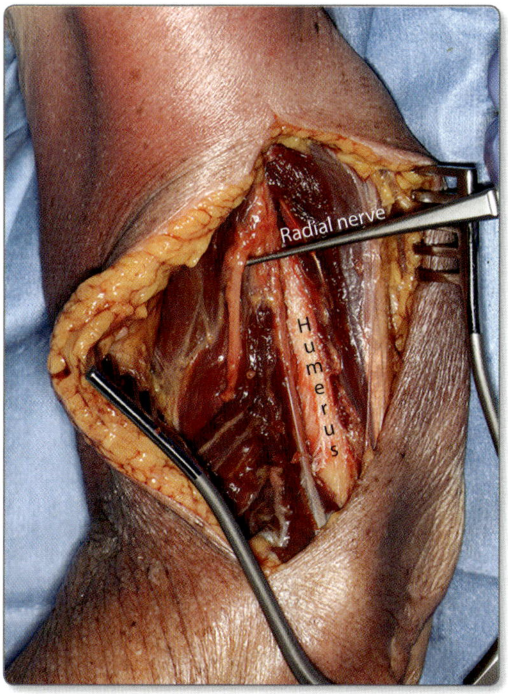

Figure 6.7 Cadaveric of distal lateral humeral exposure and orientation of radial nerve.

Rehabilitation

- Early active range of motion under physiotherapy supervision, as per surgeon's instructions
- Sling use when mobilizing for comfort

Avoiding postoperative complications

- Be aware of the medial coronoid fracture (**Figure 6.8**). This injury often looks benign but has a complex natural history. Loss of the medial buttress of the coronoid in combination with lateral ligament injury can result in gradual collapse into varus and rapid development of post-traumatic arthrosis. Restoring the coronoid medial buttress converts the injury to a simple elbow dislocation
- Avoid overstuffing the radiocapitular joint when a radial head replacement is needed (**Figure 6.9**)
- Never expose past the annular ligament to see the radial head/neck. If more exposure is required then the posterior interosseous nerve needs to be formally exposed
- Always expose the ulnar nerve when on the medial side. Be wary of self-retaining retractors when near nerves
- Early postoperative redislocation is not uncommon. A few simple measures can assist with stability in the early postoperative period
  - Avoid sustained intraoperative paralysis. Co-contraction of the biceps and triceps will help confer stability
  - The author prefers a postoperative sling to plaster. Regardless of how plaster is applied, it creates weight on the forearm which translates to a distraction force across the elbow. A sling, however, hangs the weight of the forearm off of the neck and shoulder creating a compression force at the elbow. Place the sling prior to the patient waking on the table. They are probably most at risk during wake-up and transfer. Stay with the arm through this process

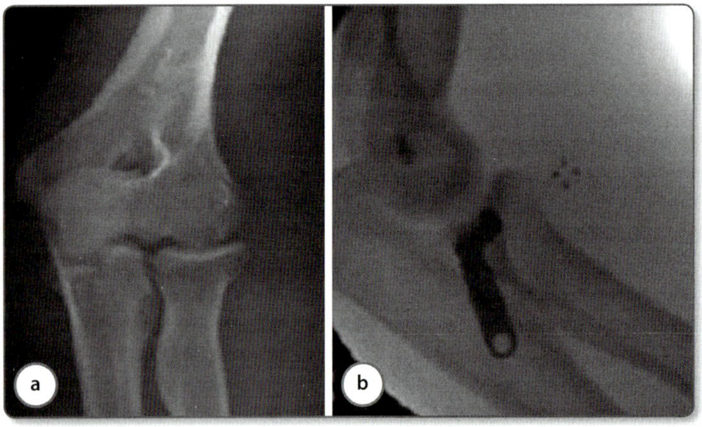

Figure 6.8 (a) A 27-year-old man fell from a ladder sustaining medial coronoid fracture. This elbow will predictably collapse into varus with loss of medial buttress and lateral tension band (lateral ligaments). If left untreated, there will be a rapid progression of post-traumatic arthritis. (b) Intraoperative views showing restoration of the medial buttress and lateral ligament repair.

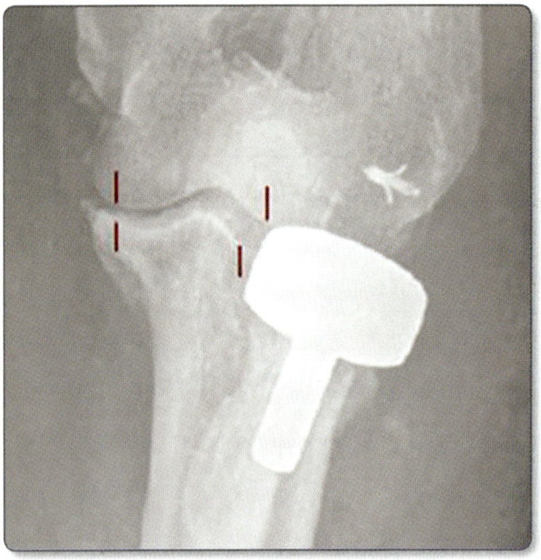

Figure 6.9 Asymmetric joint offers a clue that the radial head is oversized strutting the lateral aspect of the joint too far open, and will result in impaired function.

- If uncertain, repeat post operative X-rays in the recovery room
- During the operation, do not be tempted to accept an elbow that is barely stable at 90° of flexion. Take steps to improve stability

Summary of learning points

- Work in a logical step-wise manner approaching the structures that need repaired to confer stability
- Obtain orthogonal X-rays by moving the C-arm and not rotating the shoulder and elbow internally or externally to avoid undue stress on ligamentous structures
- A spanning external fixator may be needed on the elbow to maintain reduction and the case be referred to a specialist colleague

Further reading

Huh J, Krueger CA, Medvecky MJ, Hsu JR. Skeletal Trauma Research Consortium. Medial elbow exposure for coronoid fractures: FCU-aplit versus over-the-top. J Orthop Trauma 2013; 27:730–734.

Mathew PK, Athwal GS, King GJ. Terrible triad injury of the elbow: current concepts. J Am Acad Orthop Surg 2009; 17:137–151.

Wiss DA. Fractures (Masters Techniques in Orthopaedic Surgery), 3rd edn. Philadelphia: Lippincott Williams & Wilkins, 2013.

7 Forearm fractures

Phillip Johnston

Introduction

Forearm injuries are relatively common, although the majority comprise, or include, injuries at the distal radius and wrist, or to a lesser extent, at the elbow. Apparently isolated forearm fractures should therefore be considered in the context of potential injury at the joints above and below, including the joints connecting the two forearm bones: proximal radioulnar joints (PRUJ) and distal radioulnar joints (DRUJ) and the interosseus membrane. Similar to fractures in the lower limb below the knee, there is a relatively high incidence of open injury and of compartment syndrome. Vascular and neurologic injury must also be actively excluded.

Incidence

A large series from Edinburgh reported in 1998 has provided the most accurate estimate of fracture rates. Incidence varied according to sex and age, up to 4.49 per 10,000 patients per annum. Other groups have reported rates of forearm fractures, as a proportion of all fractures presenting to secondary care, to range between 5% and 44%. In one series, only 35% of forearm diaphyseal injuries were isolated and a further 40% were sustained in combination with multiple other injuries (polytrauma). Part of the uncertainty in knowing the 'true' rate of such fractures lies in the fact that isolated radius and ulna fractures represent only a subset of all forearm injuries. Ulnar shaft fracture with PRUJ disruption (Monteggia pattern) and radial shaft fracture with DRUJ disruption (Galleazi pattern) may be reported in published series as either within, or separate to, this overall category. Of course the commonest injury of all to the forearm is that of distal radius fracture, considered in the next chapter.

Mechanism of injury

During a fall onto the outstretched hand, the body usually turns away from the injured limb, leading to a supination (external rotation), valgus and often an extension (dorsally directed) force applied. Thus, the common fracture patterns will exhibit a short oblique or spiral configuration (with the fractures at different levels in each bone). A direct blow to the forearm will lead to a short oblique fracture with or without associated radioulnar joint disruption; the ulnar 'night-stick' fracture being a classic example. As with all fractures, the greater the energy transferred to the limb, the greater the degree of bone fragmentation (comminution) and of associated soft tissue injury.

Initial management/ prioritization

Following general considerations for patient resuscitation and stabilization, the most pressing associated injury is that of vascular compromise. An arterial disruption will occur at the time of maximal limb deformation and, as knowledge of warm ischemic time is crucial in decision-making with regard limb salvage or amputation, the time between injury and assessment must be known. If distal pulses are 'thready' or impalpable, then Doppler vascular assessment is essential. Angiography remains the gold-standard to assess distal vessel run-off but where perfusion remains clinically satisfactory, and therefore collateral flow is predicted to be sufficient for limb viability, there is less urgency to intervene.

Rates of compartment syndrome in the forearm have been reported as higher following soft tissue, than bony, injury. Predictably, this risk is greatest in young males, sustaining higher energy-transfer injuries. As elsewhere, the diagnosis is clinical, with reliance on invasive monitoring only an adjunct, and most useful in the anesthetized patient on ITU. Pain out of proportion to what is expected from the injury, especially once the limb is splinted, and with opiate analgesia administered, pain on passive stretch of the digital flexor and extensor muscles should prompt urgent review and consideration of myofascial compartment decompression (fasciotomy). In addition, acute carpal tunnel syndrome (and more rarely other acute nerve entrapments) – which presents with painful loss of function of the affected nerve, as opposed simply to dysesthesiae in its territory – requires combined fasciotomy and carpal tunnel release.

Open injuries are treated with the same principles as for an open injury of the lower limb. British guidelines, supported by extensive evidence, recommend a joint orthopedic-plastic surgical approach to all severe open limb injuries with formal debridement of the wound performed with more emphasis on presence of appropriately skilled surgeons, than on the time that the first debridement is performed. However, it should be remembered that, with increasing delay to first debridement, the rate of bacterial contamination, and therefore infection, will increase. Hence there is a balance to be struck to ensure the first wound debridement is effective but also timely.

Neurological assessment should comprise confirming integrity of the four motor nerves (median, anterior interosseus, ulnar and posterior interosseus) and three sensory (median, ulnar and radial). Penetrating or open injury, evolving neurological signs and neurologic deficit accompanied by vascular injury should all suggest nerve exploration. Where a nerve lesion

Case example: Diaphyseal both-bone forearm fracture

A 29-year-old female radiographer fell at work, striking the X-ray table and then landed on her outstretched hand. Initial clinical assessment showed that there was vascular compromise, no compartment syndrome, the fracture was closed and there was no neurological compromise. X-rays (**Figure 7.1**) revealed a spiral-pattern fracture of both forearm bones (with the fracture at different levels in each bone). This, unstable injury pattern was selected for operative stabilization. Using a high arm tourniquet both bones were approached separately and stabilized using absolute stability principles: inter fragmentary lag screw compression and compression plating (**Figure 7.2**).

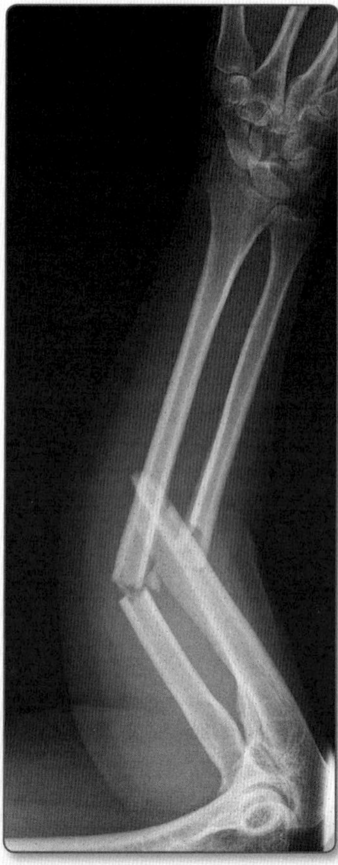

Figure 7.1 X-ray of unstable both-bone diaphyseal forearm fracture.

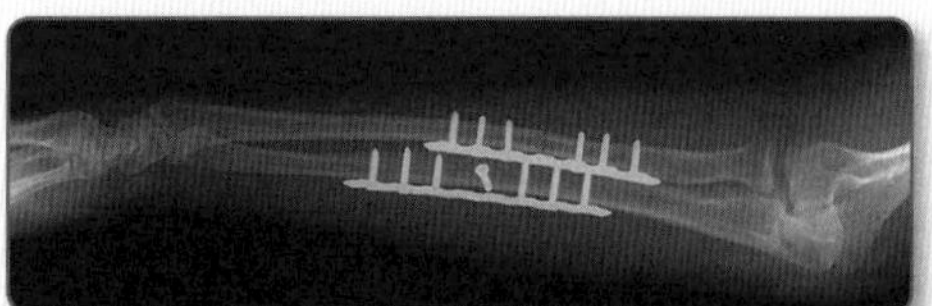

Figure 7.2 Postoperative fixation both-bone forearm fractures from the case illustrated in Figure 7.1.

is identified in the absence of these risk factors, it may be reasonable to monitor the deficit initially but not to intervene.

Considerations for surgery

Timing, as always, depends on clinical prioritization and skill-mix of the available surgical team. Most forearm injuries, which do not have one or more of the serious associated pathologies discussed above, can safely be splinted in a plaster slab and brought back for operative treatment on a semi-elective operating list.

As the forearm bones are connected throughout the entire limb, although such fractures are rarely truly intra-articular, all forearm fractures should be considered to disrupt this 'pseudo' articulation. Importantly, the radius is bowed to allow rotation about the ulna for forearm prono-supination. Malunions, or fixation of long segments of radius with a straight plate, will affect this movement, reducing range of motion significantly.

Thus, operative fixation must restore the natural curvature of the radial shaft, and reduce and stabilize the ulnar shaft, to allow optimal rotation. Further, specific fracture-dislocations (Monteggia and Galleazi patterns, as above) are 'true' intra-articular injuries and almost always require operative management. Finally, for isolated fractures (e.g. ulnar night-stick) the amount of displacement in the early weeks after injury will provide a guide to fracture stability. Non-operative management of an unstable such fracture has a high-rate of nonunion (mostly due to rotational shear forces at the fracture site).

As above, therefore, nonoperative management of adult forearm fractures is rarely appropriate, and relative contraindications to anesthesia or patient preference represent the commonest reasons to avoid surgery.

Theater layout and patient positioning

The patient is placed supine on the operating table. An arm table is used and a tourniquet applied for the approach. The author uses an adhesive U-drape to protect against surgical preparation-fluid ingress under the tourniquet.

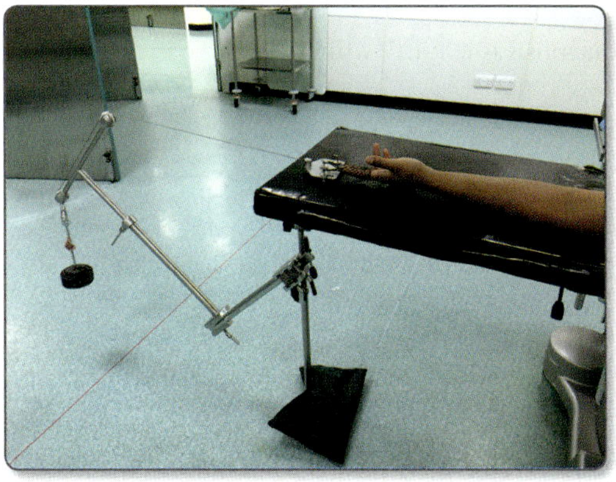

Figure 7.3 Finger traps and pulley system attached to arm table to help stabilize the limb with traction.

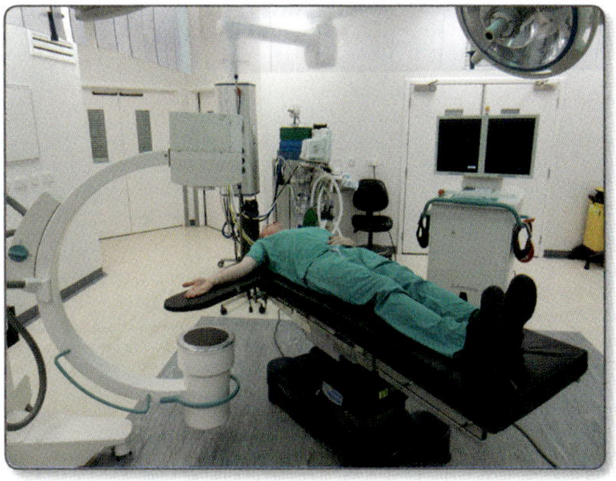

Figure 7.4 Positioning of operating table, arm board and image intensifier to the surgeon's preference.

To help stabilize the limb in some fractures, traction can be applied through the use of finger traps and a T-bar pulley system or equivalent (**Figure 7.3**).

In general, for forearm fracture fixation it is usual to sit adjacent to the patient's pelvis ('in the patient's axilla') and for the fluoroscopy C-arm, when required, to be positioned next to the assistant, brought in from the cranial end. Bipolar diathermy, suction and warming machines are positioned on the patient's contralateral side. The table may need to be eccentrically placed in the laminar flow hood, to centralize the limb under the laminar flow and also to protect the instruments under the hood (**Figure 7.4**).

Review of surgical approaches

Henry approach

- This approach employs the internervous plane between median and radial nerves
- Surface landmarks are the distal biceps tendon proximally and the radial styloid distally
- Cutaneous nerves potentially at risk include the lateral cutaneous nerve of the forearm (terminal branch of the musculocutaneous, and emerging from the radial border of brachialis, just above the elbow) and the palmar branch of the median nerve which pierces the distal forearm fascia in the midline, in the region of palmaris longus tendon (if present) or otherwise between flexor carpi radialis and flexor digitorum superficialis (**Figure 7.5a**)
- Often, this straight line is not the line of skin incision, especially if a concomitant fasciotomy and carpal tunnel release is planned, or if the incision is expected to extend above the elbow or below the wrist for some other reason
- Under these circumstances, the skin incision starts over the brachial artery proximally, medial to the distal biceps tendon, then swings obliquely radially across the limb toward the proximal radial musculature ('mobile wad'), longitudinally distally, and then obliquely toward the ulnar neurovascular bundle at the wrist before swinging obliquely radially again to run longitudinally distally over the carpal tunnel
- Superficial dissection is between the flexor muscles (pronator teres the most radial) and the 'mobile wad', comprising brachioradialis and the radial wrist extensors

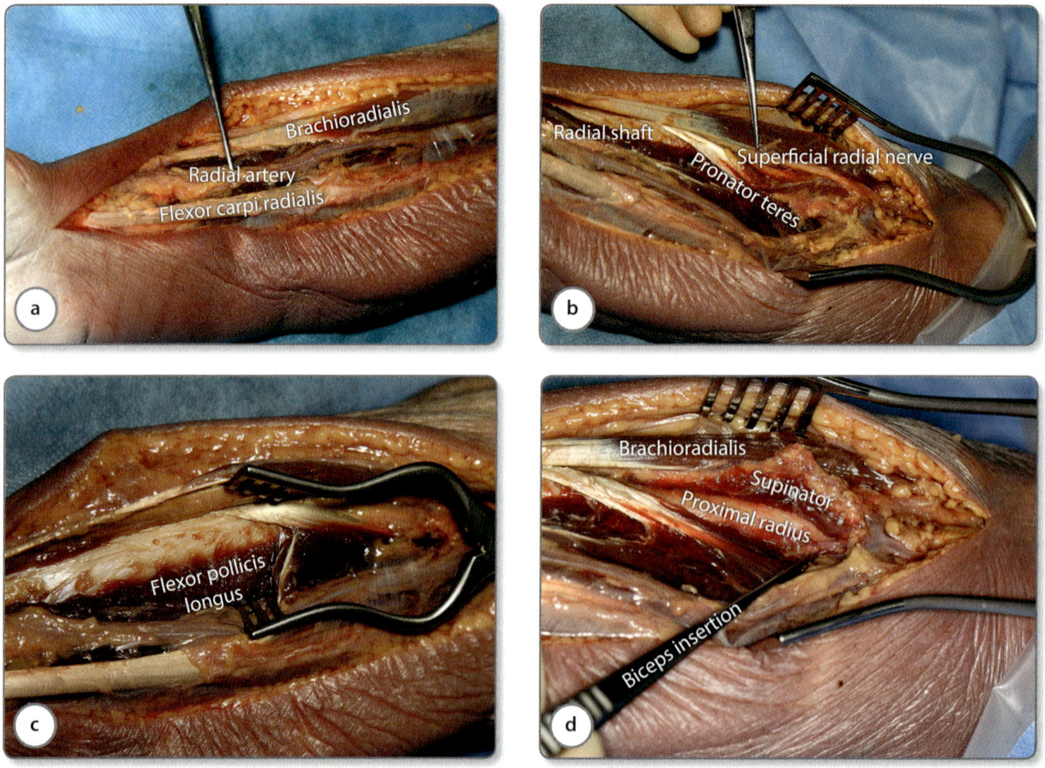

Figure 7.5 (a) Volar incision over flexor carpi radialis, with identification of radial artery. (b) Superficial radial nerve just under cover of brachioradialis. (c) Subperiosteal dissection of flexor pollicis longus giving access to anterior radial surface. (d) Proximal access to radius gained by careful subperiosteal elevation of supinator.

- The superficial radial nerve runs as the continuation of the radial nerve 'proper' once the posterior interosseus nerve has been given off in the proximal forearm. This sensory nerve runs under the tendon of brachioradialis (**Figure 7.5b**)
- Depending on the segment of radius required to be accessed, the radial artery will be reflected in an ulnar direction (for more proximal access) but may require radial reflection more distally. For accessing the entire radial shaft, there may be 'windows' above and below the point at which the artery crosses the radius bone. The 'true' Henry approach reflects the artery toward the ulna for the entire dissection but, as the artery wraps around the radial side of the wrist joint, deep to the first and third compartment tendons to the thumb and distal to the radial styloid, it is necessarily tethered relatively distally. Hence, this modification of the Henry approach as described above
- Deep dissection to access the mid-shaft of the radius is between pronator teres and supinator
- The forearm is pronated to access the most radial insertion of the pronator, performing subperiosteal dissection and releasing this muscle proximally and toward the ulna. The forearm is then supinated to access the most ulnar insertion of the supinator more proximally, which is then released toward the radial side. Proximal to this will be the biceps tendon, attaching to the radial tuberosity. Distally, flexor pollicis longus will require subperiosteal release in an ulnar direction to complete the exposure (**Figure 7.5c, d**)

Ulnar approach

- This approach employs the internervous plane between the ulnar-sided forearm flexors (ulnar nerve) and the ulnar-sided forearm extensors (posterior interosseous nerve)
- Surface landmarks are a straight line between the olecranon proximally and the ulnar styloid distally (**Figure 7.6a**)
- The ulnar shaft is palpable throughout its length, being subcutaneous (**Figure 7.6b**). The only cutaneous nerve at risk is the dorsal sensory branch of the ulnar nerve, given off at a variable position (mid- to distal ulnar shaft) in the flexor compartment and running around the ulnar side of the wrist joint, usually distal to the ulnar styloid where it may be palpable over the extensor carpi ulnaris tendon
- It can often be difficult to find a plane proximally between the two muscle bulks (flexors and extensors) but distally, this plane is usually obvious (**Figure 7.5b**)
- Bone levers, carefully inserted around the ulnar shaft, can help with this dissection, but it must be remembered that these can exert a large local force around neurovascular structures and should be used with care

Thompson's approach

- This approach employs the internervous plane between those forearm extensor muscles

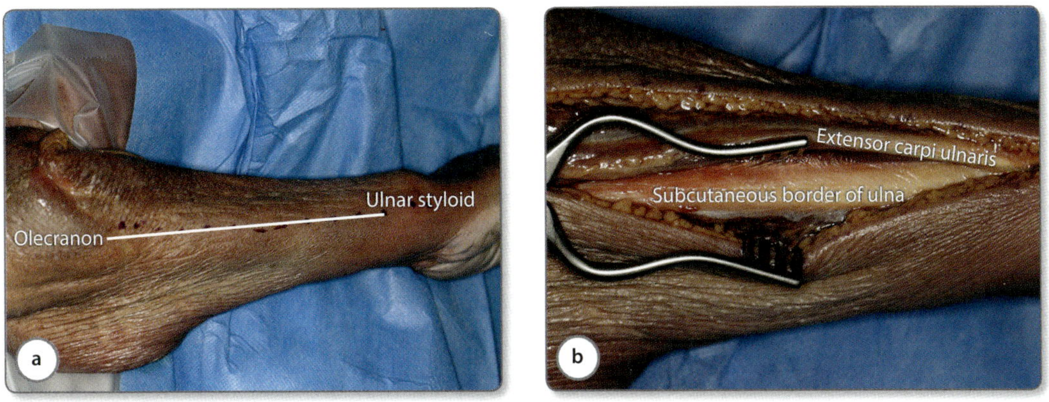

Figure 7.6 (a) Proposed skin incision for ulna approach. (b) Separation of extensor and flexor muscles giving access to subcutaneous border of ulna.

supplied by the radial nerve (above its bifurcation) and by the posterior interosseous nerve (beyond the supinator tunnel)
- Surface landmarks are the lateral epicondyle of humerus proximally and Lister's tubercle of the radius distally (**Figure 7.7a**)
- Cutaneous nerves at risk include the posterior cutaneous nerve of the forearm (which runs around the elbow on its lateral side in the region of the lateral epicondyle of the humerus) and the superficial radial nerve, after it has pierced the fascia under brachioradialis to enter the extensor compartment of the forearm
- The posterior interosseous nerve runs between the two layers of the supinator muscle to enter the extensor compartment of the forearm. Thus, those muscles in the 'mobile wad' are usually supplied by branches of the radial nerve above this division. These comprise brachioradialis and the radial sided wrist extensors [extensor carpi radialis longus (ECRL) and brevis (ECRB)]. The ECRB may be supplied by a branch from the posterior interosseous nerve, but this branch arises proximal to the supinator tunnel and, therefore, this muscle may still be reflected radially with its fellows and separated from these in the forearm as below
- Proximal superficial dissection is therefore between the ECRB and extensor digitorum communis (**Figure 7.7b**). In the bed of this plane lies the supinator
- Mid-shaft dissection reveals abductor pollicis longus (APL) and extensor pollicis brevis (EPB) in the bed. Distal dissection is between ECRB and extensor pollicis longus (**Figure 7.7c**)
- For deeper dissection proximally, as per the Henry approach to the flexor aspect of the forearm, supinating the forearm protects the posterior interosseous nerve as the nerve is moved toward the ulna within supinator, and the most ulnar fibers of muscle can be dissected off the radial shaft and reflected dorsally and toward the ulna

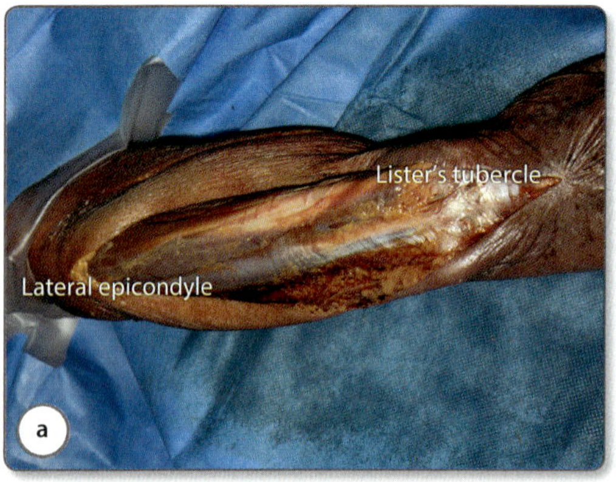

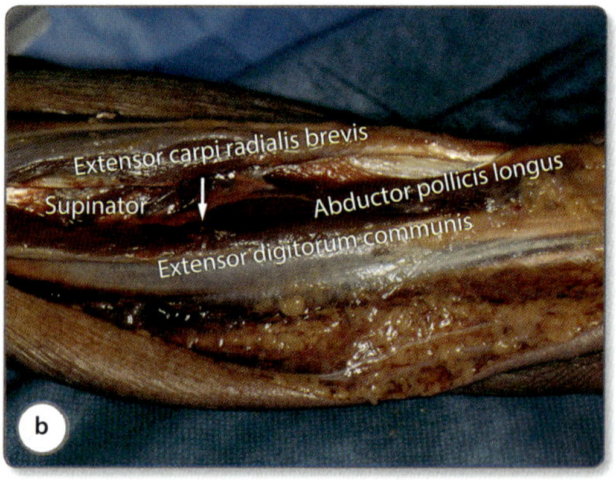

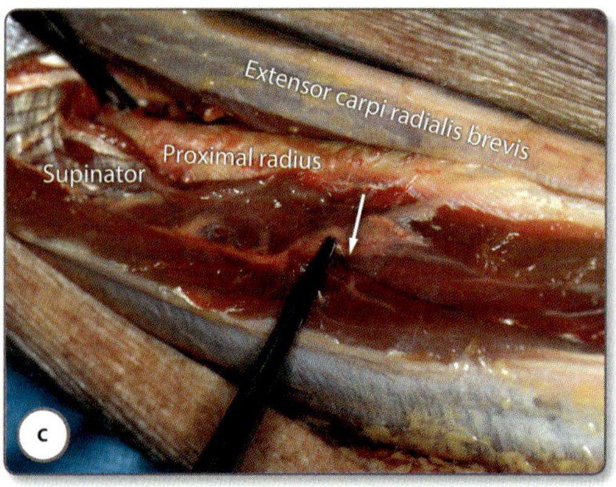

Figure 7.7 (a) Dorsal skin incision with exposure of posterior forearm muscle. (b) Dorsal muscle groups, with arrow localizing posterior interosseous nerve (arrow shows pin). (c) Proximal radial exposure with elevation of the supinator (the arrow shows the localizing posterior interosseous nerve).

- In the mid-shaft of the radius, APL and EPB arise from the ulnar surface of the radius and the interosseous membrane. They run obliquely radially and distally, crossing superficial to the radial wrist extensors. Thus, access to the section of the bone requires 'windows' above and below these muscles which must be mobilized accordingly

Equipment requirements

- A tourniquet should be applied and inflated for dissection, but may sometimes be deflated for the remainder of the fixation and also before closure, to minimize tourniquet time and optimize hemostasis
- Bipolar diathermy should be used, given the number and proximity of neurovascular structures
- Most fracture systems now provide for locking, and nonlocking screw-plate interface. Thus, dynamic compression may be achieved but fixed-angle construct completion may also be performed, using the same plate. Plates designed specifically for the proximal ulna (olecranon, coronoid), proximal radius (radial neck) and distal radius and ulna are often of a smaller gauge, and again precontoured. It is not unreasonable to fix segmental fractures with two separate plates
- Segmental fractures can be stabilized during fixation using a temporary external fixator or finger-trap traction as above

Reduction and stabilization methods

Fix the simpler fracture pattern first to use as a guide for forearm length, especially if there is bone loss in the other bone. In any case, once the first bone has been fixed, this incision is left open for subsequent adjustment as necessary when fixing the second. Two incisions should be used if possible, to minimize the risk of subsequent heterotopic ossification (synostosis).

If compression plating is employed, an eccentric screw, beyond the planned plate position, may be used to augment the compression, either using a plate- or screw-holding forceps, or with an articulated tensioning device.

When fixing oblique fracture patterns, creating an 'axilla' between the bone and the plate will allow the other fragment to be compressed into this space, minimizing translational displacement during compression. In addition, some oblique fractures lend themselves to interfragmentary compression (lag) screw placement, either through, or separate to, the plate.

Depending on which surface of the radius the fixation is placed, the plate may require precontouring, to restore the natural radial bow. When plating the entire ulna, again ulnar-specific plates may be used, which recognize that the ulna has a bend in the junction between the proximal and middle thirds of its diaphysis. Short segments of the radial and ulnar shafts may be fixed with a straight plate.

If bridge-plating is planned, then precontoured plates are at their most useful, as they can be used as a template to reduce the various fragments to. For highly comminuted segmental fractures, passing a small titanium elastic nail along the intramedullary canal of each fragment may help to maintain some stability prior to fixation. Lag-screw or K-wire fixation of larger fragments may also help simplify the overall fracture pattern, even if these are subsequently removed following fixation (**Figure 7.2**).

Grafting materials

Managing bone loss in radial or ulnar shaft fractures is no less challenging than in other parts of the appendicular skeleton. As elsewhere, acute shortening is an option, which can be combined either concomitantly or subsequently with distraction osteogenesis to restore length. Scant evidence exists to guide the amount of shortening in the forearm which may be accepted without significant functional loss of the digital flexor and extensor muscles. For defects less than 2.5 cm, no functional deficit is expected and therefore lengthening techniques are probably not necessary under these circumstances.

For larger defects, the Masquelet technique may be used in combination with bridge-plating, with bone graft material applied secondarily into the cavity, following removal of the temporary cement spacer, once the Masquelet membrane has been induced. This bone graft may be autologous cancellous chips, cadaveric bone graft or one of the several forms of calcium phosphate synthetic grafts available.

Free vascularized grafts have been used, the commonest being free fibular graft, which have the advantage of immediate structural stability. This is probably most appropriate for the largest bone defects.

With regard to the abovementioned significant open injuries, management of bone loss is rarely a situation that should be tackled by an inexperienced surgeon and should be undertaken in conjunction with a team skilled in the regular management of such problems.

Rehabilitation

Directed physiotherapy with specific attention to:

- Wrist excursion (flexion/extension)
- Forearm supination/pronation
- Hand intrinsic muscles
- Shoulder movement

Avoiding postoperative complications

- A written step-by-step operative plan, displayed within the operative theater, will serve as a holistic team brief and aide-mémoire for the various pieces of extra equipment which may make the process of fracture fixation simpler or more efficient
- Meticulous soft tissue technique can reduce the risk of postoperative adhesions and myotendinous tightness
- Employing two separate incisions to fix the two forearm bones is almost always mandatory, as this will be associated with a lower rate of heterotopic bone formation and synostosis formation
- Attention to the patient as a whole (avoiding hypothermia and generalized or localized limb hypoperfusion) is equally important, hence minimize duration of the tourniquet
- A stable construct which can facilitate immediate or early mobilization is associated with fewer complications with regard stiffness
- A tourniquet is used throughout the dissection and fixation, released before wound closure. This has two benefits: firstly ischemic time is minimized (wound closure can take some time) and secondly vessels which bleed appreciably can be identified and cauterized before closure. Hematoma formation will increase the risk of postoperative infection and that of swelling, and swelling-associated complications
- Wound closure is as important as the remainder of the procedure and closure under tension should be avoided, as this can lead to ischemia, secondary wound dehiscence and infection. If the injury leads to such significant swelling that the wound edges cannot be approximated, then involvement of a plastic surgeon may be necessary to discuss the need for alternative techniques such as temporary negative-pressure wound therapy with subsequent skin grafting, or other local (and sometimes distant) flaps

Salvage options

Principles behind treating nonunion include recognizing the cause(s) and altering the environment to remove, or minimize, the effect of these. For example, following open fractures, low-grade infection is a common cause for nonunion. The biomechanical environment will have a significant influence and the role of soft tissue cover should not be underestimated.

It is therefore incumbent on the nonunion surgeon to be familiar with techniques which address these issues, and a multidisciplinary approach is often required, with input from infectious diseases physicians and reconstructive (plastic) surgeons, in addition to the orthopaedic surgeon.

In situations where low-grade infection is present, segments of bone may need to be debrided and certainly no necrotic native material should be left in situ. The secondary defect thus created will need to be addressed using methods outlined above, along the lines of managing a primary bone defect due to trauma. Skeletal stability is paramount and suppressing infection to allow bone union, even in the presence of contaminated metalwork, is always preferable to removing metalwork (and therefore losing construct stability). For this reason, surgeons treating infected nonunions may employ external fixation techniques, such as use of hybrid or circular frames, to maintain skeletal stability despite removing internal fixation implants.

Where infection is not present, the biomechanics of the fracture site must be addressed.

If the strain at the fracture is low (< 3%), there is a tendency for direct bone healing, which cannot occur if the fracture gap is greater than 50–100 μm. Thus, a poorly reduced fracture, or one in which the bone ends have resorbed, e.g. due to loss of vascularity, will not unite if treated with 'absolute stability' techniques.

Conversely, bridge-plating – allowing the bone to heal with callus – requires a greater strain (5–10%) which only becomes likely with increasing comminution, as the strain is shared between the various fragments. Implants that are too stiff (e.g. stainless steel plates with a relatively short 'working length', or distance between the nearest screws on opposite sides of the fracture) may not favor such a strain environment. Optimizing the working length may require appreciable dissection above and below the zone of injury to fix the plate well away from the fracture zone, although minimally invasive percutaneous fixation techniques can reduce the soft tissue insult of long plate placement.

Treating nonunion where absolute stability is required, but where a fracture gap exists or has developed, is relatively straightforward: without opening the fracture ends, reducing the strain and fracture gap leads to union. This usually requires significant compression, only achievable using eccentrically-placed equipment such as the articulated tensioning device and/or interfragmentary lag-screw(s). The compression afforded using an eccentrically drilled screw in a dynamic compression plate is rarely sufficient under these circumstances.

Where nonunion follows bridge-plating, often the segmental fracture has become simpler with union between some of the fragments. Thus ongoing strain experienced at the fracture site(s) is concentrated at fewer points and is therefore greater. This situation can be treated along the lines described above, with compression plating. If nonunion occurs in combination with a short plate (three or fewer screws per segment), this again may relate to suboptimal mechanical stability afforded by the construct, which may be ameliorated by using a longer plate.

In situations where nonunion relates to overlying soft tissue loss, local or distant (free) flaps of soft tissue may be required to bring with them increased vascularity.

Summary of learning points

- Neither bone is straight, and reduction of either bone to a straight plate will alter the natural curvature of each, which will reduce the potential rotation of one about the other
- Second to the tibia, the forearm is the most common region to develop compartment syndrome after injury
- Vascular injury is also not uncommon, especially after elbow or proximal forearm fractures
- Open fractures need consideration along the same lines as those for the lower limb, and evidence supports urgent, but not emergency, debridement and fixation, usually on the first available daytime operating list
- The most common nerve lesion seen following forearm fractures is that of acute carpal tunnel syndrome
- Most forearm fractures are optimally treated by open reduction and internal fixation

Further reading

Hertel R, Pisan M, Lambert S, Ballmer FT. Plate osteosynthesis of diaphyseal fractures of the radius and ulna. Injury 1996; 27:545–548.

Jayakumar P, Jupiter JB. Reconstruction of malunited diaphyseal fractures of the forearm. Hand (NY) 2014; 9:265–273.

Kapandji A. Biomechanics of pronation and supination of the forearm. Hand Clin 2001; 17:111–122.

Rehim SA, Maynard MA, Sebastin SJ, Chung KC. Monteggia fracture dislocations: a historical review. J Hand Surg Am 2014; 39:1384–1394.

Rupasinghe SL, Poon PC. Radius morphology and its effects on rotation with contoured and noncontoured plating of the proximal radius. J Shoulder Elbow Surg 2012; 21:568–573.

8 Distal radial fractures

Alan Johnstone, Iain Stevenson

Introduction

Distal radial fractures are commonly encountered in the daily practice of an orthopaedic surgeon. Their management is often dependent on surgeons' education and past clinical experience with a careful assessment of patient functional demands.

Incidence

In adults, recent epidemiological studies suggest that their incidence is approximately 18% and that the distribution of injury is bimodal affecting principally young adults and the elderly.

Mechanism of injury

Younger adult patients tend to have higher energy injuries most commonly resulting from sports and road traffic accidents. In the elderly, multiple factors contribute to the increased incidence of these injuries, including a higher proportion of elderly people within Western populations, extreme age, osteoporosis, significant co-morbidities resulting in falls, and for a select group, higher activity levels.

Initial management/ prioritization

A complete history should be obtained and a full examination performed on all patients with a distal radial fracture remembering the potential for injury to other sites in the ipsilateral limb. In particular, the neurovascular status of the patient's forearm and hand should be assessed to identify signs of median nerve injury or an evolving acute compartment syndrome. Gross anatomical abnormalities should be reduced to alleviate symptoms, especially if there is neurovascular compromise, and splinted prior to obtaining routine imaging. A minimum standard radiographic examination should include a posteroanterior (PA) and a true lateral X-ray of the wrist.

The treatment strategies vary depending upon several factors including the age of the patient, premorbid function, mechanism of injury, associated skeletal injuries affecting other sites, status of the soft tissue envelope, and fracture complexity.

The majority of distal radius fracture results from simple low energy falls and can be treated satisfactorily by conservative treatment in a well molded cast.

Considerations for surgery

Absolute indications

- Open fractures
- Associated neurovascular injuries including compartment syndrome

Compartment syndrome (CS) is more common than is currently appreciated. High energy injuries and segmental fractures should increase suspicion of compartment syndrome. Compartment syndrome should be also considered in the patient who has sustained a number of injuries resulting in systemic hypovolemia or hypoxia. Open fractures do not preclude CS and once diagnosed, patents should undergo urgent open decompression of the carpal tunnel and fasciotomies as necessary.

Relative indications

- Fracture mal-alignment resulting in any of the following:
  - Greater than 10° of dorsal angulation
  - Less than 15° of radial inclination
  - Greater than 3 mm of radial shortening
  - Intra-articular step or gap of greater than 2 mm
  - Complex or inherently unstable fracture patterns

Case example: Distal radial fracture

A middle-aged woman fell getting out of the shower, injuring her non-dominant wrist (**Figure 8.1**). She underwent a focused neuromuscular examination of the injured upper limb before a manipulation under hematoma block was undertaken. This reduction was suboptimal and she was admitted for further surgical management. She underwent reduction and fixation via a bed of flexor carpi radialis approach and application of a volar plate (**Figure 8.2**).

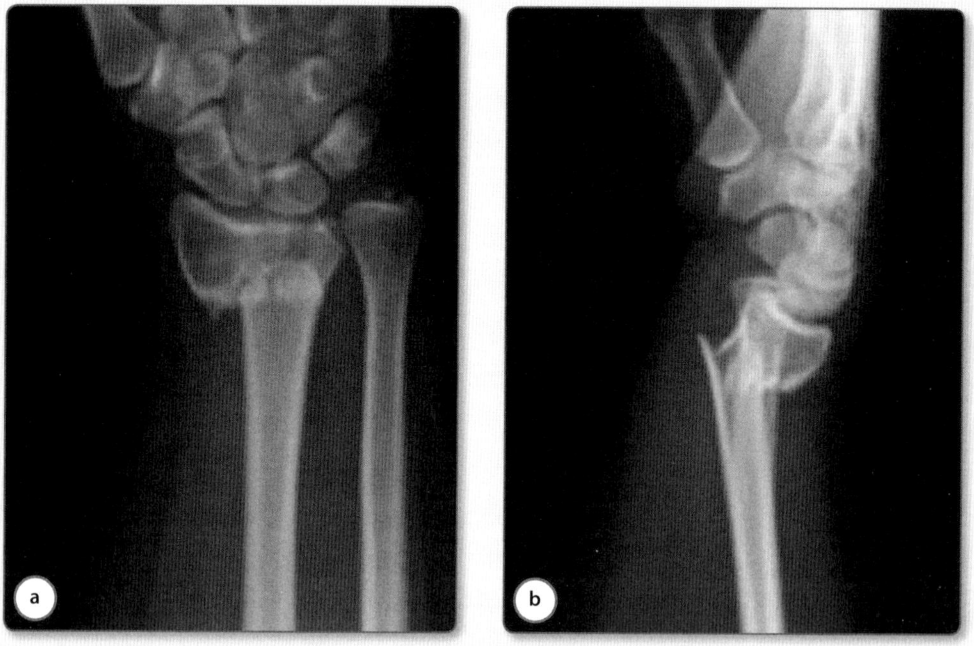

Figure 8.1 (a, b) X-rays of a wrist injury in a middle-aged woman.

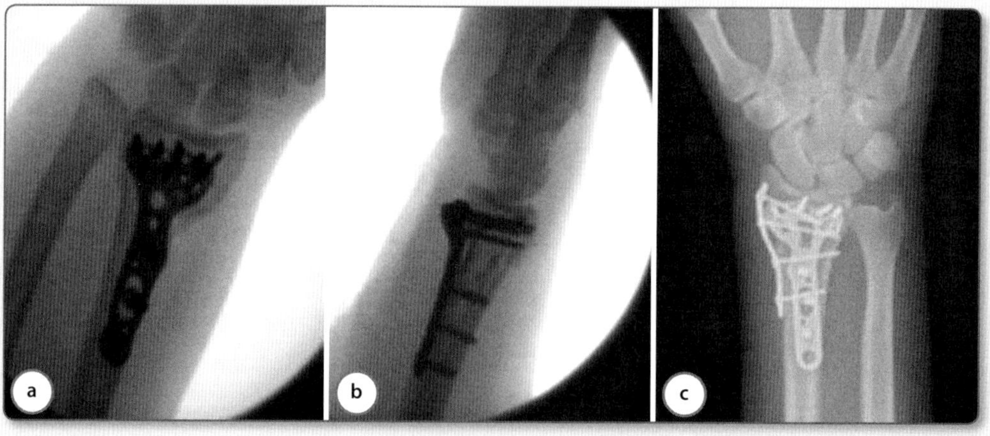

Figure 8.2 (a, b) Postoperative images of case example. (c) X-ray of radial styloid plate and volar locking plate in situ.

Theater layout and patient positioning

Position patient supine and use a radiolucent arm board or table (**Figure 8.3**). An upper limb tourniquet should be used (sterile if proximal forearm or elbow injury suspected) although a tourniquet is beneficial for any form of open reduction and internal fixation, tourniquet time should be minimized. Where possible, the tourniquet pressure should be reduced in line with each patient's preoperative blood pressure to minimize ischemic damage and tourniquet crush. As a rule, tourniquets must be deflated at 120 minutes and not re-inflated for at least 10–15 minutes thereafter. Sit in axilla of patient for surgical access. Position the C-arm and screens appropriately for unobstructed visualization.

Review of treatment options

Kirschner wiring (K-wiring)

The recent distal radius acute fracture fixation trial (DRAFFT) study which was a randomized controlled trial comparing K-wire fixation versus volar locking plate fixation in dorsally displaced distal radial fractures, has renewed the popularity of K-wire fixation. The main techniques use either extrafocal or intrafocal wire placement although a combination can be used if considered necessary. Extrafocal wires cross from one bone segment to the other after the wrist has been manipulated into a satisfactory position. Intrafocal wires are inserted into the fracture site and are used to partly lever open the collapsed fracture prior to being drilled into intact volar cortical bone maintaining the fracture position (Kapandji technique).

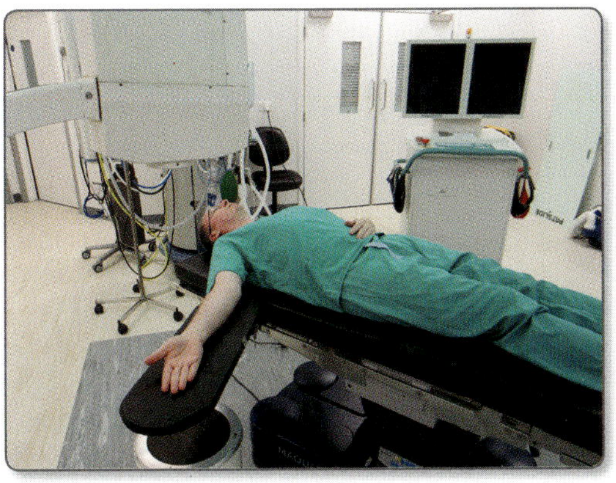

Figure 8.3 Proposed theater layout and positioning.

Extrafocal technique

A useful tip is to place a wire along the axis of the radius in line with Lister's tubercle as visualized on the anteroposterior (AP) intensifier image and to mark the skin with a pen.

Similarly, on the lateral intensifier image, place a wire along the optimal position and again mark with a pen. This can act as a handy perioperative reference tool for wire placement in both the coronal and sagittal planes.

Via stab incisions and blunt dissection to avoid iatrogenic nerve or tendon injury, the wires are advanced. In our institution, we prefer to bend and bury the wires to reduce the risk of infection and some studies suggest that rate of infection can be reduced from 20% to 4% by adopting this technique although it does necessitate another operation to remove them once the fracture has healed.

Intrafocal technique

The dorsal wire(s) is placed through the fracture site. In the original description of the technique, the dorsal wire was initially passed percutaneously through the fracture site at 90° to the axis of the radius. With the tip of the wire at the midpoint of the canal the wire was angled distally by approximately 45° and then advanced proximally through the volar cortex. A styloid wire was passed to augment the fixation and then the wires cut, bent and dressed with a cast being applied.

Bridging external fixation

Joint bridging external fixation can be utilized as either a definitive or temporizing treatment.

The three potential perioperative complications that are of concern surgically are:

- Tethering of the extensor tendons
- Damage to the superficial radial nerve
- Fracture of the metacarpal

Ways to avoid these complications include:

- 3 mm metacarpal pins should be placed bicortically in the metaphyseal flare and the shaft of the 2nd metacarpal via an open approach and should be inserted at 45° to the dorsoradial plane

- Excellent anatomical knowledge and familiarity with topical landmarks, pin placement in the diaphysis is again via an open technique between the extensor carpi radialis longus and brevis interval
- Predrilling of the radial shaft and the index finger metacarpal prior to insertion of Schantz screws

Unless the skin incisions are excessive, they should be left open, but if wounds do need to be closed, this should be undertaken at this stage before the clamps and connected bars are attached.

Once the frame construct has been loosely applied, the fracture is reduced and the clamps tightened.

- Excessive palmar flexion of more than 10° must be avoided as is associated with increased carpal tunnel syndrome
- Ulnar deviation of more than 20° should be avoided due to excessive strain on the triangular fibrocartilage complex
- if either excessive palmar flexion or ulnar deviation is required to maintain fracture reduction then alternative frame construct, possibly including additional pins placed in the 4th metacarpal, should be considered

After tightening the frame, the fingers should flex easily to the palm. Failure to achieve this passively or if it is associated with excessive rebound, may indicate over distraction of the fracture with excessive tensioning of the extensor digitorum tendons that can result in long term functional deficit.

The radiocarpal and midcarpal joints should be assessed radiographically to avoid over distraction. Over distraction of 5 mm or more should be avoided as this is associated with a poor clinical outcome.

Nonbridging external fixation

- Allows mobility of the wrist in the early postoperative period
- Two half threaded 3 mm Schantz pins are inserted into the distal fragment under image intensifier control The intervals between 1st and 2nd extensor compartment and in the 3rd compartment after retracting the extensor pollicis longus tendon are used
- Volar cortical purchase must be achieved
- A good tip is to pass the pins parallel to the joint on the lateral view and subsequently use these to reduce the fracture
- Proximal pins are placed in a similar fashion to the bridging technique described above

Internal fixation

Volar locking plate (VLP) fixation is thought by many to be the 'gold standard' but even these implants need to be used properly to achieve the desired aims.

Indications for internal fixation with a VLP are:

- Failed conservative management
- Marked comminution of the metaphyseal region of the volar cortex
- Oblique fracture configuration involving the metaphysis
- Segmental fracture pattern

Review of surgical approaches

Volar approach – flexor carpi radialis (FCR)

- Supinate the forearm
- Perform longitudinal incision over FCR tendon (**Figure 8.4a**)
- Retract to ulnar side
- Incise bed of FCR, to reveal flexor pollicis longus, retract this to ulnar side (**Figure 8.4b**)
- Identify pronator quadratus (PQ) in bed of incision
- Sharply dissect PQ from radial border of radius to expose volar aspect of distal radius (**Figure 8.4c**)
  - Care must be taken not to open the radiocarpal joint (RCJ)
  - After reflecting the PQ, the distal radioulnar joint (DRUJ) should be easily palpable but should not be opened
  - A hypodermic needle can be used to identify the RCJ
  - Complex fractures may require increased exposure to facilitate fracture reduction and/or supplementary plate fixation along the radial border of the radius. In these instances it is necessary to open the carpal tunnel by extending the incision into the palm. The incision is curved ulnar wards over the transverse wrist crease and

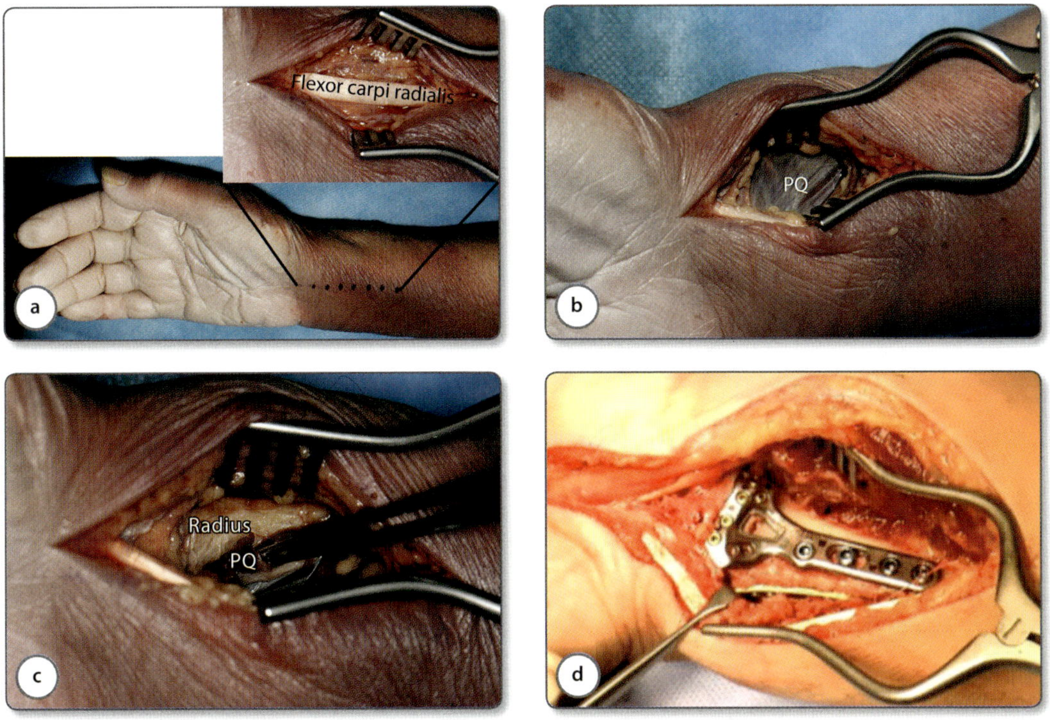

Figure 8.4 (a) Palmar incision over flexor carpi radialis tendon. (b) Incise bed of FCR and retract to ulnar side with flexor pollicis longus to expose pronator quadrates (PQ). (c) Sharply dissect PQ from radial border of radius to reveal volar surface of distal radius. (d) Intraoperative image of extended carpal tunnel release and volar locking plate in situ.

extended longitudinally in line with the long finger metacarpal taking care to identify and protect the median nerve, the motor branch of the median nerve and the palmar cutaneous branch of the median nerve (**Figure 8.4d**).

Dorsal approach

- Pronate the forearm and perform longitudinal incision in line with the long finger metacarpal extending from the midpoint of the metacarpal, across the wrist crease centered on Lister's tubercle, and extended approximately 10 cm proximal to the RCJ (**Figure 8.5a**). This length of incision is required to permit adequate mobilization of the extensor tendons to expose the fracture adequately
- Open the extensor retinaculum through the 3rd extensor compartment, containing the extensor pollicis longus (EPL) tendon. The tendon is dislocated from the compartment and allowed to adopt a position overlying the 2nd extensor compartment
- Using sharp dissection, the remaining long finger extensor tendons, contained within the extensor retinaculum, are elevated both radially and ulnar wards to expose the dorsal radius (**Figure 8.5b**)
- Usually, it is also necessary to expose the RCJ to facilitate restoration of the joint surface via an arthrotomy. This is undertaken by sharp dissection placed 2–3 mm distal to the rim of the distal radius exposing the scaphoid and lunate. Exposure of the joint is improved by palmar flexing the wrist and also enables the surgeon to assess any damage to the scapholunate ligament
- In extreme cases, where patients have sustained extensive carpal injuries in addition to a distal radius fracture, the dorsal capsule can be reflected from the dorsal aspect of the proximal and distal rows using sharp dissection. The method described by Berger is

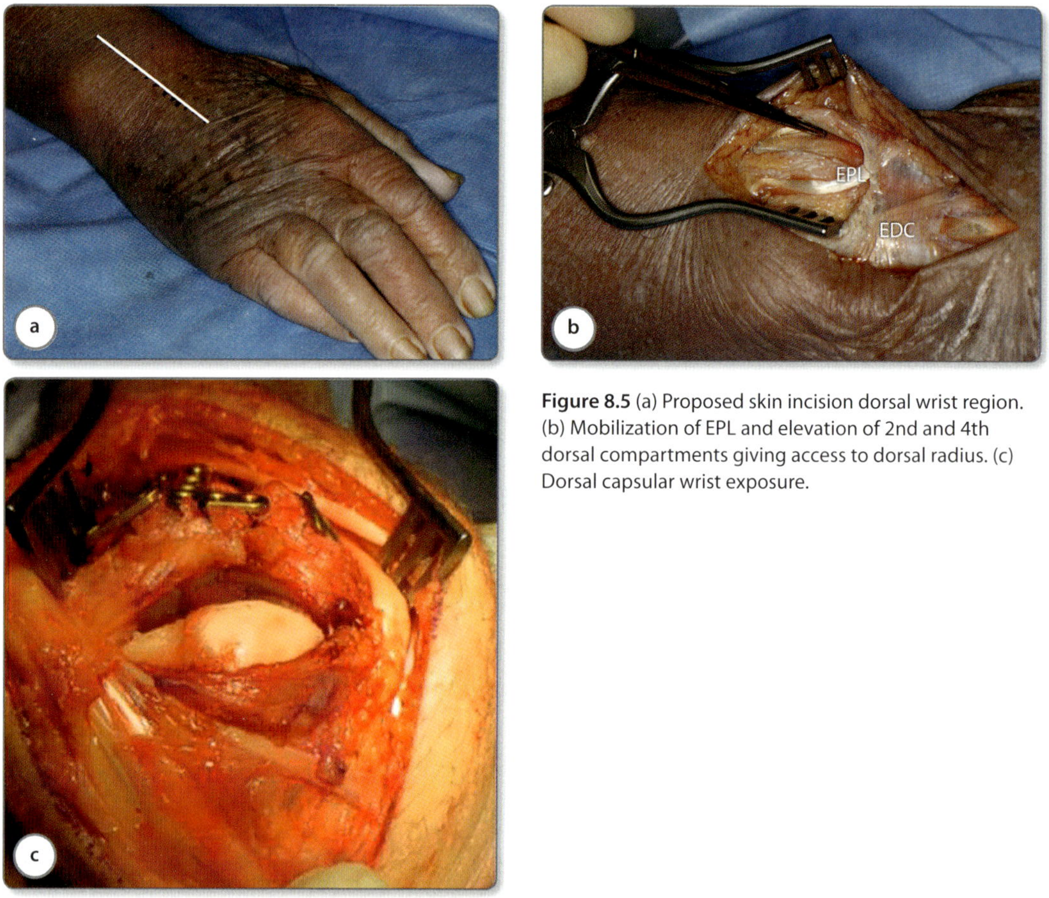

Figure 8.5 (a) Proposed skin incision dorsal wrist region. (b) Mobilization of EPL and elevation of 2nd and 4th dorsal compartments giving access to dorsal radius. (c) Dorsal capsular wrist exposure.

probably advantageous over other exposures since it is least disruptive to the dorsal wrist ligaments and provides excellent exposure (**Figures 8.5c**)

Timing of surgery

Definitive treatment for the majority of distal radius fractures that have occurred following low energy injuries can usually be undertaken within 24–48 hours following the injury.

One other exception to this is when the surgeon believes that a combined approach, using both volar and dorsal approaches, will be necessary to restore bone alignment. In these circumstances, it is essential to permit soft tissue swelling to resolve over a period of several days and not uncommonly 10–14 days. During this period, it may be necessary to apply a bridging external fixator to maintain overall length of the radius if cast immobilization is insufficient. Care must be taken to apply the external fixator in a way that will prevent the pin sites from communicating with the future definitive internal fixation.

Equipment requirements

- 1.6 mm K-wires
- Wiring set including wire cutters and benders
- Wrist specific plating systems and implants/ small fragment system
- Battery drill
- Wrist external fixator systems

Reduction and stabilization methods

Utilizing open exposures as necessary the joint surface needs to be recreated and the bones held out to length before being stabilized as appropriate.

Fracture reduction of dorsally angulated and/or displaced fractures can usually be performed by palmar flexion of the distal radius and hand. The position can be maintained by resting the dorsum of the wrist/hand on several packs prior to a suitable volar locking plate being applied.

Additionally temporary fixation using K-wires or spanning external fixator can be utilized to maintain fracture reduction prior to the plate being applied.

Fracture reduction of volarly displaced fractures can usually be performed by direct pressure applied to the fracture while applying a volar buttress plate (**Figure 8.2**).

The distal locking screws need to be placed close to the articular surface if good stability is to be achieved permitting early active mobilization.

The surgeon also has to be certain that the VLP is providing adequate stability of all of the fracture fragments. One common mistake is to assume that large styloid fracture fragments, especially if the fracture line is oblique, are adequately supported by the VLP. In these circumstances, the surgeon should consider the use of a second-plate, placed along the radial border of the radius to buttress the styloid fragment (**Figure 8.2c**).

It is necessary to carry the dissection sufficiently radially to release part of the insertion of Brachioradialis and to open the first dorsal extensor compartment.

Predictors of instability

- Fractures that over displace, i.e. are easily overcorrected so that the distal fragment is translated volar to the radial shaft
- Metaphyseal or radial column comminution
- Associated ulnar column fractures involving the distal shaft of the ulna
- Elderly patients

Grafting materials

Bone graft is rarely required since carefully placed plates and screws can usually support the elevated bone fragments. Where bone graft is required, it is usually possible to obtain sufficient cancellous bone from the shaft of the radius, either accessing the canal of the radius through the fracture or through a separate cortical window after predrilling the cortex. We have little experience with using artificial graft materials although others advocate their use, usually combining them with limited percutaneous fracture fixation methods. In these circumstances, injectable calcium phosphate cements are advantageous since they conform well to the shape of the fracture cavity and harden to give good resistance to longitudinal loading of the forearm although torsional stability is limited.

Rehabilitation

- Request physiotherapy review and input early
- Elevation of limb
- Encourage finger/elbow/shoulder range of movement if patient casted
- Undertake strengthening and wrist range of motion exercises with progression of union

Avoiding postoperative complications

Infection/wound healing problems

- Careful soft tissue handling
- Tension-free wound closure
- Consideration to inserting buried K-wires
- Prescription of antibiotics

Loss of reduction

- Appropriate fracture reduction
- Properly applied implants and/or K-wires

Complex regional pain syndrome

One apparent advantage of VLP fixation over conventional cast +/– K-wire fixation has been the reduction in cases of CRPS-I that occur following treatment of a distal radius fracture. Presumably this reflects the ability of the patient to undertake early active movements of the forearm, hand and wrist postoperatively.

Salvage options

The majority of distal radius fractures heal adequately and patients function sufficiently well and without significant symptoms. However, problems that may require further treatment are:

- Post-traumatic osteoarthritis of the RCJ
- Disruption of the DRUJ resulting in significant limitation of forearm rotation

Post-traumatic RCJ arthritis requiring surgical intervention is uncommon and tends to be most troublesome in young manual workers. In these

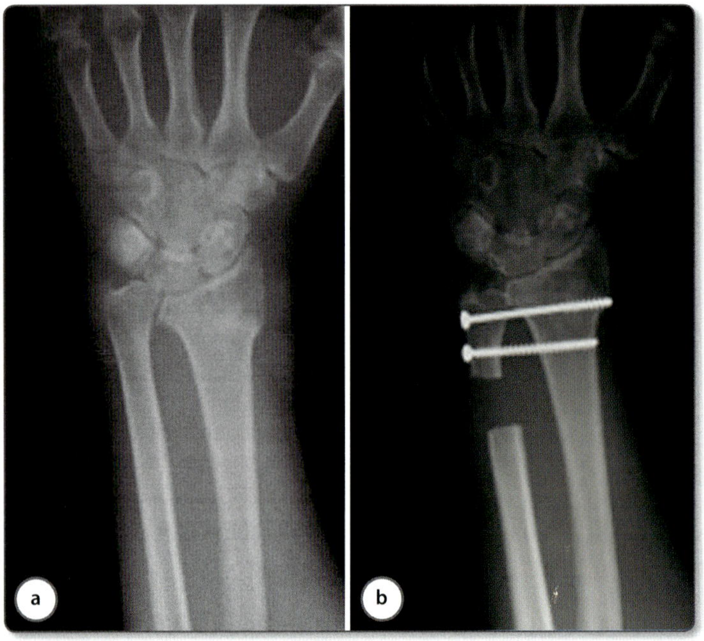

Figure 8.6 An example of Sauvé-Kapandji procedure: (a) pre- and (b) postoperative X-rays.

circumstances a wrist fusion, performed using one of the anatomical wrist fusion plates gives a predictably good result.

DRUJ disruption is common and usually results from excessive shortening of the radius following the conservative management of fractures, but the majority of these patients do not have significant functional restriction. However, for those whose function is poor, usually due to marked restriction of forearm rotation, consideration should be given to performing a modified Sauvé-Kapandji procedure (**Figure 8.6**). From our experience, this is a good method for restoring function and minimizing symptoms, although care must be taken to maintain the soft tissue envelope between the shaft of the ulna and the distal end of the ulna to prevent 'chop-sticking' of the ulna shaft against the radius.

Summary of learning points

- Accurate neurovascular documentation both pre- and postoperatively is mandatory
- Presurgery CT scans may be necessary in complex fracture management planning
- Be prepared to decompress the median nerve as necessary, but avoid damaging the recurrent branch (motor) and the palmar cutaneous branch (sensory) in extended carpal tunnel release.
- Be familiar and proficient with the above techniques in order to manage the vast spectrum of distal radial fractures
- Dorsally protruding screws will result in extensor tendon ruptures
- Early rehabilitation improves function and reduces the incidence of chronic pain

Further reading

Berger RA. A method of defining palpable landmarks for the ligament-splitting dorsal wrist capsulotomy. J Hand Surg Am 2007; 32:1291–1295.

Capo JT, Swan KG Jr, Tan V. External fixation techniques for distal radius fractures. Clin Orthop Relat Res 2006; 445:30–41.

Costa ML, Achten J, Parsons NR, et al. Percutaneous fixation with Kirschner wires versus volar locking plate fixation in adults with dorsally displaced fracture of distal radius: randomised controlled trial. BMJ 2014; 349:g4807.

Fujita S, Masada K, Takeuchi E, et al. Modified Sauve-Kapandji procedure for disorders of the distal radioulnar joint in patients with rheumatoid arthritis. Surgical technique. J Bone Joint Surg Am 2006; 88:24–28.

Kapandji A. Ostéosynthèse par double embrochage intra-focal traitement fonctionnel des fractures non articulaires de l'extrémité inférieure du radius. Ann Chir 1976; 30:903–908.

Rafique A, Ghani S, Sadiq M, Siddiqui IA. Kirschner wire pin tract infection rates between percutaneous and buried wires in treating metacarpal and phalangeal fractures. J Coll Physicians Surg Pak 2006; 16:518–520.

Hemorrhage control

The pelvis is next evaluated in the emergency department. Following Advanced Trauma Life Support (ATLS) guidelines, pelvic injuries are addressed during the 'circulation with hemorrhage control' part of the primary survey. Springing or stressing the pelvis is now discouraged if an injury is suspected. It is both unreliable and risks disturbing the retroperitoneal clot. A pelvic X-ray used as an adjunct to the primary survey should be obtained early.

If a pelvic ring injury is identified, resuscitation should continue with the pelvic binder in situ. Log rolling the patient is strongly discouraged, if a pelvic ring injury is identified as this also risks disturbing a retroperitoneal clot. The best clot is the first clot and every effort should be made to preserve it.

Damage control resuscitation (DCR)

The concept of DCR, which started in the military, is now well accepted and is being adopted in civilian trauma centers. Initial resuscitation for severely injured patients is based on a strategy of permissive hypotension and blood product resuscitation guided by patient's physiologic response. In severely injured trauma patient with on-going major hemorrhage, there is improved outcome from early hemostatic resuscitation compared to large volume clear fluid resuscitation. In the UK, National Institute for Health and Care Excellence (NICE) recommends that crystalloid fluid therapy should only be administered to a trauma patient if there is an absent radial pulse. Boluses of 250 mL of crystalloid should be given while the patient is being transported to hospital without delay and the radial pulse intermittently checked. Hemostatic transfusion (also referred to as massive transfusion protocols across trauma centers) should be initiated early. Most transfusion protocols will contain plasma and platelets as well as packed cells in an attempt to replenish the clotting factors that have been lost in the retroperitoneal hematoma. Tranexamic acid has also been shown to be effective in reducing mortality as a result of significant bleeding. It is most effective when administered as a 1 g bolus within the first 3 hours following the injury.

In approximately 90% of hemodynamically unstable patients with pelvic ring injuries, the previously outlined measures should be sufficient to control hemorrhage and stabilize the patient. In the remaining 10% of patients who continue to exsanguinate, more aggressive intervention is needed.

In a major trauma center, a combination of surgical stabilization, pelvic packing and angiographic embolization can be used if general resuscitative measures are unable to control the bleeding. The management algorithm is dependent on available local resources. The use of cell-savers and other auto-transfusion devices has become standard practice during pelvic and acetabular surgery.

The lethal triad

The 'bloody vicious cycle' of coagulopathy, hypothermia and acidosis should be corrected simultaneously to give the patient the best chance of survival. Surgical intervention to stabilize the pelvis has been shown to help control hemorrhage and avoid late complications. The timing of surgery is based on the patient's physiological state. A traffic light system of monitoring venous lactate, in conjunction with correcting acidosis, hypothermia and coagulopathy, has been shown to be effective in guiding management. A venous lactate > 2.5 mmol/L is a 'STOP' sign for surgical intervention, as the surgery will provide another physiological insult that a compromised patient may not tolerate. A venous lactate of < 2 mmol/L is 'GO' for surgical stabilization. If the venous lactate is 2–2.5 mmol/L, then the trend is observed, with a descending pattern being favorable for surgery.

Dynamic assessment and observing of trends during resuscitation with regular communication between the decision-making clinicians has been demonstrated to improve overall safety and team effectiveness.

Urinary and bowel injury

The incidence of urethral lacerations and bladder ruptures in complex pelvic injuries appears to be 5% to 10%. Urinary catheterization should also be used as a guide for resuscitation. The perineum should be inspected for any external signs of a urological injury. Blood at the external meatus is a sign of potential urethral or bladder injury. One catheterization attempt by an experienced practitioner should be performed along with a retrograde urethrogram. Early urological consultation should be sought if an injury is suspected or a failed catheterization. A suprapubic catheter or complete urinary diversion may have to be undertaken in severe cases.

Open injuries

In addition to inspection of the perineum, an open pelvic ring injury is not excluded until rectal and vaginal examinations have been performed. If this is not possible in the emergency department, it should be documented as 'outstanding' and eventually performed once the patient is stabilized or prior to surgery. Early administration of intravenous antibiotics with gram positive and negative cover is now considered lifesaving in these injuries. If a rectal or bowel injury is suspected, a diverting colostomy with placement in the upper abdomen is advised.

Considerations for surgery

In injuries where a mild amount of energy is absorbed, the pelvic ring tends to fail anteriorly first; symphysis pubis diastasis or pubic rami fractures of different configurations occur at the front. This is usually accompanied by some degree of strain to the sacro-spinous and sacro-tuberous ligaments.

With the continued application of force, the pelvic ring then goes on to fail posteriorly. This can occur at the sacroiliac joint, through a sacral fracture or through the posterior aspect of the iliac wing (crescent fracture). Sacral fractures can be difficult to identify on plain radiographs and the exact configuration is better appreciated on CT scans.

Hemorrhage following a pelvic ring injury can be life-threatening. Most of the pelvic bleeding is venous arising mainly from the presacral and paravesical venous plexus posteriorly and from bleeding cancellous surfaces. Blood will quickly fill up the retroperitoneal space and the formation of a clot in that space is essential to stop further bleeding from the disrupted veins. In approximately 10% of cases with significant pelvic bleeding, an arterial injury will be the cause. The mechanism of injury has been directly linked to the amount of blood loss.

The bony pelvis also provides protection and soft tissue attachments for intrapelvic organs. The integrity of the pelvic floor is an important consideration and the direction of displacement can give an indication of associated soft tissue injury. Urogenital injuries are most common with APC and LC injuries while neurovascular injuries are more common in vertical sheer type injuries. More than 80% of patients with unstable pelvic fractures have additional musculoskeletal injuries. Associated injuries have been closely linked to functional outcome measures.

Open fractures

Although a rare occurrence, open pelvic fractures are very serious injuries and carry a mortality of up to 50%. The open nature of the fracture can be due to penetration of rectum or vagina as well as through external wounds. Open injuries are frequently missed and often only discovered at time of surgery.

Theater layout and patient positioning

The decision to position the patient prone or supine depends on what is needed to reduce and stabilize the posterior part of the ring. A radiolucent carbon fiber table enables adequate image intensifier access (**Figure 9.2**). Inlet and outlet views require the image intensifier to achieve quite severe angles under the table. Visualization can sometimes be quite poor due to bowel gas and certain body habitus. Having

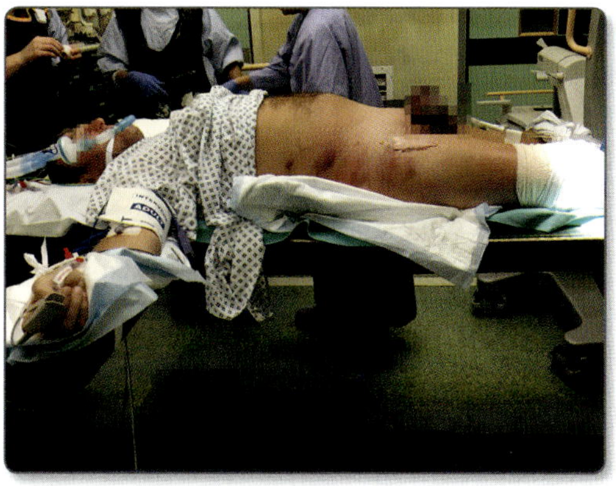

Figure 9.2 Carbon fiber table with clear space below for image intensifier; arms out at right angles to body.

Case example: Vertically unstable pelvic fracture

A 32-year-old man fell off a climbing wall from a height of approximately 12 m, landing mainly on his right lower limb. Initial management took place in accordance with ATLS guidelines. He was initially hemodynamically unstable but stabilized following one major trauma transfusion pack. Following this he underwent an initial AP pelvis X-ray (**Figure 9.3a**) and CT scans (**Figure 9.3b,c**). He was taken to theater and placed supine on a radiolucent table before anterior pubic stabilisation was undertaken via a Pfannenstiel skin incision and separation of the rectus sheaths allowing reduction and plating of the pubic rami. Then, still in the supine position, the posterior pelvis was stabilized with bilateral percutaneous cannulated sacral screws (**Figure 9.4**). Note suture anchors for rectus sheath reattachment, damaged at the time of injury.

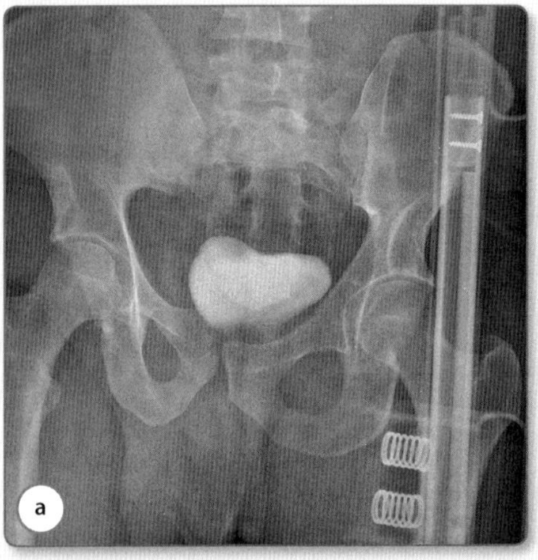

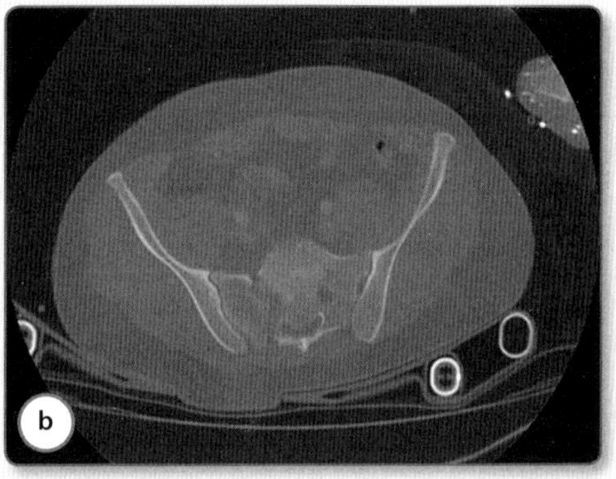

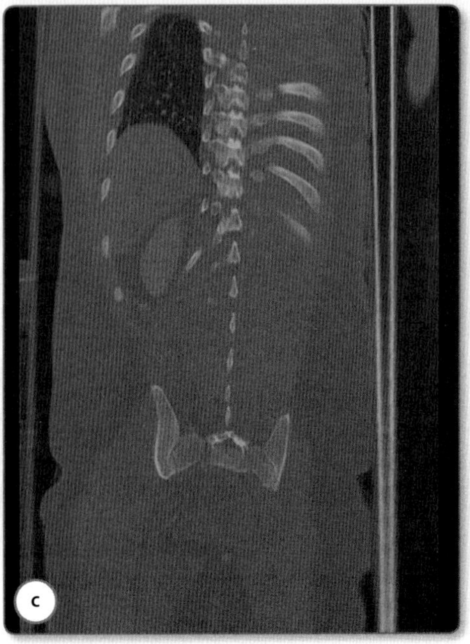

Figure 9.3 (a) Initial AP pelvic X-ray showing anterior ring disruption at symphysis: contrast in bladder. (b, c) Axial and coronal CT images showing bilateral sacral fracture posteriorly.

Case example: *continued.*

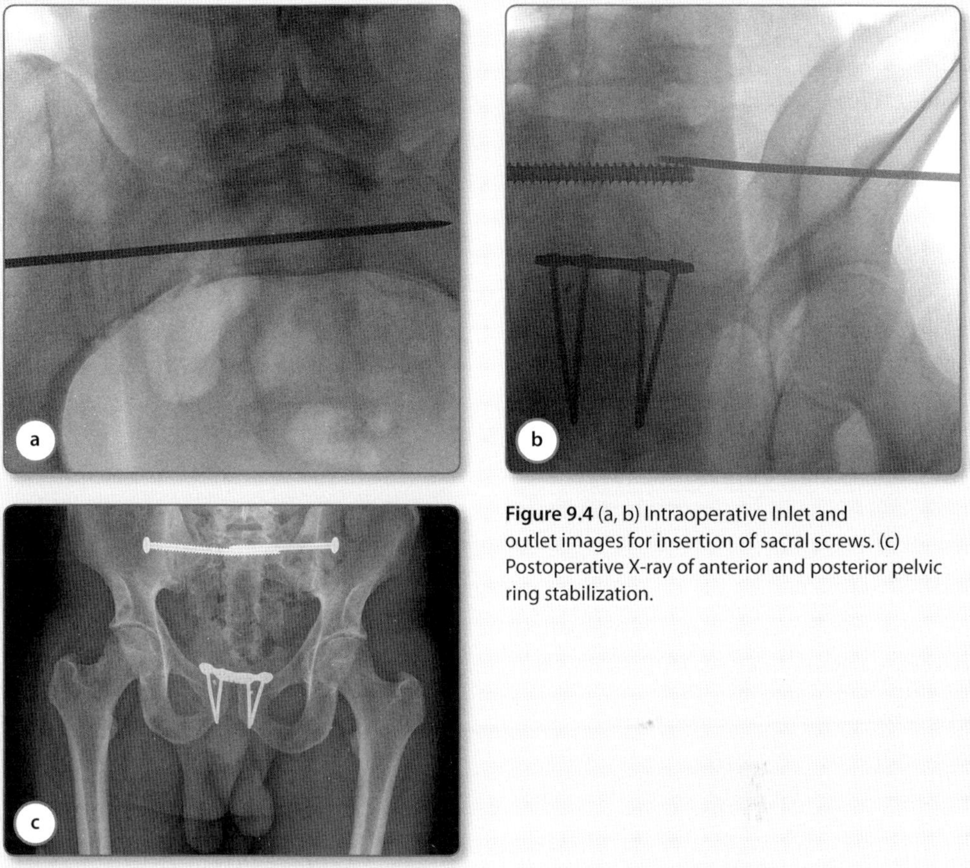

Figure 9.4 (a, b) Intraoperative Inlet and outlet images for insertion of sacral screws. (c) Postoperative X-ray of anterior and posterior pelvic ring stabilization.

a table with metal extension will compromise visualization. It's imperative that adequate image intensifier visualization is checked before prepping and draping and the radiographer marks out the position of the intensifier on the floor and the angles identified for the different views.

Review of surgical approaches

Anterior ring

Symphyseal diastasis is best treated by open reduction and internal fixation. The type of fixation used will be determined by the pattern of injury the options available include plate fixation and column screws.

Anterior plating (**Figure 9.5a**) for a symphyseal diastasis normally only requires a Pfannenstiel-type incision and it is common to discover that the insertion of the rectus abdominis muscles has been avulsed from the anterior aspect of the pubis, making dissection relatively straight-forward.

Surgical approach

- Horizontal incision 1 cm proximal to symphysis, through skin and subcutaneous tissue down to anterior rectus sheath (**Figure 9.5b**)
- The rectus sheath is then split vertically in the linea alba allowing separation of the recti giving access to the space of Retzius (**Figure 9.5c**)
- Where injury to the anterior part of the pelvic ring is complex and involves the pubic rami,

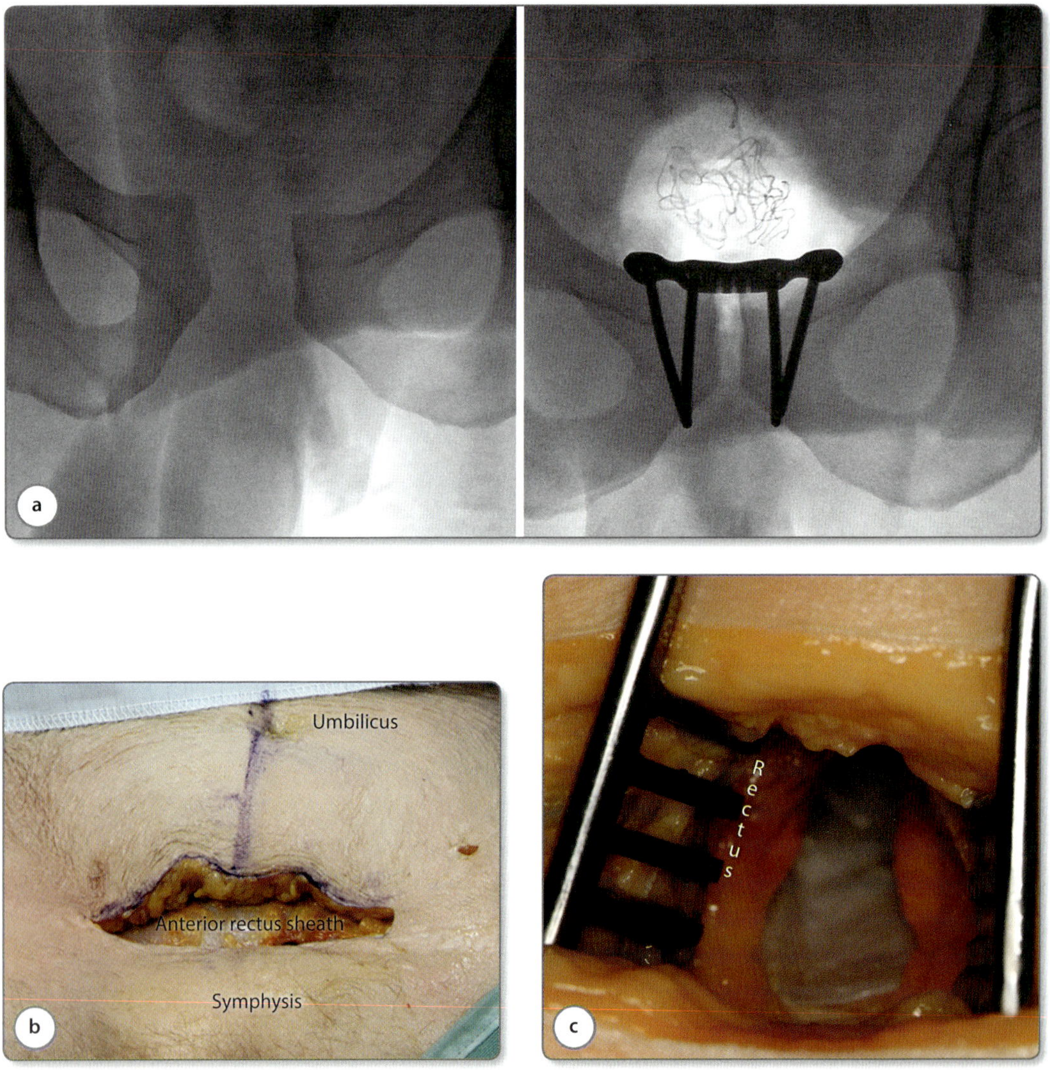

Figure 9.5 (a) Symphyseal disruption treated with reduction and plating (b) Cadaveric image of surgical dissection, showing skin marker line from umbilicus to symphysis outlining linea alba position. (c) Cadaveric image following splitting of rectus abdominis along linea alba and retraction. Pointed Holman retractors can be placed over pubic tubercles for further retraction of the recti.

additional access for longer plates may be required. Image-guided column screws (**Figure 9.6**) may be used if the fracture is minimally displaced after closed reduction

Equipment requirements

- Radiolucent flat top table
- Suitable image intensifier to acquire diagnostic images
- External fixator set, half pins and T-handle
- Small fragment set and plates, +/- pelvic specific plates
- Cannulated screw set
- Reduction clamps
- Cell salvage device for open surgery

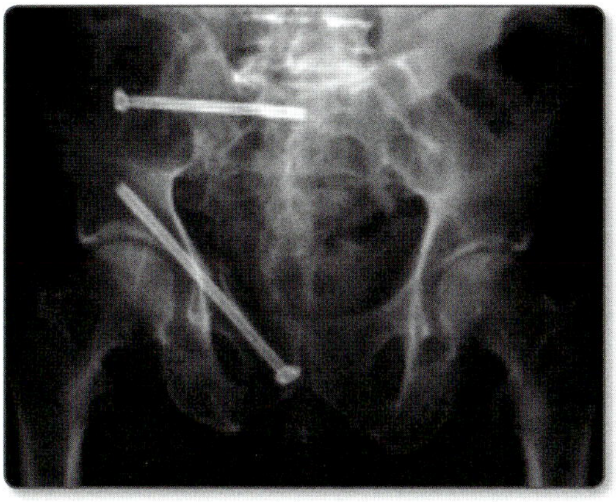

Figure 9.6 Column screw fixation to anterior ring.

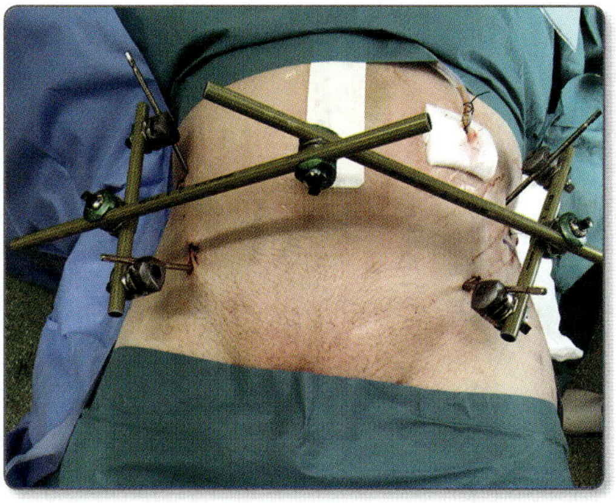

Figure 9.7 The author's preferred configuration of anterior standard external fixture showing orientation of supra-acetabular and iliac crest pins.

Reduction and stabilization methods

The aim of sophisticated reconstruction of the pelvis is the prevention of deformity. Deformity can occur as a result of fracture displacement at the time of injury or develop over time because of loading through unstable fractures or disrupted ligaments. Unequal leg length, rotational inequality of the legs and asymmetry of the ischial tuberosities resulting in a sitting deformity, are sequelae of malunited fractures of the pelvis.

Pelvic external fixation is a good method of surgical pelvic stabilization. It can be used in the emergency setting or as definitive fixation. Several pin and bar configurations can be utilized but the authors' preferred method is the use of two supra-acetabular pins and two iliac crest pins with either a low or a high bar configuration (**Figure 9.7**). If severe pelvic displacement is present, skeletal traction through a distal femoral pin can also be utilized in combination with the external fixator.

Posterior ring

Stabilization of the posterior structures of the pelvic ring can be achieved by a combination of closed or open reduction, percutaneous screw fixation (**Figure 9.3a, b**) or plate fixation.

Rehabilitation

- Early protected mobilization under physiotherapy supervision
- Input from specialist urinary/stoma teams as necessary
- Pain team input to reduce neuropathic symptoms
- Occupational therapy and joint splintage in patients with neurological damage

Avoiding postoperative complications

Complications can be divided into those of the injury and of the treatment. The clinician should be aware of the likely complications that this challenging group of patients might encounter and be prepared to deal with them in a timely fashion.

Venous thromboembolism

Pelvic fractures have been identified as a risk factor for increased incidence of venous thromboembolism. Currently, the natural history of pelvic vein thrombosis is not known, but evidence suggests that more proximal clots are more likely to embolize. Pulmonary embolism is a potentially lethal complication in patients with pelvic and acetabular fractures, and has been reported as the most common fatal complication after operation or trauma to the lower extremities.

Patients should commence low molecular weight heparin (LWMH) without delay.

Authors current practice is to use LMWH and compression stockings pre- and postoperatively for a period of 6 weeks.

Another alternative for prophylaxis is vena cava filters. Filters are recommended in patients with a contraindication to chemical anticoagulation (e.g. traumatic brain injury, patients managed nonoperatively for splenic or liver laceration) or in patients with pelvic or acetabular fractures that warrant surgical management and are considered high risk for a thromboembolic event. Patients who are transferred or present late should be screened for DVT preoperatively. If a clot is identified, a vena cava filter should be used prior to surgery. The use of filters is not without its complications and should only be advocated when necessary.

Sexual and urinary dysfunction

In a prospective cohort study of 151 patients with surgically treated pelvic ring injuries, the incidence of new sexual dysfunction was 43% and the incidence of urinary dysfunction was 41% with similar rates in males and females. LC injuries are less likely to cause new onset sexual or urinary dysfunction compared with APC or vertical sheer injuries.

Functional outcome

There is a significant discrepancy in the reporting of functional outcomes after fractures of the pelvis. Different authors have reported many factors associated with worse functional outcome including open fracture, urological injury, neurological injury, fractures requiring open reduction and internal fixation posterior displacement, injury pattern and psychological problems.

Suzuki et al. found that the Majeed score, Iowa pelvic score and Medical Outcomes Study Short Form 36-item Health Survey (SF-36) are each altered after fractures of the pelvis and correlate closely with the presence of a neurological injury.

What is well recognized is that these are serious injuries and this group of complex patients will require prolonged physical, psychological and nutritional rehabilitation as well as vocational support until they return to their maximal level of function.

Summary of learning points

- Regional protocols are mandatory for the management of these complex injuries
- Pelvic binders should be available both in the pre-hospital setting and in all emergency departments
- Early CT scanning and hemorrhagic resuscitation protocols with appropriate blood products should be available
- A high index of suspicion for genitourinary and open fractures needs to be maintained
- Early transfer to a specialist center with surgical expertise, urological, general surgical, pain team and specialist rehabilitation availability is mandatory

Further reading

Costantini TW, Coimbra R, Holcomb JB, et al. Current management of hemorrhage from severe pelvic fractures: Results of an American Association for the Surgery of Trauma multi-institutional trial. J Trauma Acute Care Surg 2016; 80:717–723.

Grotz MR, Allami MK, Harwood P, et al. Open pelvic fractures: epidemiology, current concepts of management and outcome. Injury 2005; 36:1–13.

Manson T, O'Toole RV, Whitney A, et al. Young-Burgess classification of pelvic ring fractures: does it predict mortality, transfusion requirements, and non-orthopaedic injuries? J Orthop Trauma 2010; 24:603–609.

Sathy AK, Starr AJ, Smith WR, et al. The effect of pelvic fracture on mortality after trauma: an analysis of 63,000 trauma patients. J Bone Joint Surg Am 2009; 91:2803–2810.

Schulman JE, O'Toole RV, Castillo RC, et al. Pelvic ring fractures are an independent risk factor for death after blunt trauma. J Trauma 2010; 68:930–934.

Smith W, Williams A, Agudelo J, et al. Early predictors of mortality in hemodynamically unstable pelvis fractures. J Orthop Trauma 2007; 21:31–37.

Suzuki T, Shindo M, Soma K, et al. Long-term functional outcome after unstable pelvic ring fracture. J Trauma 2007; 63:884–888.

Yoshihara H, Yoneoka D. Demographic epidemiology of unstable pelvic fracture in the United States from 2000 to 2009: trends and in-hospital mortality. J Trauma Acute Care Surg 2014; 76:380–385.

10 Acetabular fractures

Paul Duffy, Brad Meulenkamp

Introduction

Fractures of the acetabulum are among the most complex of orthopaedic injuries. They are a cause of significant morbidity with multiple important complications associated with both the injury itself, as well as surgical management. The goals of surgical management are to obtain and maintain a stable hip joint with congruent articulation under the weight-bearing dome of the acetabulum, allowing for early mobilization.

Incidence

Acetabular fractures account for approximately 10% of pelvic fractures, or 3.7 per 100 000 fractures overall. There is a predilection for the male population, with 69.4% of fractures occurring in men with an average age of 38.6 years.

Mechanism of injury

Direct impaction of the femoral head into the acetabulum results in fracture of the articular socket. These are often high-energy injuries resulting from motor vehicle collisions, however with an aging population, low energy osteoporotic fractures are providing a second demographic spike.

Variations in fracture pattern are subsequent to position of the hip as well as the vector of force at the time of impact. Axial load through the femoral shaft are more likely cause fracture of the posterior wall and/or posterior column, whereas direct lateral impact is more likely to result in fractures of the anterior wall and column, transverse, T-typed and associated both column fracture, depending on hip rotation at the time impact.

Initial management/ prioritization

Patients presenting with acetabular fractures are often polytraumatized and should undergo a full Advanced Trauma Life Support (ATLS) evaluation and resuscitation when appropriate. Combined injuries to the pelvic ring and acetabulum are not uncommon with high energy trauma and may be associated with hemodynamic instability. Up to 56% of patients present with associated injuries including head, visceral and other extremity trauma.

Limb-specific physical examination should include overall limb posture, motor and sensory examination with particular attention to the sciatic nerve, as well as careful assessment of the soft tissue envelope. The Morel-Lavallée lesion is a severe 'internal degloving' injury usually located over the greater trochanter, associated with a high risk of infection. When encountered, aggressive debridement and dead space management with suction drains or VAC should be employed, with bony fixation delayed until soft tissues are amenable. Ipsilateral knee examination is critical, particularly when the acetabular fracture is a result of a dashboard injury.

In cases of associated hip dislocation, urgent reduction should be performed and confirmed radiographically to decrease the risk of avascular necrosis and cartilage injury. Skeletal traction should be used for fractures difficult to maintain reduction, or fracture patterns with point loading on the femoral head.

Considerations for surgery

The majority of displaced acetabular fractures will undergo open reduction and internal fixation. Nonoperative management is indicated for minimally displaced fractures with articular step of less than 2 mm or poor surgical candidates with secondary congruity. Successful surgical outcomes are most dependent on a thorough understanding of the complex, three-dimensional (3D) anatomy of the acetabulum. The work of Letournel and Judet has been instrumental in classifying acetabular fractures, and in turn planning appropriate surgical strategy. Through their work, five elementary fracture patterns and five associated fracture patterns were grouped (**Figure 10.1**). Elementary patterns have the unique feature of a part or all of a single column being detached from the acetabulum, whereas associated patterns are more complex and comprised of combinations of elementary fractures.

Elderly patients with acetabular fractures provide a unique challenge due to overall poor bone quality, comminution, and a predisposition for roof impaction seen as the 'Gull sign' (**Figure 10.2**). These fracture characteristics, patient factors and surgeon experience should all be considered when managing acetabular fractures in this population due to the known failure rate of up to 45%.

It is important to obtain, study and understand the imaging. This should include anteroposterior (AP) pelvis, Judet views, as well as 2D and 3D CT images where available. A thorough understanding of the fracture pattern is necessary to plan your surgical approach and reduction strategy.

Theater layout and patient positioning

- Patient positioning will depend on fracture pattern and planned surgical approach
- In any case, the radiolucent fracture table is used

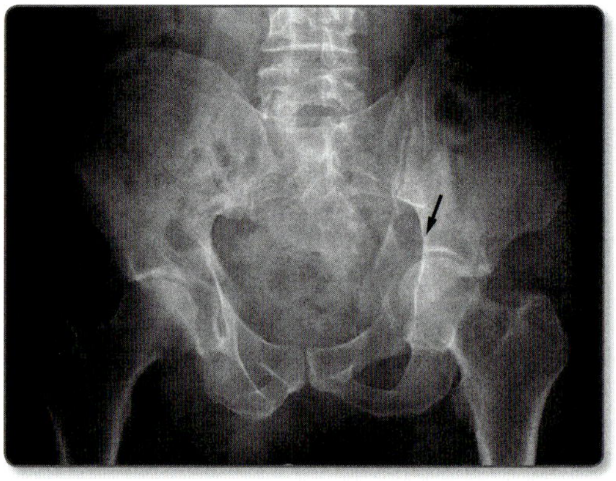

Figure 10.2 Example of the 'Gull sign' (arrow) characteristic of osteoporotic acetabular fractures with dome impaction.

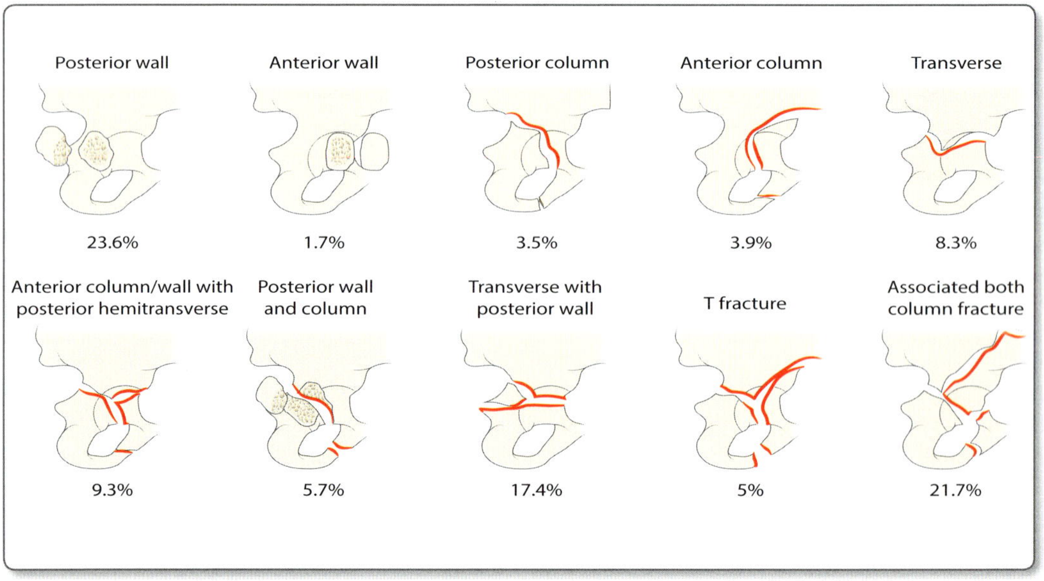

Figure 10.1 The classification scheme of Judet and Letournel with prevalence.

Case example: Fracture dislocation of native hip joint

A restrained seat passenger was involved in a motor vehicle collision. He sustained an isolated injury to his right hip region, with an AP X-ray showing a dislocated right hip joint (**Figure 10.3a**). The patient had no sciatic nerve involvement on examination prior to, and following, closed reduction. A CT scan post-reduction confirmed no fragments in the joint but a comminuted posterior wall (**Figure 10.3b**). The hip was unstable on screening and the patient proceeded to posterior wall stabilization via a Kocker-Langenbeck approach utilizing a combination of third tubular spring and 3.5 mm reconstruction buttress plates (**Figure 10.4**).

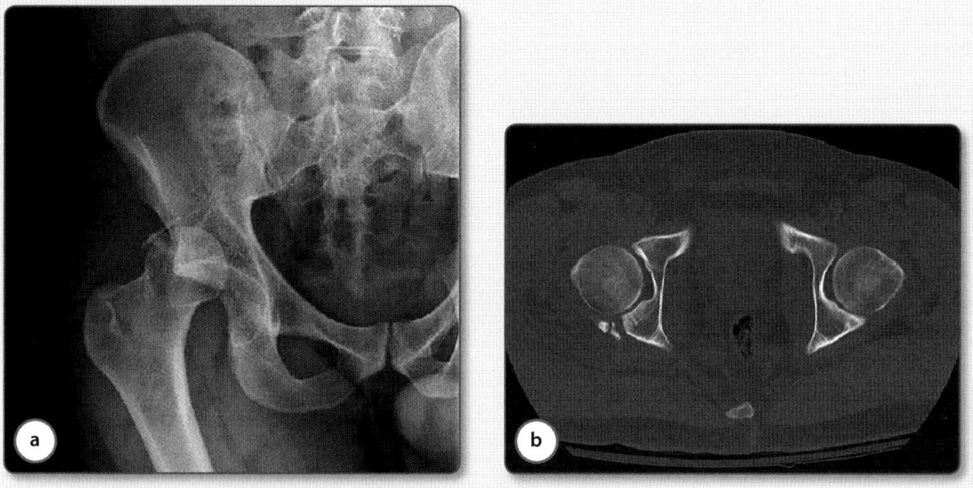

Figure 10.3 (a) Posteriorly dislocated right native hip. (b) Post-reduction CT showing comminuted posterior wall.

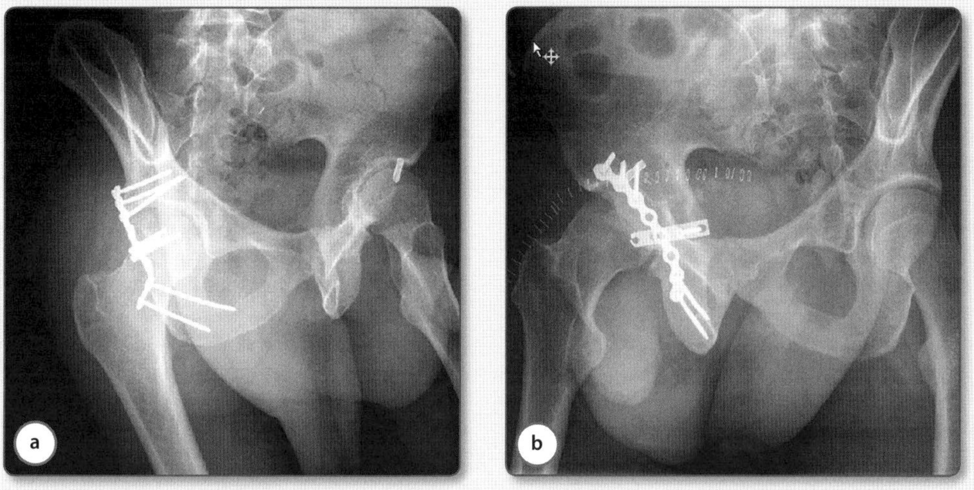

Figure 10.4 (a) Obturator oblique Judet view showing fixation technique with combination spring and buttress plate. (b) Corresponding iliac oblique Judet view.

- For the Kocher-Langenbeck approach, we prefer the patient be positioned in lateral decubitus on a radiolucent suction beanbag
- For the ilioinguinal or Stoppa approach, the patient is positioned supine. We prefer a sandbag under the ipsilateral buttock with a wide prep to allow appropriate soft tissue excursion with use of the lateral window
- We have c-arm in from the contralateral side as the surgeon, ensuring appropriate imaging prior to skin incision

Review of surgical approaches

Ilioinguinal/Stoppa approach

The ilioinguinal and Stoppa approaches are used primarily for access to the anterior column, although indirect reduction of the posterior column is possible. Gentle hip flexion to relax the iliopsoas is helpful for these approaches, and foley catheter is essential to deflate and protect the urinary bladder.

- Patient is positioned in the supine position on the radiolucent table
- The incision is made from two fingerbreadths proximal to the pubic symphysis, extended laterally to the anterior superior iliac spine (ASIS) and proximally along the iliac crest for 5 cm (**Figure 10.5a**)
- Laterally, the tendinous insertion of the abdominal muscles are incised along the iliac crest, with subperiosteal elevation of the iliacus muscle to reveal the inner table of the ilium (**Figure 10.5b**). This will expose the SI joint, running anteriorly along the pelvic brim (**Figure 10.5c**)
- Medially, the aponeurosis of the external oblique is opened, exposing the superficial inguinal ring
- The spermatic cord or round ligament are identified and protected with a Penrose drain, allowing access to the posterior wall of the inguinal canal (**Figure10.5d**)
- The internal oblique and transversus abdominus muscles form the posterior wall of the inguinal canal, and are now divided. Care is taken to identify and ligate the corona mortis when present
- The iliopectineal fascia will be found separating the femoral nerve from the femoral vessels. This must be divided to the pectineal eminence, and then from the pelvic brim to the anterior SI joint. This exposes the true pelvis and allows access to the quadrilateral plate (**Figure10.5e**)
- The femoral nerve and iliopsoas are mobilized together with a Penrose drain, as are the femoral vessels
- The rectus abdominus insertion is then divided from the superior pubic ramus, and the space of Retzius is entered (see **Figure 9.5c**)
- The three windows of the ilioinguinal approach are now accessible:
  - The lateral window runs from the anterior SI joint to the iliopsoas/femoral nerve. It gives access to the entire iliac fossa and pelvic brim
  - The middle window is developed between the iliopsoas/femoral nerve and the femoral vessels, also giving access to the pelvic brim and also the quadrilateral plate
  - The medial window is medial to the femoral vessels and allows access to the superior pubic ramus to pubic symphysis
- Careful closure of the posterior inguinal ring is essential to prevent inguinal hernia

Modified Stoppa approach

The modified Stoppa approach provides much of the versatility and exposure of the ilioinguinal approach. It has the advantage of avoiding use of the middle window, thereby preventing dissection of the inguinal canal and mobilization of the femoral nerve and iliac vessels.

- The patient is positioned supine as in the ilioinguinal approach
- The surgeon will typically stand on the contralateral side as the injury to improve visualization of the true pelvis
- A Pfannenstiel incision is created and the rectus abdominus is split in its midline
- Transversalis fascia is opened 1 cm proximal to the pubic symphysis
- The space of Retzius is entered and bladder protected with a sponge
- Subperiosteal dissection along the superior ramus and pelvic brim is then performed, with gentle retraction of the psoas and iliac vessels
- The corona mortis is ligated when encountered, and care must be taken to protect the obturator nerve and artery as they run inferior to the superior pubic ramus

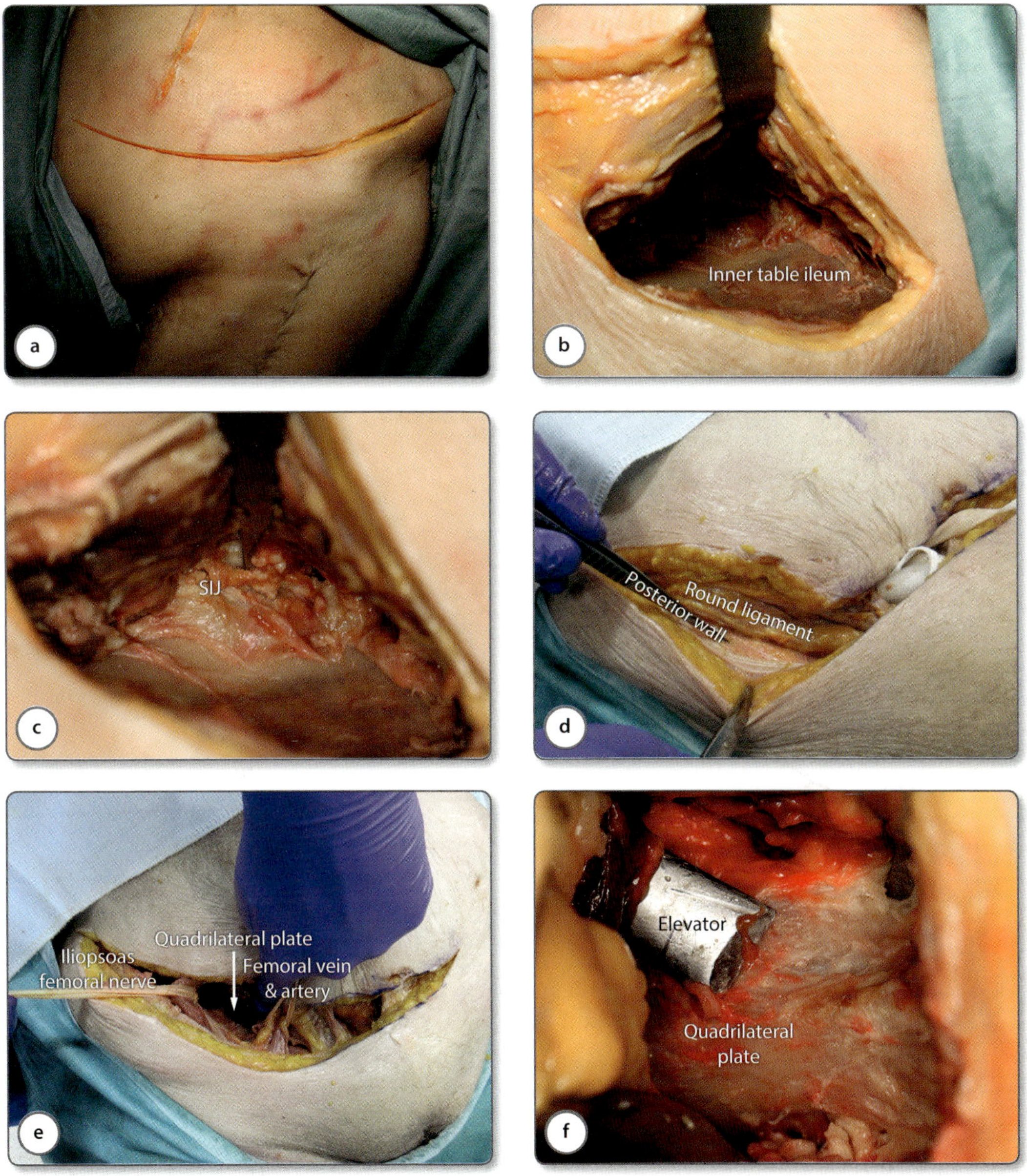

Figure 10.5 (a) Skin incision for ilioinguinal or Stoppa approach. (b) Lateral window exposure following elevation of iliacus of internal iliac wing. (c) Exposure of anterior aspect of sacroiliac joint. (d) Posterior wall of inguinal canal. (e) Division of iliopectineal fascia giving access to true pelvis: pubic rami and quadrilateral plate. Femoral vein and iliopsoas retracted laterally with femoral artery and vein retracted medially. (f) Dissection along the pubic ramus toward the quadrilateral surface, care being taken with the corona mortis anastomoses. Elevator pass from proximal to distal submuscularly can be seen also: aids passage of anterior column plates.

- Dissection may be continued along the pelvic brim expose to the anterior SI joint
- Hohman retractors can be variably placed to assist with exposure of the quadrilateral plate (**Figure 10.5f**) and medial aspect of the posterior column
- The lateral window is often used as an adjunct to this approach to assist with fixation of high anterior column fractures and screw placement posteriorly along the pelvic brim (**Figure 10.5b**)

Kocher-Langenbeck approach

This approach allows visualization of the full exterior aspect of the posterior column, including the greater and lesser sciatic notches. The greater sciatic notch allows for indirect access to the quadrilateral surface.

- The patient is positioned in the lateral decubitus position
- Incision in line with the femur to the tip of the greater trochanter (GT), then angled 45° toward the posterior superior iliac spine (PSIS) (see **Figure 12.3a**)
- The fascia lata is incised with proximal blunt division of the gluteus maximus (GMax) in line with the muscle fibers. This proximal split should be planned based on the specific fracture pattern, with higher splits needed for fracture extending higher on the column
- The proximal half the GMax insertion may be released
- The sciatic nerve is palpated and inspected for an anomalous course through the piriformis. The piriformis is tagged and released to reveal the sciatic nerve. The nerve should be followed to the sciatic notch, and may be tagged with a Penrose drain to keep it in view
- The tendonous insertion of the obturator internus (OI) is then tagged and released 1.5 cm away from the femur (**Figure 10.6a**), revealing the synovial obturator bursa. This is an important landmark for safe retractor placement over the ischium, used to retract the short external rotators, protecting the sciatic nerve
- The remaining short external rotators are released, avoiding the quadratus femoris to protect the medial femoral circumflex branch
- The column is now exposed and the fracture can be identified, debrided and reduced (**Figure 10.6b**)
- Release of the proximal hamstrings from the ischial tuberosity may be necessary for plate placement

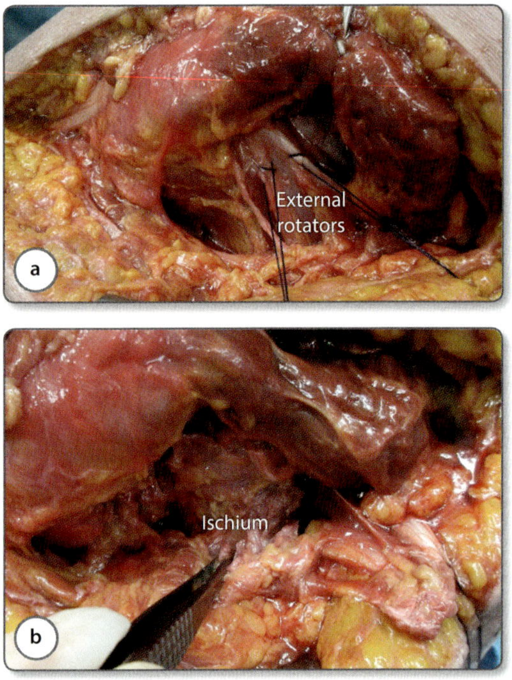

Figure 10.6 (a) Tagging of short external rotators, prior to division. (b) Exposure of posterior wall and column.

- Proximal exposure is limited by the superior gluteal bundle and must be kept in mind throughout surgery to prevent inadvertent tearing leading to massive intrapelvic bleeding
- For fractures extending higher or into the anterior column, a digastric slide or trochanteric flip of the GT can be performed, allowing improved visualization or possible surgical dislocation of the hip for irrigation of loose bodies.

Post-operative X-rays of the clinical case example **Figure 10.3** treated using Kocher-Langenbeck approach are shown in **Figure 10.4**.

Iliofemoral approach

The iliofemoral approach will not be discussed in detail as it is infrequently used due to complications of abductor weakness and necrosis, heterotopic bone formation, and potential compromise of future arthroplasty incisions. Nonetheless, it should be considered for complex both column fractures where alternative approaches prove difficult or impossible to obtain anatomic articular reduction.

Equipment requirements

It is important to ensure appropriate clamps and reduction adjuncts are available prior to surgery. Exact clamps and instruments will depend on patient and surgeon preference, but may include:

- Clamps: Jungbluth, Farabeuf, offset and Weber clamps, and co-linear reduction clamp (**Figure 10.7**)
- K-wires, Shantz pins, and ball-spiked pelvic pusher
- Small-fragment instrumentation and screws with lengths up to 150 mm
- Pelvic-reconstruction plates and plate bending forceps
- The large AO distractor

Reduction and stabilization methods

The key to reduction and fixation of acetabular fractures is to thoroughly understand the 3D anatomy of the fracture. It is important to anticipate what aspects of the fracture will be able to be visualized directly, as well as indecently through palpation. Potentially helpful tips and tricks include:

- Incomplete fractures may need to be completed prior to allowing reduction
- The reduction is almost always multi-planar, including flexion/extension as well as rotation:
  - Joysticks will assist in multiplanar reductions
- Careful planning of clamp placement is essential so as not to 'box yourself out' when placing fixation:
  - Lag screws or provisional Kirschener wires should be used where possible to allow clamp removal
- Ensure that clamps are placed perpendicular to fracture lines to prevent rotational malreduction

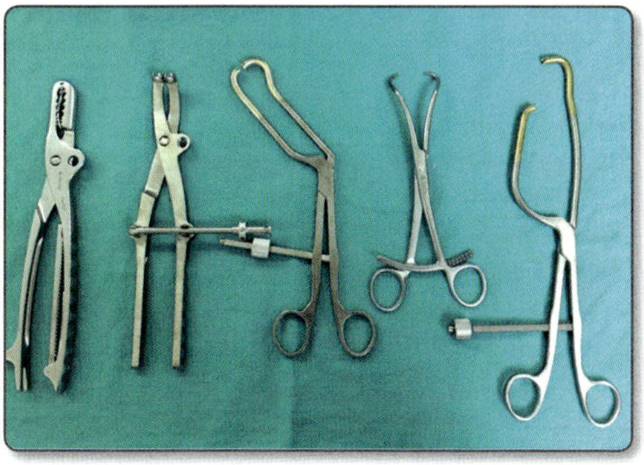

Figure 10.7 Examples of reduction clamps and tools. From left: Farabeuf clamp, Jungbluth clamp, angled pelvic reduction clamp, pointed reduction clamp, offset pelvic reduction clamp.

Rehabilitation

Patients are made toe-touch weight-bearing in the immediate postoperative period until 6 weeks. Full weight-bearing is advised at 6–8 weeks. Patients are encouraged to begin early hip, knee and ankle motion exercises without restriction.

Avoiding postoperative complications

Complications may be divided into general complications and fracture specific complications.

General complications

Infection

- Postoperative infections rates are approximately 5%
- Prevention is key with meticulous soft tissue handling and dead space management
- Aggressive management of the Morel-Lavallée lesion with serial debridement, application of negative pressure wound dressing or suction drain, and definitive surgery delayed until soft tissues are amenable
- Established infection taken for irrigation and debridement with culture specific antibiotic treatment

Venous thromboembolism

- Despite prophylaxis, DVT has been demonstrated in up to 12% of patients with acute pelvis and acetabular fractures
- Our practice is to use low molecular weight heparin in patients without contraindications to anticoagulation or pneumatic compression devices in patients with contraindications

Fracture-specific complications

Nerve injury

- Several nerves are at risk with acetabular fractures and surgery
- Thorough knowledge of applied surgical anatomy with meticulous dissection is the key to prevention
- The lateral femoral cutaneous nerve may be injured during the ilioinguinal approach itself as it exits the pelvis through the inguinal ligament
- The femoral nerve may be injured from errant retractor placement, specifically when using the middle window of the ilioinguinal approach
- The obturator nerve may become injured from intrapelvic dislocation of the femoral head, or by errant retractor placement in the Stoppa approach as it passes just medial to the quadrilateral plate
- Injury to the sciatic nerve is a devastating complication, reported at 16.4%, but up to 40.3% in cases of posterior hip dislocation, and may also be injured due to errant retractor placement:
  - The nerve should be protected intraoperatively by extending the hip and flexing the knee
  - It is our preference to tag the sciatic nerve with a Penrose drain during exposure so as to keep it in view throughout the case
  - Sciatic nerve injury should be treated with fitting of a foot drop splint and physiotherapy to prevent contracture
  - Posterior tibial tendon transfer may be considered once recovery is deemed unlikely

Heterotopic ossification

- Matta reported incidences of 20% for iliofemoral approach, 12% for Kocher-Langenbeck, and 2% for ilioinguinal
- May be prevented by minimizing soft tissue stripping
- Prevention with either indomethacin for 3 weeks postoperatively, or with radiation delivered between 12 hours prior to and 72 hours following surgery
- Functionally limiting bone should not be allowed to mature prior to excision.

Post-traumatic arthrosis

- Post-traumatic hip arthritis is the most common complication following acetabular fracture with a clinically significant incidence of 20%
- Several risk factors for poor outcome include femoral head chondral injury, malreduction > 2 mm, dome impaction, and age > 40 years

Salvage options after failed fracture fixation

The failed acetabular fracture will be most frequently salvaged with total hip arthroplasty. There are several challenges to anticipate in post-traumatic arthroplasty and preoperative planning is essential.

- Rule out infection with serology and if joint serologic markers are elevated, infection must be managed aggressively with a staged reconstruction
- Management of bone deficits with allograft or augments should be anticipated and are critical for appropriate cup placement in the context of pelvic deformity
- Porous metal cups and cups with multiple screw options are helpful to ensure stable implantation and ingrowth
- Pelvic discontinuity should be managed with column plating, or with the use of a cup-cage type construct
- Large head options, typically 32 mm or 36 mm, can be used to decrease dislocation risk

Summary of learning points

- Acetabular fractures are often associated with the multi-injured patient and great care must be given to primary, secondary and tertiary survey of these patients
- These are complex injuries that must be managed by surgeons trained and proficient in the appropriate exposures and fixation techniques
- Understanding complex fracture patterns are of utmost importance as this will guide operative approach to the fracture
- Workhorse exposures include the ilioinguinal or modified Stoppa approaches for anterior column exposure and fixation, and the Kocher-Langenbeck approaches
- Complications are not uncommon and include infection, neurovascular injury, heterotopic bone formation and post-traumatic arthrosis
- Salvage options are limited with total hip arthroplasty being the most common method. Infection must be ruled out prior to intervention and thought should be given to large head options to minimize dislocation risk

Further reading

Anglen JO, Burd TA, Hendricks KA, Harrison P. The "Gull sign": a harbinger of failure for internal fixation of geriatric acetabular fractures. J Orthop Trauma 2003; 17:625–634.

Ferguson TA, Patel R, Bhandari M, Matta JM. Fractures of the acetabulum in patients aged 60 years and older: an epidemiological and radiological study. J Bone Joint Surg Br 2010; 92:250–257.

Ganz R, Gill TJ, Gautier E, et al. Surgical dislocation of the adult hip a technique with full access to the femoral head and acetabulum without the risk of avascular necrosis. J Bone Joint Surg Br 2001; 83:1119–1124.

Hak DJ, Olson SA, Matta JM. Diagnosis and management of closed internal degloving injuries associated with pelvic and acetabular fractures: the Morel-Lavallée lesion. J Trauma 1997; 42:1046–1051.

Judet R, Judet J. Letournel E. Fractures of the Acetabulum: Classification and Surgical Approaches for Open Reduction. Preliminary Report. J Bone Joint Surg Am 1964; 46:1615–1646.

Matta JM. Fractures of the acetabulum: accuracy of reduction and clinical results in patients managed operatively within three weeks after the injury. J Bone Joint Surg Am 1996; 78:1632–1645.

Sierra RJ, Mabry TM, Sems SA, Berry DJ. Acetabular fractures: the role of total hip replacement. Bone Joint J 2013; 95-B:11–16.

Stannard JP, Singhania AK, Lopez-Ben RR, et al. Deep-vein thrombosis in high-energy skeletal trauma despite thromboprophylaxis. J Bone Joint Surg Br 2005; 87:965–968.

Tannast M, Najibi S, Matta J. Two to twenty-year survivorship of the hip in 810 patients with operatively treated acetabular fractures. J Bone Joint Surg Am 2012; 94:1559–1567.

11 Thoracolumbar spinal fractures

George Mataliotakis, David Fender

Introduction

Thoracolumbar fractures range from low-energy injuries in osteoporotic older patients to high-energy fracture/dislocations with neural injury in younger active individuals. A large number of low-energy fractures without neurological involvement are treated conservatively. High-energy fractures can be challenging, requiring surgical treatment and may be associated with neurologic deficits, deformity, chronic pain and long-term disability.

Incidence

The incidence of spinal fractures in adults is of the order of 0.05–0.10% per year. Lumbar fractures are most common, with 50% of all thoracic and lumbar fractures occurring at the thoracolumbar junction (T11–L2), where there is a transition from relatively mobile lumbar to less mobile thoracic spine.

Mechanism of injury

High-energy trauma such as road traffic accidents, falls from heights and horse riding are frequent mechanisms of injury, with fractures often occurring in the polytrauma patient. The three-column Denis classification concept still dominates our understanding regarding the anatomical disruption of the spinal column following injury. The thoracic cage and sternum provide additional stability in the thoracic spine and together are often termed the 'fourth-column'. The spine may fail in flexion/extension, axial compression/distraction, rotation/translation or a combination of each mechanism.

High-energy thoracolumbar fractures may be associated with visceral injuries, particularly to retroperitoneal structures such as the great vessels, the second part of the duodenum and the pancreas. Spinal fractures at noncontiguous levels occur in approximately 15% of cases, with compression injuries being associated with calcaneal, tibial plateau, acetabular and C1 fractures. Assessment of the injury mechanism, the stability of the fracture pattern, the presence of other spinal fractures and the identification of neurologic injury are all mandatory.

Initial management

A high-velocity mechanism of injury leads to a high index of suspicion to the presence of multiple injuries. Life-threatening injuries are prioritized and managed according to Advanced Trauma Life Support and local protocols. A detailed history of the mechanism of injury needs to be gathered from the patient and witnesses, including members of the emergency services who attended the scene.

Full spinal precautions including log-rolling, inline immobilization with a collar, sandbags and tape is needed until a complete spinal assessment with imaging has been performed. Examination of the back requires full exposure and log-rolling of the patient. Assessment includes looking for external evidence of injury (swelling, bruising, wounds, focal deformity) and feeling for tenderness, 'bogginess' (indicating a hematoma) steps or gaps in the posterior elements. With the patient still in the lateral position, a rectal examination assessing for tone, perianal sensation, active sphincter contraction, and internal bleeding is mandatory. A complete assessment of neurological function is performed and documented in a standard fashion [the American Spinal Injury Association (ASIA) chart allows comprehensive and reproducible neurological assessment and monitoring]. If there is evidence of complete neurologic injury, the bulbocavernosus reflex must be documented to assess whether spinal shock is ongoing. Until this primitive reflex returns, the injury should not be termed complete. Neurogenic shock must be suspected in a hypotensive patient with bradycardia. Frequent re-examinations and documentation are necessary to establish a neurological deficit and any evidence of progression or recovery.

Spiral computed tomography (CT) scanning of the spine is the 'gold standard' imaging modality, with plain radiographs an essential addition for patients going to theater. CT imaging should cover the whole spine with coronal and sagittal reconstructions and include the chest wall and sternum. Such imaging helps to identify the levels of fracture, confirm the pattern/mechanism of injury, assess stability and guide management. Magnetic resonance imaging (MRI) is indicated to assess neural injury and to establish soft tissue injury to the intervertebral disc or posterior ligamentous structures if doubt remains after clinical and CT examination.

Fracture classification

The AO classification is comprehensive and widely used. It is based on a two-column theory and the forces resulting in failure. There are three groups of fracture:

- **Type A:** compression-failure of the anterior structures under compression
- **Type B:** distraction-failure of the posterior or anterior tension band
- **Type C:** rotation-failure of all elements leading to dislocation/displacement

Each type is further divided into subtypes (1.1–3.3) according to fracture morphology and complexity (**Figure 11.1**). The types and subtypes progress from simple to severe injury patterns: the higher the number of the subtype, the greater the instability of the fracture and the higher the risk of neurologic injury.

Considerations for surgery

Indications for surgery are spinal instability and neurological dysfunction. Unstable injuries without neurological involvement or complete neurological deficit are an indication for urgent stabilization. Injuries with incomplete or progressive neurologic deficit are an indication for emergency decompression and stabilization.

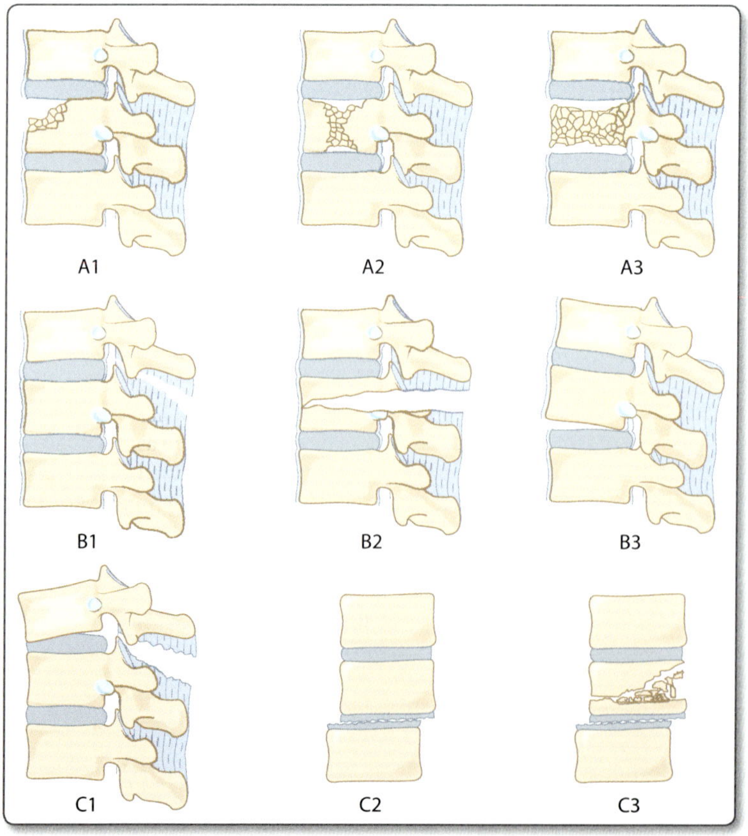

Figure 11.1 The AO classification.

AO type B and C fractures represent unstable fracture patterns and require surgical stabilization. A1 fractures are stable injuries and may be treated conservatively. A2 (split/pincer) fractures are often stable, yet may be treated operatively due to the high likelihood of nonunion secondary to disc impaction across the fractured vertebral body. A3 (burst) fractures are a source of debate with regard to stability, with a spectrum of opinions existing. 'Unstable' burst fracture patterns may lead to secondary deformity or neurological impact and require close radiological follow up if treated nonoperatively. Factors in favor of operative management include kyphosis angulation > 30° and loss of anterior body height > 50%. The extent of canal

Case example: Type A injury

A 45-year-old man fell 5 meters onto hard ground. Hemodynamically stable, upper lumbar pain without posterior tenderness and normal neurological examination.

Sagittal, coronal and axial CT scans of whole spine confirmed an isolated burst fracture of L1 vertebra (AO A3) (**Figure 11.2a**).

After adequate analgesia, the patient regained trunk control and was able to stand without obvious structural deformity or neurological deterioration. Standing AP and lateral radiographs confirmed maintenance of coronal and sagittal alignment (**Figure 11.2b**).

The injury was deemed stable and the patient was treated nonoperatively with close clinical and radiological follow up 3 months' post-injury the patient had returned to most activities including work. Standing AP and lateral radiographs showed maintenance of alignment (**Figure 11.2c**).

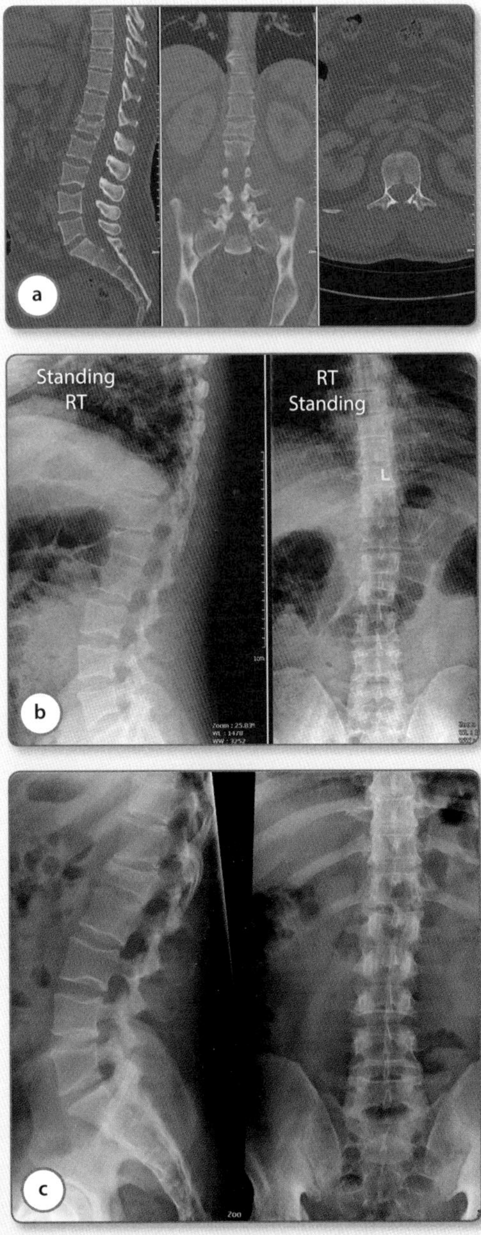

Figure 11.2 (a) Sagittal, coronal and axial CT scans of whole spine confirmed an isolated burst fracture of L1 vertebra. (b) Standing AP and lateral radiographs confirmed the maintenance of coronal and sagittal alignment. (c) Standing AP and lateral radiographs 3 months post-injury.

Case example: Type B injury

A 22-year-old woman driver was in a high-velocity vehicle collision with a lamp post.

Ambulance to district hospital A&E, hemodynamically stable, with thoracolumbar and upper abdominal pain, posterior midline tenderness, gap in the interspinous space and normal neurological examination.

Plain radiographs were interpreted as showing compression fractures (AO A1) of L3 and L4 (**Figure 11.3a**). Neurosurgical advice was to obtain an MRI (CT scanner broken in district hospital) with subsequent opinion to treat as stable injuries with mobilization as pain allows. Due to persistent abdominal pain and tenderness (and lack of CT availability) patient was transferred to tertiary center for further investigation under a general surgeon.

CT scan with contrast confirmed a pancreatic injury with subsequent reconstructed images showing an unstable flexion distraction injury at L1 (AO B2/Chance fracture) (**Figure 11.3b**).

Retrospectively the injury was evident on the initial plain radiographs (**Figure 11.3a**) which showed the interspinous widening and fractured pedicles.

Such an injury should have been suspected given the posterior tenderness and gap in the interspinous ligament on examination. Final images show posterior instrumentation (**Figure 11.3c**).

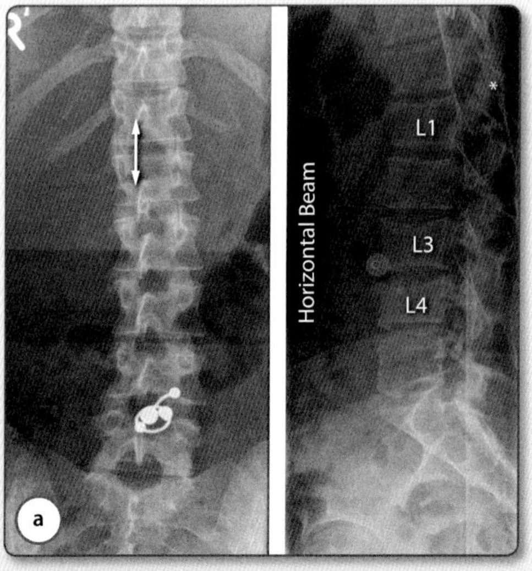

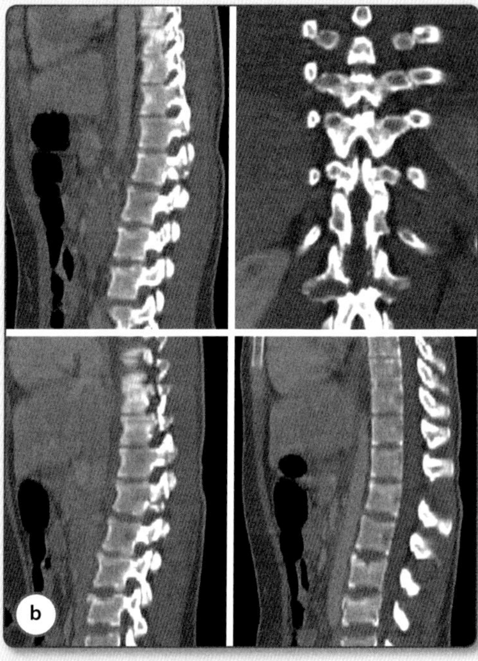

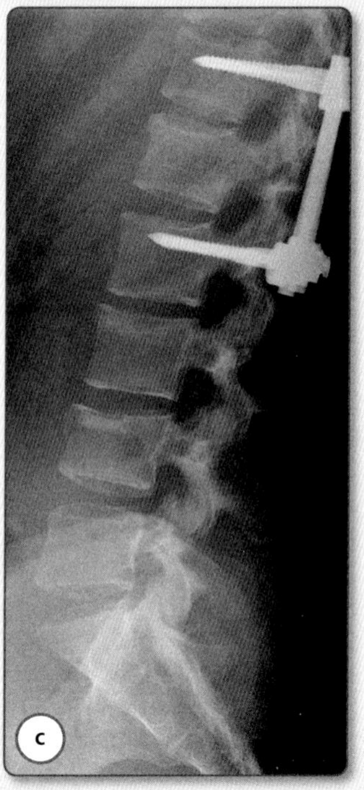

Figure 11.3 (a) X-rays were interpreted as showing compression fractures (AO A1) of L3 and L4. But note increase in interspinious distance between T12 and L1 (arrows). Lateral X-ray shows abnormality at posterior elements (*). (b) CT scan images showing an unstable flexion distraction injury at L1 (AO B2/Chance fracture). (c) Lateral X-ray post instrumentation of unstable L1 injury pattern.

compromise on CT imaging is controversial and in isolation should not be used as a guide to fracture stability.

Patient comorbidities influence treatment, with a lower threshold to stabilize the spine of an uncooperative patient or those with multiple injuries in order to simplify rehabilitation.

Other injuries (e.g. to the head, thorax, abdomen, limbs) need to be evaluated and a surgical plan formulated on the basis of damage control or total care. The 'second hit' phenomenon needs to be considered when planning the timing of any extensive spinal intervention in polytrauma patients. Incomplete spinal cord injuries should be stabilized within 24 hours of injury. It is mandatory for patients with neurological injury to have spinal precautions including catheterization, pressure area care and prophylaxis for infection and thrombosis.

Theater layout and patient positioning

- Lamina flow theater, monopolar and bipolar diathermy, suction, pneumatic stockings and relevant imaging
- The patient is positioned prone with the face down, with eye protection (soft padding and foam block)
- The abdomen is free to reduce pressure and therefore venous bleeding
- The spine should be in a neutral position, maintaining lumbar lordosis
- The upper and lower limb should be positioned to avoid pressure areas with foam gutters for the upper limbs
- Shoulder and elbow flexion/abduction should be less than 90°

Review of surgical approaches

The mainstay approach is the midline posterior approach.

Posterior midline surgical approach

- Level confirmation should be undertaken with fluoroscopy, followed by preparation and draping, and a midline skin incision centered at fractured level (**Figure 11.4a**)
- The length of the incision depends on the preoperatively-planned length of posterior fixation
- Subperiosteal muscle is stripped to expose the facet joints, pars interarticularis and transverse processes of vertebra to be instrumented (**Figure 11.4b**)
- The facet joint capsules of levels not being fused should be preserved

Equipment requirements

- Spinal table (i.e. OSI Jackson) with appropriate positioning supports
- C-arm image intensifier with 360° access
- All of the appropriate instruments/retractors for the posterior or anterior thoracolumbar approach
- Comprehensive instrumentation/fracture system (i.e. DePuy Synthes USS)

Posterior reduction and stabilization methods

Principles

In compression injuries (type A) the ligaments are intact. The reduction of the fracture is based on ligamentotaxis, which reduces the angulation and height of the fractured segment. It also reduces any retropulsed fragment back into its original position, restoring the patency of the canal and relieving any pressure on the neural elements.

In distraction and rotational injuries (types B and C), the ligamentotaxis principle cannot be applied as the posterior tension band is disrupted. Removal of any interposed ligament remnants is necessary to allow reduction, avoidance of pressure on the neural elements and to allow bony contact for healing. Finally, gradual compression, restoration of anatomical relationships and posterior stabilization (restoration of posterior tension band) is achieved.

Technique

For safe freehand pedicle screw placement, the transverse process, facet joint and pars interarticularis need to be visualized. There are slight variations to the entry point and trajectory for each region of the spine (**Figure 11.4c**).

An awl or bone nibbler is used decorticate the entry point (**Figure 11.4d**). If the anatomy is distorted or the pedicle is obviously small on

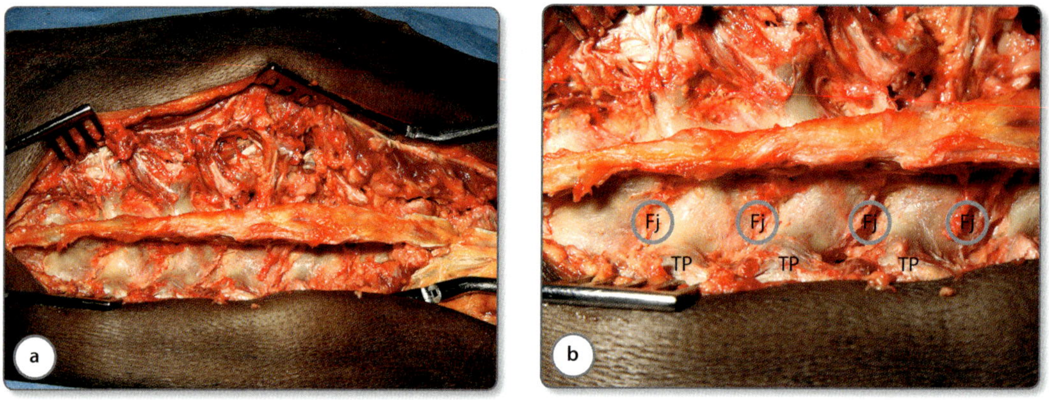

Vertebrae		Entry points Transverse angle	Trajectories Sagittal angle	
T1, T2, T3	T12	Junction of the bisected TP and lamina at the lateral border of the pars.		
T4, T5	T11	Junction of the proximal 1/3 of the TP and lamina just medial to the lateral border of the pars.		
T6	T10	Junction of the upper laminar ridge and lamina just medial to the lateral border of the pars.	0° at T12 increasing proximally to 30° at T1	Parallel to the endplate
T7, T8, T9		Junction of the proximal edge of the TP and just lateral to the mid portion of the base of the SF (usually just 2-3 mm medial to the lateral border of the pars).		
L1-L5		Junction of the bisected transverse process at the lateral border of the SF, in line with the lateral border of the pars.	0°-5° (L1) 10° (L2) Increasing to 25° at L5	Parallel to the endplate
S1		Junction of the Sacral alar and the Lateral border of the S1 facet at the level of the base if the S1 facet; in line with the pars if the exposure allows its visualization.	40°	Parallel to S1 endplate or towards promontory

c

SF, superior facet; TP, transverse process

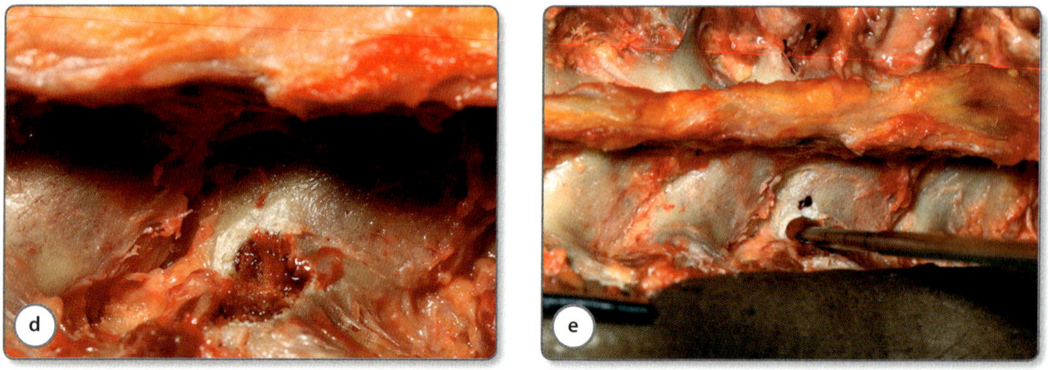

Figure 11.4 (a) Midline posterior approach centered over area of surgery. (b) Subperiosteal elevation bilaterally of muscles to expose facet joints and transverse processes of vertebrae. (c) Table of pedicle screw insertion sites and trajectories. (d) A bone nibbler is used to decorticate the entry point prior to using a pedicle probe. (e) Pedicle probe inserted into vertebral body.

imaging, the surgeon should have a low threshold to use fluoroscopy. A pedicle probe is then used bimanually to open the cancellous bone of the pedicle into the vertebral body (**Figure 11.4e**). The integrity of the bony walls and bottom of this tract are confirmed with the pedicle feeler. A soft wall indicates breeching of the tract and repositioning is necessary.

CT imaging can be used to plan screw size. Typically, adult lumbar pedicles will accommodate a screw of 6 mm or 7 mm in diameter with lengths varying from 40–55 mm. Thoracic pedicles are likely to require screws of 5 mm or 6 mm in diameter with the length dropping to 35 mm. Final screw position is confirmed with multiplanar fluoroscopy. Rods are cut to the required length and reduced into the pedicle screw-heads but not fully tightened. Further reduction is achieved via the instrumentation either by distraction, compression or rotation maneuvers.

Once coronal alignment and sagittal alignment is confirmed with fluoroscopy, the implants are finally tightened. A cross-connector bridges the two rods in order to enhance the torsional stability and pull-out strength of the construct. A bone graft may be applied.

Anterior reduction and stabilization methods

Most of the trauma is adequately dealt with by posterior surgery, but for completeness, anterior surgery should be considered if:

- There is residual anterior canal compromise after posterior fixation
- There is residual instability or increasing kyphosis despite posterior stabilization
- Anterior column restoration is required, e.g. for highly comminuted body fractures or for body fractures unlikely to heal (AO A2/ 'pincer' type injury)

Principles for anterior surgery

- Canal clearance
- Restoration of the anterior column height and support
- Stabilization and graft to allow fusion

Positioning

- Lateral decubitus position, usually left side up
- An anterior support at the pubic symphysis and posterior support at the sacrum
- Left leg slightly bent to relax the psoas
- The left upper limb should be supported in a comfortable position
- All bony prominences must be well padded

Method of stabilization: anterior approach

- The incision should be centered over the level of the fracture (typically two ribs proximal to the fracture, 10th rib for T12 and L1 to allow thoracoabdominal approach, 12th rib for lower lumbar fractures)
- In line with rib length
- Subperiosteal excision of the rib (used in combination with fracture vertebral body for bone graft) and a retroperitoneal approach to the lateral aspect of the spine. The diaphragm should be divided for fractures at the thoracolumbar junction
- Identify the fracture and expose the adjacent intervertebral discs and vertebral bodies. Subperiosteal exposure anteriorly with division of segmental vessels is needed to allow a swab to be packed into the interval between the spine and great vessels for protection
- Complete discectomy above and below the fracture followed by removal of the fractured vertebral body back to the spinal canal. Profuse epidural bleeding is often encountered
- Reconstruction with a cage packed with graft to restore coronal and sagittal alignment. This can be confirmed by fluoroscopy
- Neutralization of the construct with screw/plate instrumentation into adjacent vertebral bodies
- Closure should be in layers in a retrograde fashion over a chest drain

Rehabilitation

- Prophylactic antibiotics should be given according to the normal hospital protocol
- Any drains should be removed 24–48 hours postoperatively
- The patient can be mobilized with physiotherapy once trunk control is established. External bracing is seldom required
- Standing whole spine AP and lateral radiographs should be taken pre-discharge
- Regular and frequent outpatient review (clinical and radiological), should continue until healing/fusion is confirmed or instrumentation removed
- A return to work can be made from 6 weeks postoperatively, in a graduated fashion

- Contact sports or heavy manual work should only be undertaken after confirmation of healing/fusion
- Longer-term follow up is necessary for patients with secondary problems such as sagittal imbalance, neurological dysfunction or delayed/nonunion

Avoiding postoperative complications

- **'Wrong' indication:** understand the mechanism of injury and fracture pattern in order to formulate the correct operative plan
- **'Wrong' patient:** ensure that the patient is fit to undergo the planned operation with adequate cardiorespiratory reserve and appropriate physiological paramaters such as clotting and renal function. Other injuries need to be considered with regard to prioritization and final functional recovery
- **Wrong timing:** in neurologically intact patients with unstable spinal injuries and patients with nonprogressive neurological injuries, operative intervention should be made as soon as it is safe, to optimize the potential recovery and simplify rehabilitation. Progressive neurological dysfunction is an indication for urgent surgical intervention
- **'Wrong' operation:** once the indication for surgical stabilization is established, meticulous preoperative planning with regard to the approach, the extent and type of instrumentation and bone graft material needs to be performed
- **Wrong level:** ensure adequate preoperative imaging with obvious anatomical reference points (e.g. lumbosacral junction, 12th rib morphology) which can then be referenced by fluoroscopy intraoperatively
- **Implant misplacement:** ensure adequate exposure of anatomical landmarks to allow a safe two-handed technique for pedicle tracts and multiplanar fluoroscopy
- **Implant failure:** ensure adequate size and extent of instrumentation; reduce/reconstruct the fractured segment and employ meticulous fusion technique. Be aware of poor bone quality in the elderly/patients with osteoporosis and patients with comorbidities
- **Avoid infection:** give prophylactic antibiotics, use a laminar flow theater and meticulous operative technique, including wound closure and dressings
- **Anticipate potential problems:** have a 'bailout plan' in mind should the intervention not go as planned

Summary of learning points

- Careful assessment must be made of a polytrauma patient with spinal injuries, with regard to the severity of other injuries, the presence of neurology, the mechanism of injury and the stability of the spinal fracture
- Adequate imaging including plain radiographs and CT scan (with coronal and sagittal reconstruction) is necessary to allow detailed fracture classification and operative planning
- Specialist spinal theater staff, anesthetists, equipment, and theater set up are vital
- The posterior approach is the mainstay of spinal fracture surgery. It can be used as a definitive treatment or for initial realignment and stabilization followed by staged anterior column reconstruction
- Attention to detail in every step of decision making and surgical technique is the key to avoiding complications

Further reading

Denis F. The three column spine and its significance in the classification of acute thoracolumbar spinal injuries. Spine 1983; 8:817–831.

Magerl F, Aebi M, Gertzbein SD, et al. A comprehensive classification of thoracic and lumbar injuries. Eur Spine J 1994; 3:184–201.

Pneumaticos SG, Triantafyllopoulos GK, Giannoudis PV. Advances made in the treatment of thoracolumbar fractures: current trends and future directions. Injury 2013; 44:703–712.

Wood KB, Li W, Lebl DS, Ploumis A. Management of thoracolumbar spine fractures. Spine J 2014; 14:145–164.

12 Proximal femoral fractures

Faiz Shivji, Daren P Forward

Introduction

Hip fractures are common, representing the culmination of an aging, osteoporotic population with significant medical co-morbidities. They are associated with a high mortality, morbidity, and significant financial cost.

Incidence

In the UK, the National Hip Fracture Database (2016) reported at least 64,864 patients were admitted over a 1-year period (2015), with a 30-day mortality of 7.1% and mean length of stay of 20 days.

Mechanism of injury

Simple falls from standing height commonly lead to hip fractures in the elderly population due to osteopenic bone.

Hip fractures in young patients are the result of high-energy trauma leading to a large axial load placed through the femoral neck, or low-energy trauma through bone infiltrated with metastatic lesions.

Initial management/ prioritization

Full medical evaluation, investigation and management should be conducted, including hematological and radiological tests. An assessment of the patient's cognitive function should be performed. Adequate analgesia should be provided, including local anesthetic blocks. Orthogeriatric input should be sought within 72 hours of admission and preferably prior to surgery. The national 'best practice tariff' for hip fractures has provided a financial incentive for institutions to improve care against national standards. A reduced morbidity and mortality rate has been demonstrated as a result.

Advanced Traume Life Support assessment must be conducted for young patients suffering a hip fracture.

Considerations for surgery

Patients should have any reversible medical conditions, such as concurrent infections, electrolyte imbalance, anemia, or anticoagulation treated prior to operative management. Surgery should take place within 36 hours of admission. Surgical treatment must allow patients to fully weight bear in the immediate postoperative period.

Young patients suffering a hip fracture should undergo surgical fixation on the next available planned trauma list with a named orthopedic consultant. The surgery should be performed to a high standard by a capable surgeon.

Theater layout and patient positioning

Proposed theater layouts for internal fixation and arthroplasty are illustrated in **Figure 12.3**.

Review of surgical approaches

Lateral (modified Hardinge) approach

- Incise over greater trochanter (GT) in line with the femoral shaft (**Figure 12.4a**)
- The iliotibial band is split in line with the skin incision distally, while proximally the gluteus maximus is split. This exposes the gluteus medius proximally and vastus lateralis distally
- Using diathermy, vastus lateralis can be elevated just distal to the trochanter, moving proximally to elevate gluteus medius, minimus and the capsule as single layer (**Figure 12.4b**)

Case example: Impacted intracapsular hip fracture

A 45-year-old man slipped in his kitchen and sustained an isolated injury to his right hip region (**Figure 12.1**). He had no pre-existing hip pain and no significant past medical history. He had a full medical workup to exclude any associated injuries and concurrent medical conditions. He was taken to theater, placed on a traction table and underwent percutaneous pinning in situ of his right valgus impacted intracapsular neck of femur fracture (**Figure 12.2**).

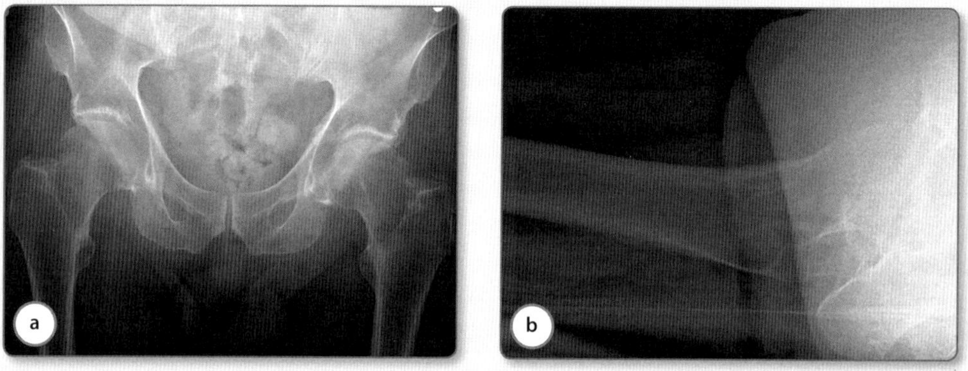

Figure 12.1 (a, b) AP pelvis and lateral radiograph of right hip. Minimally displaced right intracapsular neck of femur fracture.

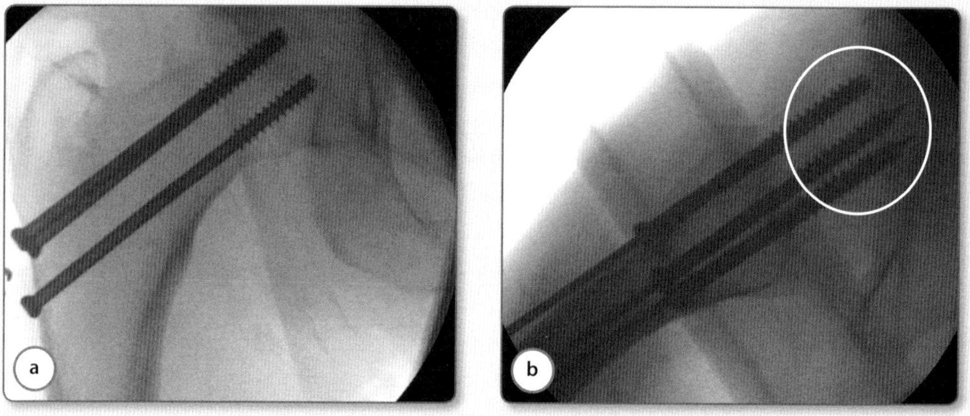

Figure 12.2 (a, b) Intraoperative AP and lateral radiographs showing cannulated screw fixation. Note the inverted triangle position of the screws.

in the line of their fibers, from the anterior part of the GT, leaving a cuff of the tendon behind to aid re-attatchment. Positioning the leg in external rotation places the muscle under tension and facilitates this approach. The capsule can be split appropriately and the hip then dislocated (**Figure 12.4c**)

Anterolateral (Watson-Jones) approach

- Incise in line from the anterior-superior iliac spine of the iliac crest to the GT, then down femoral shaft (**Figure 12.5a**)
- Incise the fascia lata over the femur and extend

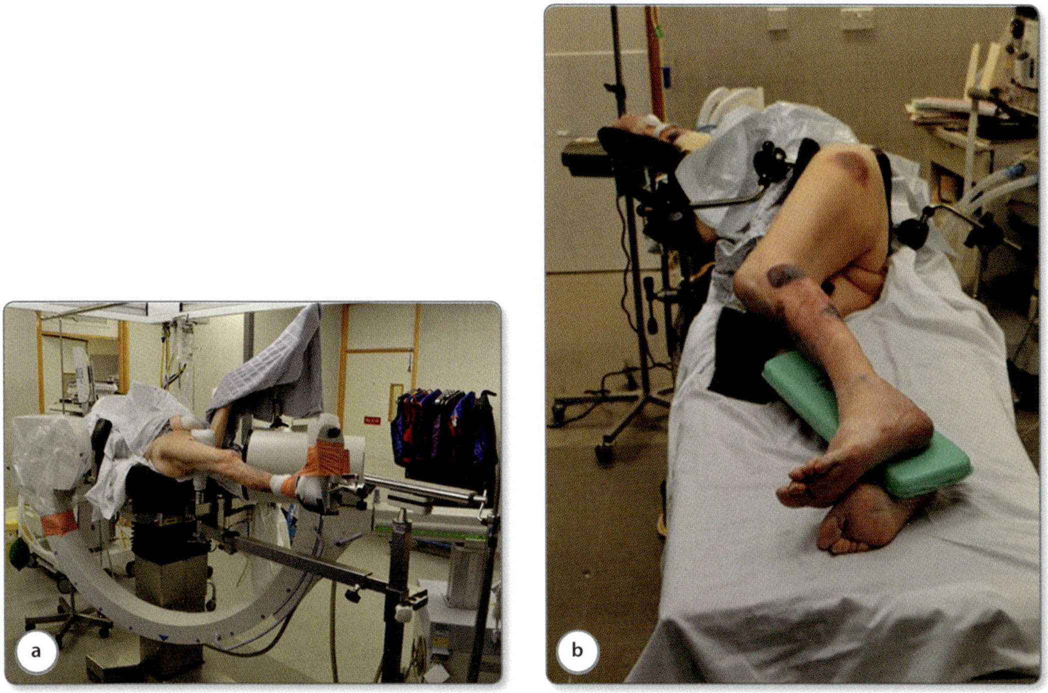

Figure 12.3 (a) Theater layout for cannulated screws/DHS/IM nail fixation. A traction table is used with the affected leg placed in the traction boot. Counter traction is produced by placing a padded post against the perineum. For IM nail fixation, the affected leg can be slightly adducted to allow ease of nail insertion. The contralateral leg is placed in hip flexion and abduction to remove it from fluoroscopic field as shown or placed in the 'scissors position'. (b) Theater layout for lateral position used in arthroplasty. The patient is held by anterior and posterior supports with a pressure relieving pad between legs. DHS, dynamic hip screw; IM, intramedullary

this incision proximally along the posterior border of the muscle

- Retract the tensor fascia lata anteriorly and the gluteus medius muscle posteriorly. Expose this interval using blunt dissection, paying careful attention to crossing blood vessels (**Figure 12.5b**)
- External rotation of the leg improves access to the hip capsule, with appropriately placed retractors. A GT osteotomy or partial release of the anterior gluteus medius may be used occasionally to aid access
- A capsulotomy is performed demonstrating the femoral head and neck, care being taken not to damage the labrum (**Figure 12.5c**)
- Using pointed reduction forceps, the intracapsular fracture can then be reduced prior to suitable stabilization

Dangers of the lateral and anterolateral approaches

- **Superior gluteal nerve:** runs between the gluteus medius and minimus approximately 5 cm above the upper border of the GT. Be wary of proximal extension of dissection
- **Lateral circumflex artery:** usually cut when vastus lateralis is incised, and must be cauterized
- **Femoral nerve:** most lateral structure in neurovascular bundle – at risk from anterior retractors

Posterior hip approach

- Incision is centered over GT and curved slightly posteriorly proximally as shown in **Figure 12.4a**

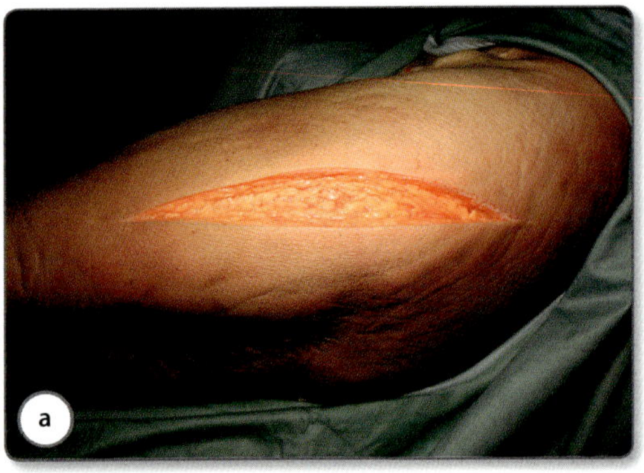

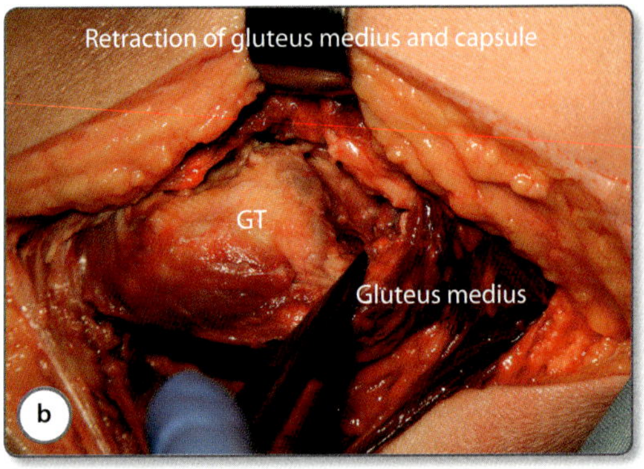

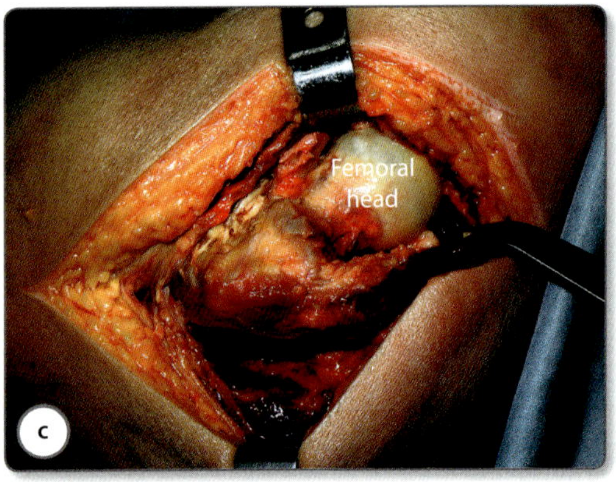

Figure 12.4 (a) Incision over greater trochanter in line with femoral shaft. (b) After splitting fascia lata and gluteus maximus, gluteus medius, minimus and capsule can be elevated in a single layer. (c) Femoral head being dislocated by externally rotating and adducting hip.

- Iliotibial band and proximal gluteus maximus is split in line with its fibers. The sciatic nerve can be identified at this stage to avoid iatrogenic damage during the procedure (**Figure 12.6a**)
- Retractors hold the anterior fibers of gluteus maximus and tensor fascia anteriorly while the posterior fibers of gluteus maximus are maintained posteriorly
- The posterior attachment of gluteus medius is released from the posterior crest of the trochanter
- The piriformis is then tagged and released before a similar technique is used on the superior gemellus, obturator internus and the inferior gemellus, which can be elevated off the posterior capsule as a continuous layer (**Figure 12.6b**)
- The posterior capsule is then excised as necessary, the hip dislocated and appropriate retractors inserted

Dangers of the posterior approach

- The sciatic nerve is at risk from malpositioned retractors, or tractional injuries
- In femoral head preserving surgery, the medial femoral circumflex artery should be preserved, so quadratus femoris should not be incised and the division of the short external rotators should be at least 1.5 cm from the femoral insertion

Anterior (Smith-Peterson) approach

- Position the patient supine. Incise from just below anterior-superior iliac spine distally for about 10 cm over the lateral border of sartorius (**Figure 12.7a**), taking care not to damage lateral cutaneous nerve of the thigh in the proximal aspect of the incision
- The tensor fascia lata laterally and sartorius medially are identified and this interval developed (**Figure 12.7b**). The ascending branches of the lateral circumflex artery and vein are also encountered and will need to be ligated (**Figure 12.7c**)
- External hip rotation will bring the femoral head anteriorly and gluteus medius and tensor fascia can be retracted laterally. The reflected head of rectus femoris is then

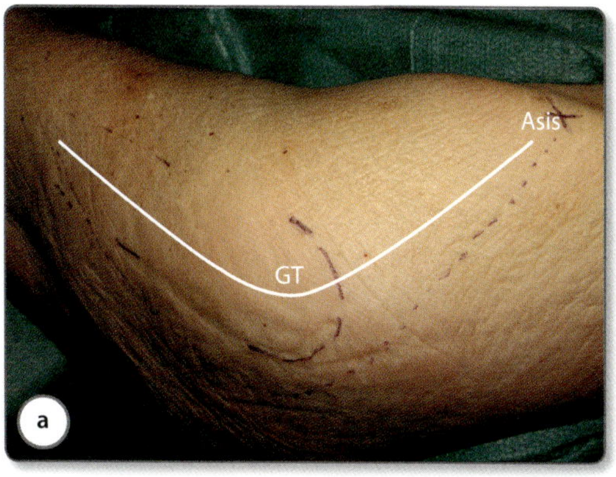

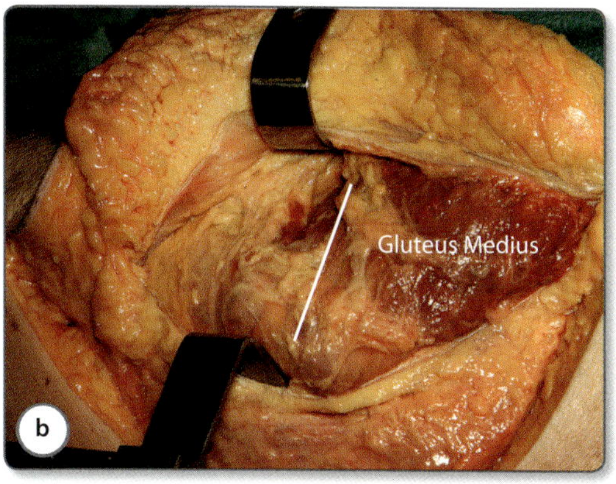

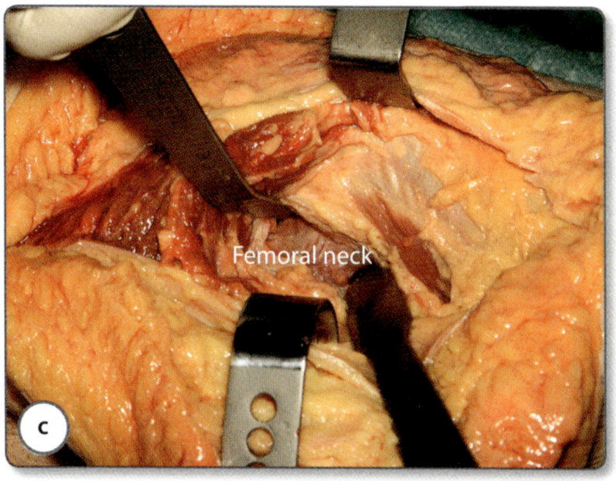

Figure 12.5 (a) Proposed skin incision for Watson-Jones approach. (b) Interval between tensor fascia lata anteriorly and gluteus medius posteriorly is identified and opened. (c) The femoral neck and head is made more prominent by externally rotating the leg, allowing a capsulotomy to be performed, exposing the femoral neck and head as necessary.

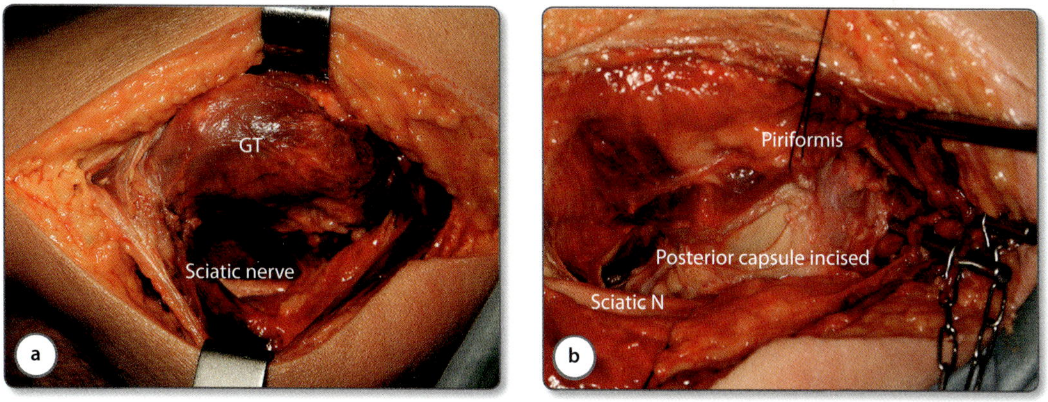

Figure 12.6 (a) Sciatic nerve identified prior to division of short external rotators of hip. (b) Stay suture in piriformis for later repair. Posterior short external rotators divided and retracted posteriorly giving access to the posterior capsular structures of the hip.

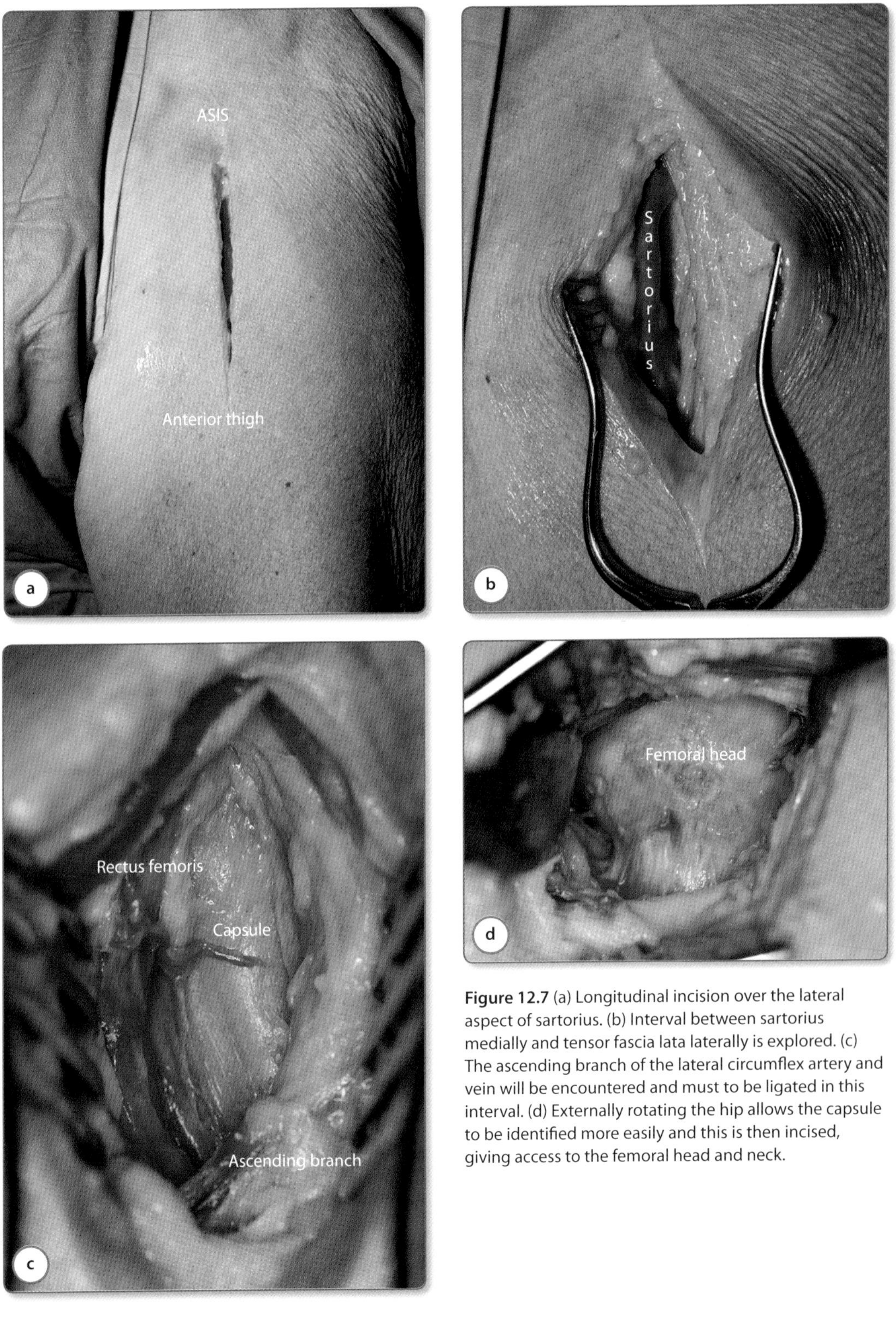

Figure 12.7 (a) Longitudinal incision over the lateral aspect of sartorius. (b) Interval between sartorius medially and tensor fascia lata laterally is explored. (c) The ascending branch of the lateral circumflex artery and vein will be encountered and must to be ligated in this interval. (d) Externally rotating the hip allows the capsule to be identified more easily and this is then incised, giving access to the femoral head and neck.

incised to allow the anterior hip capsule to be opened, exposing the femoral neck and head (**Figure 12.7d**)

Dangers of the anterior approach

- The lateral femoral cutaneous nerve of the thigh lies 2.5 cm inferior to the ASIS and is at risk

Dynamic hip screw: elevation of vastus lateralis

- Use the image intensifier to identify the appropriate entry point for the dynamic hip screw (DHS), and make a 5–8-cm incision down the lateral side of the thigh, starting at this point
- Incise the fascia in the line of the incision, exposing the vastus lateralis
- Incise along the posterior aspect of the vastus lateralis fascia and then elevate the muscle off the fascia using a periosteal instrument, allowing identification and ligation of the perforators in a controlled manner
- The lateral aspect of the femur can now be exposed and appropriate retractors inserted for wire placement, etc.

Intramedullary nail entry

- Palpate the tip of the GT
- Make a 5-cm incision centered over an imaginary point where a perpendicular line directed downward from the anterior superior iliac spine and a longitudinal line in the direction of the lateral shaft of the femur intersect
- Incise the fascia and use blunt dissection to split the fibers of gluteus maximus, and reach the tip of the GT
- Nail entry point insertion will be dictated by the implants used and the company's operative technique guide

Equipment requirements

- Traction table
- C-arm image intensifier
- Cannulated screw set
- Dynamic hip screw set
- Hemiarthroplasy instrumentation and implants
- Total hip replacement instrumentation and implants
- Intramedullary (IM) nailing equipment and implants
- Reduction aids: forceps, cables, bone holders

Reduction and stabilization methods

Displaced intracapsular fractures: young patients

Closed reduction

- The Leadbetter technique can be used: the hip is flexed to 90° with slight adduction. Traction is applied in this position, followed by internal rotation. Finally, the leg is brought into extension and slight abduction whilst maintaining traction and internal rotation

Open reduction

- Watson-Jones approach (see above)
- The anterior Smith-Peterson approach (see above) with a separate mini-lateral approach is used to surgically stabilize the fracture

Method of fixation

- Cannulated screws are placed in an inverted triangular orientation
- Intraoperative screw placement in relation to the clinical case examples illustrated in **Figure 12.1** is shown in **Figure 12.2**. Screws are parallel, inserted as an inverted triangle with a posterior neck supporting screw
- A DHS two-hole plate is also an acceptable and equally favored technique, which is often more familiar to the operating surgeon

Displaced intracapsular fractures in the elderly

Hemiarthroplasty

Hemiarthroplasty is recommended for all displaced intracapsular fractures in the elderly due to the risk of developing either avascular necrosis of the femoral head or a nonunion at the fracture site if these fractures are surgically stabilized (**Figure 12.8**). A higher patient satisfaction, lower pain scores, a lower reoperation rate, and lack of difference in mortality are consistently demonstrated when compared with internal fixation.

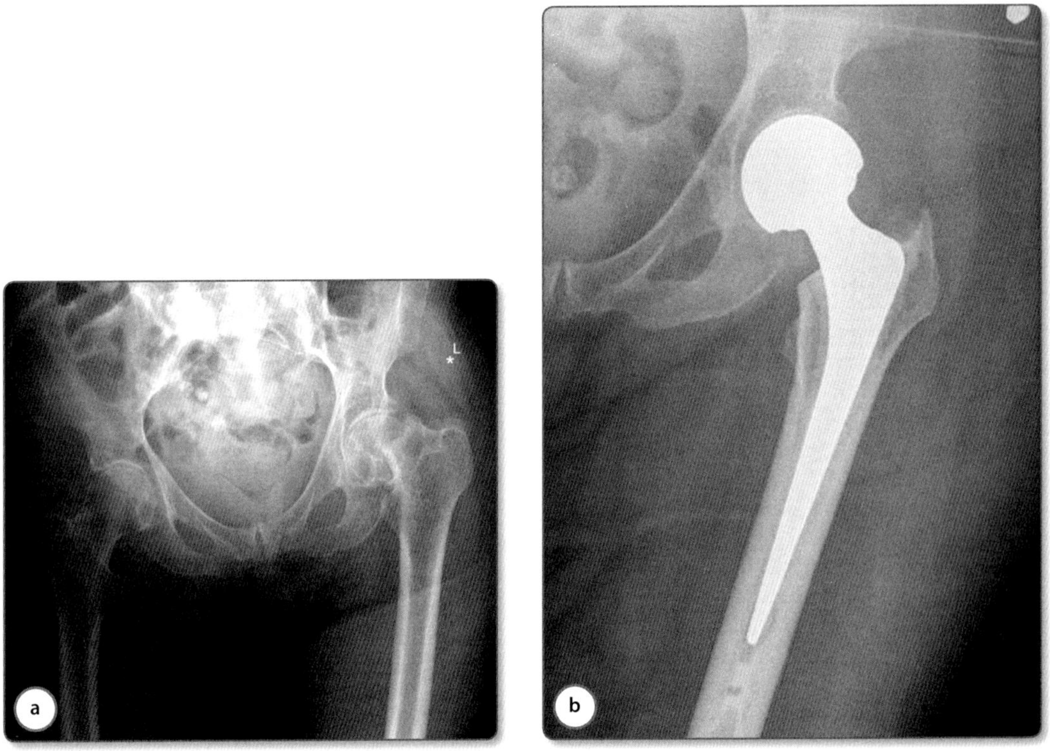

Figure 12.8 (a) AP X-ray of displaced left intracapsular neck of femur fracture in an elderly patient. (b) Postoperative management of the same patient treated with cemented hemiarthroplasty.

Total hip replacement

Total hip replacement (THR) should be considered in medically fit patients with a high premorbid function, pre-existing symptomatic osteoarthritis of the hip and pathological fractures. The National Hip Fracture Database would suggest that only 20% of patients with a displaced intracapsular fracture receive a THR.

Extracapsular fractures

Closed reduction

- The patient is positioned on a traction table with traction to the injured limb in slight flexion, abduction and internal rotation (**Figure 12.2a**)

Open reduction

- Reduction forceps or Schanz screws placed in each fragment can be used to reduce the fracture
- Reduction can be held with bone forceps/clamps and/or K-wires

Method of fixation

Closed reduction and internal fixation is recommended for extracapsular fractures. Fixation options include extramedullary fixation with a DHS – sometimes using a trochanteric support plate in fractures where the lateral wall is weak or incompetent – or intrameduallary fixation with a cephalomedullary nail (**Figure 12.9**)

Rehabilitation

- **Elderly patients:** immediate full weight bearing
- **Young patients:** partial weight bearing on the affected leg until radiographic evidence of union. At least 2 years of follow-up is necessary to exclude avascular necrosis in intracapsular fractures
- Nutritional support and input
- Ongoing medical management (e.g. orthogeriatric, combined management)

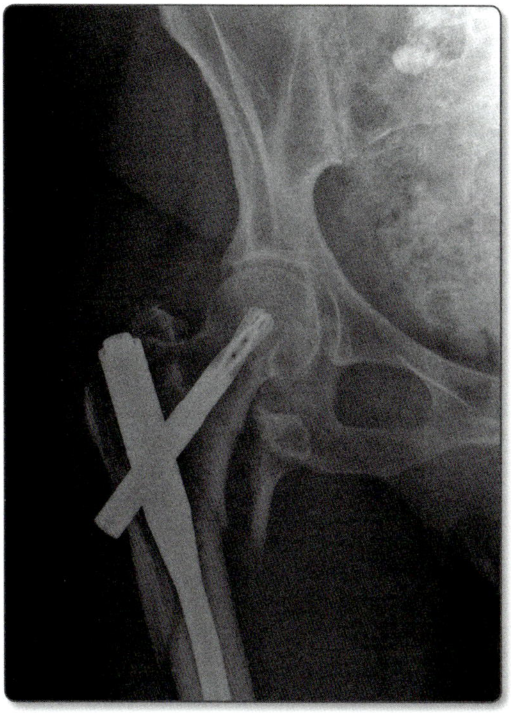

Figure 12.9 Example of an extramedullary device for extracapsular proximal femoral fracture management.

- Progressive integration with activities of daily living under physiotherapy and occupational therapy instruction

Avoiding postoperative complications

- Pre- and postoperative orthogeriatric input and active monitoring for medical complications
- Nutritional support
- Venous thromboprophylaxis and methicillin resistant *Staphylococcus aureus* (MRSA) screening
- Accurate fracture reduction
- Appropriate implant selection and correct operative technique (e.g. tip-apex distance)
- Early mobilization
- Rehabilitation input

Summary of learning points

- Joint patient care with appropriate input from care of the elderly medicine and anesthetics both pre- and postoperatively is mandatory
- Medical optimization preoperatively with HDU admission as necessary should be undertaken
- Accurate intraoperative fracture reduction prior to fracture stabilisation will reduce screw cut out and nonunion
- Correct implant selection for specific fracture configurations is necessary to reduce loss of fracture fixation and implant failure
- Surgery should be performed by a suitably qualified surgeon to reduce complications
- Patients should be mobilized early to reduce postoperative complications
- A team approach with ongoing supportive care and rehabilitation is necessary to optimize functional recovery in this often frail group of patients

Further reading

Adams C, Robinson CM, Court-Brown CM, McQueen MM. Prospective randomized controlled trial of an intramedullary nail versus dynamic screw and plate for intertrochanteric fractures of the femur. J Orthop Trauma 2001; 15:394–400.

Baumgaertner MR, Curtin SL, Lindskog DM, Keggi JM. The value of the tip-apex distance in predicting failure of fixation of peritrochanteric fractures of the hip. J Bone Joint Surg Am 1995; 77:1058–1064.

Frndak PA, Mallory TH, Lombardi Jr AV. Translateral surgical approach to the hip: the abductor muscle 'split'. Clinl Ortho Rel Res1993;295:135-141.

Garden RS. Low-angle fixation in fractures of the femoral neck. J Bone Joint Surg Br 1961; 43:647–663.

Jensen JS, Michaelsen M. Trochanteric femoral fractures treated with McLaughlin osteosynthesis. Acta Orthop Scand 1975; 46:795–803.

Moja L, Piatti A, Pecoraro V, et al. Timing matters in hip fracture surgery: patients operated within 48 hours have better outcomes. A meta-analysis and meta-regression of over 190,000 patients. PLoS One 2012; 7:e46175.

Parker MJ, Khan RJ, Crawford J, Pryor GA. Hemiarthroplasty versus internal fixation for displaced intra-capsular hip fractures in the elderly. A randomised trial of 455 patients. J Bone Joint Surg Br 2002; 84:1150–1155.

Upadhyay A, Jain P, Mishra P, et al. Delayed internal fixation of fractures of the neck of the femur in young adults. A prospective, randomised study comparing closed and open reduction. J Bone Joint Surg Br 2004; 86:1035–1040.

13 Femoral diaphyseal fractures

Rebecka Asp, Nicholas Hancock

Introduction

Femoral fractures are classified according to the anatomical location. They can either be located in the proximal, middle or distal third of the shaft or at the junctions between these locations. The geometry of the fracture is described according to the fracture pattern, e.g. oblique, transverse, comminuted or spiral.

Incidence

The incidence of femoral diaphyseal fractures is about 10 per 100 000 population. They are seen more frequently in regions where there is a high prevalence of road traffic accidents and high energy trauma.

Mechanism of injury

There is a bimodal distribution to femoral shaft fractures plotted against age. These typically occur in the younger male population attributed to high energy trauma, e.g. in road traffic accidents or in the elderly female population, associated osteopenia or osteoporosis.

During normal activities, the femur can be subjected to bending, axial and torsional forces that exceed up to four times body weight. Torsional forces cause spiral fractures whereas axial loading and bending results in transverse and bending wedge fractures. The amount of comminution is proportional to the kinetic energy imparted to the limb.

In the high energy group there is a high incidence of associated ipsilateral femoral neck fractures (up to 10%) and an increased mortality rate from pulmonary complications with bilateral femoral fractures. CT scans can be useful to detect ipsilateral femoral neck fractures.

Initial management/ prioritization

The evaluation and management to femoral shaft fractures has evolved over the last century to reduce the sequelae of shortening, mal- and nonunion. This was profoundly affected by Kuntsher's introduction of the 'marrow nailing method' around the time of the Second World War.

Identification of life-threatening injuries should be the initial approach to patients with femoral shaft fractures as they can be associated with serious injuries.

Palpation of distal pulses or use of the Doppler ultrasound to evaluate the ankle-brachial pressure index (ABPI) can be useful. An ABPI < 0.9 has been found to have a high sensitivity and specificity for a major arterial injury.

Injuries to the obturator and femoral nerves are uncommon but sciatic nerve injury does occur, therefore, the peroneal and tibial nerves should be carefully evaluated.

Circumferential evaluation of soft tissues is mandatory. Any open wounds, contusion or abrasions should raise the suspicion of an open fracture. The ipsilateral hip and knee should also be evaluated for fracture, ligamentous and soft tissue injuries.

Knee ligamentous injury is found in 50% of patients following femoral stabilization. Similarly, ipsilateral meniscal injury is found in 25% of patients with femoral diaphyseal fractures.

Considerations for surgery

Early stabilization of long bone fractures reduces the systemic effect of the inflammatory response to the multiply injured patient. Early surgical

Case example: Closed femoral diaphysial fracture

A middle-aged woman fell down several steps, was unable to weight bear and had a clinically deformed thigh. She was taken to hospital by ambulance, where she was treated with appropriate analgesia and placed in traction before X-rays were taken. The X-rays showed a diaphysial fracture to her right femur (**Figure 13.1**). The patient was taken to theater, placed on a traction table and, under image intensifier control, had a reamed antegrade locked femoral nail inserted (**Figure 13.2**).

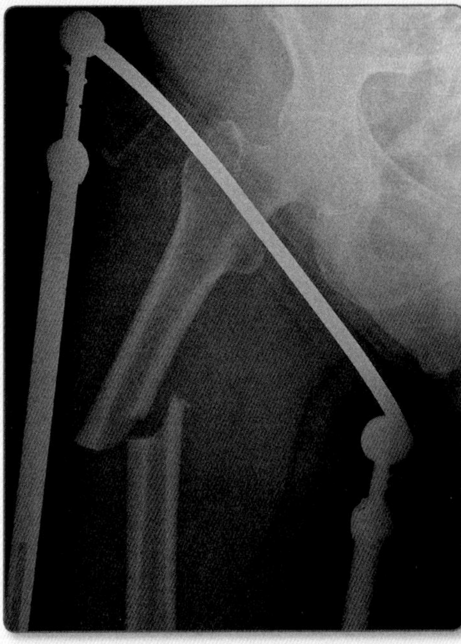

Figure 13.1 AP X-ray of injured femur with traction splint in situ.

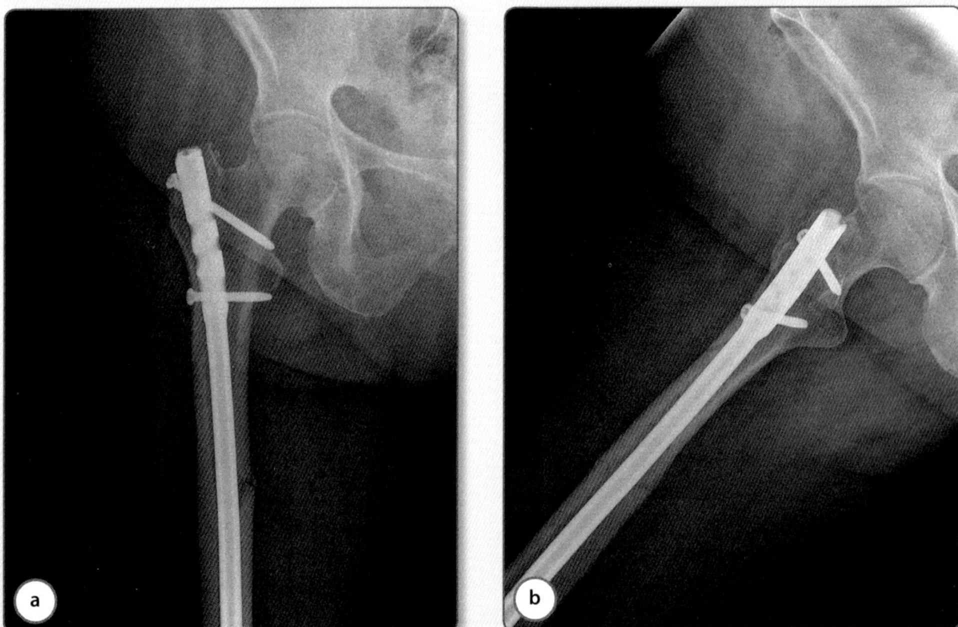

Figure 13.2 (a) AP and (b) lateral postoperative X-rays of the case example patient.

stabilization reduces bleeding, fat embolism and later mal or nonunion. Femoral shaft fractures are rarely treated nonoperatively in adults (cast braces and traction).

The mainstay of management is to restore length, axial and rotational alignment. Regardless of definitive management, initial treatment involves temporary stabilization using traction and limb realignment to a more anatomical position. This can alter vascular status but can also control pain, reduce further soft tissue damage and control hemorrhage.

External fixation is often used as a temporary measure to staged intramedullary nailing in trauma patients who are too unwell or under resuscitated. The primary indications for external fixation are severe soft tissue injury, extensive soft tissue or medullary contamination and vascular injury where arterial reconstruction or shunt placement needs to be undertaken.

Plating of femoral diaphyseal fractures can be considered where there are relative contraindications to intramedullary nailing. Typical indications for plating include patients with an extremely narrow medullary canal, fractures in the region of previous malunion and fractures extending proximally or distally into pertrochanteric and metaphyseal regions. In patients with vascular repair the extensile medial exposure may facilitate plating. However, in these circumstances nonunion is more likely due to disruption of blood supply.

Theater layout and patient positioning

Theater set up, lay out and method of obtaining the correct entry point is arguably the most important consideration intramedullary nailing method. Familiarity with theater traction table and appliances is essential. **Figure 13.3a** shows typical set up of the traction table in an open femoral fracture case.

An appreciation of the contralateral hip version preoperative on table is important in setting up the traction table position. The foot needs to be secured and the body in the 'banana' position, allowing entry to the piriform fossa or the trochanteric tip, depending on nailing kit used. The arm is positioned over the chest in order to allow rotation of the fluoroscopy C-arm and facilitate access to the proximal femoral entry point in antegrade nailing. The other leg is usually placed in a supportive gutter or in the 'scissors' position, with care of pressure areas such as the medial hamstrings and fibula head and pneumatic intermittent compression devices applied as intraoperative thromboprophylaxis.

Supine positioning for freehand femoral nailing, with the knee flexed over a bolster or Fromm triangle is usually relatively simple in retrograde femoral nailing and external fixation (**Figure 13.3b**).

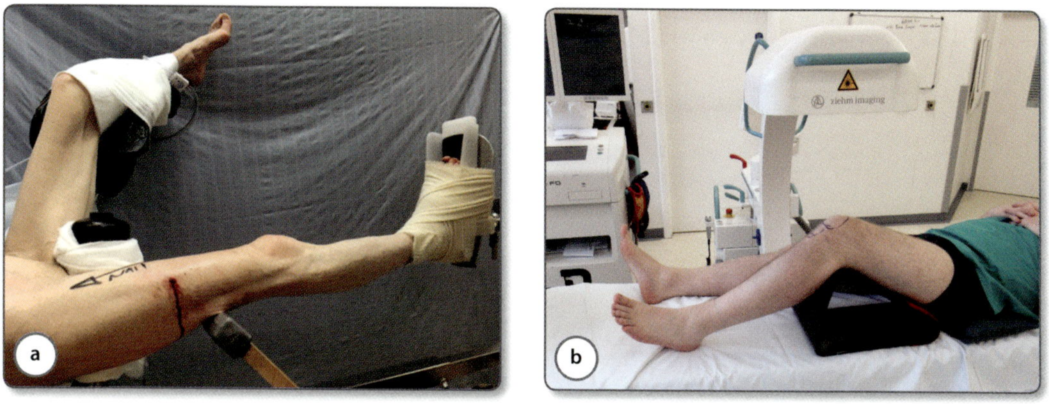

Figure 13.3 (a) Traction table set up for antegrade nailing in an open fracture: note padding, intermittent compression calf pump and securing of the foot in traction. The upper body is drawn away to allow access to the entry point. (b) Proposed setup for retrograde femoral nailing on radiolucent table.

Review of surgical approaches

External fixation

External fixation is a relatively quick and easy procedure which is beneficial to critically ill and unstable polytrauma patients as part of damage control orthopaedics. It can be utilized in patients with vascular injuries, soft tissue damage with extensive contamination, compartment syndrome, open fractures and extensively comminuted fractures. Complications include femoral shortening, angular malunion, pin site infections, knee stiffness and damage to the soft tissues the pins traverse.

Plating

Plating allows rigid stabilization, early mobilization and anatomic reduction. Length, alignment and rotation can be restored directly with plating in combination with either femoral distracters or manual traction. Indications for plating include narrow medullary canals, fractures around previous malunions and ipsilateral neck fractures requiring percutaneous screw fixation. The disadvantage is that the periosteal vascular supply to the bone beneath the plate is decreased. The surgical dissection can delay healing, cause blood loss, increase the risk of infection and further devitalize soft tissue and fracture fragments. Minimally invasive techniques for plate application can reduce these complications but may not achieve adequate reduction (**Figure 13.4**).

Intramedullary nailing

Antegrade and retrograde intramedullary nailing have succeeded other treatment options because they encompass minimal soft tissue dissection, stable realignment, rapid healing, early weight

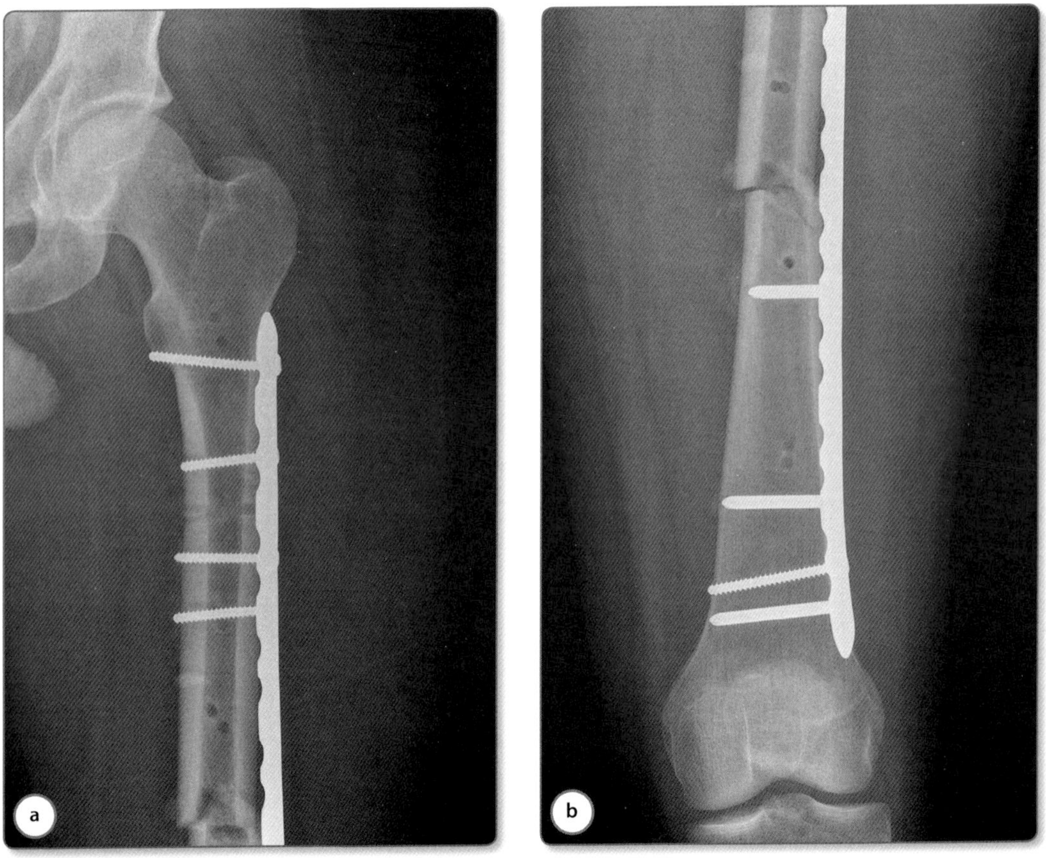

Figure 13.4 (a, b) AP X-ray showing plating of femoral fracture because of acute respiratory distress and fat embolism, this led to a nonunion and 9 months later was revised to a nailing.

bearing and functional rehabilitation. The illustrated case example shown by **Figure 13.1** is shown after treatment with an antegrade locked femoral nail, allowing early functional rehabilitation (**Figure 13.2**).

The incidence of pulmonary complications (acute respiratory distress syndrome), thromboembolic events and mortality are reduced with early stabilization. The use of locking screws prevents shortening and malrotation and increases the working length of the construct. Reaming the medullary canal increases the rate of union, reduces implant failure and allows for an appropriately sized implant to be inserted. Although intramedullary nailing and reaming is associated with fat and marrow embolism, there is no clear clinical evidence that shows that patients with pulmonary injuries should not undergo reamed intramedullary nailing if anesthetically stable and fully resuscitated. Correct entry point localization for nail insertion is paramount for successful nailing and review of the implant company's surgical technique is mandatory prior to surgical positioning.

Equipment requirements

- Traction table or radiolucent table
- Reduction clamps
- Half pins and T-handle
- F-shaped reduction tool
- Radiolucent bolsters
- Axillary crutch
- Intramedullary nailing systems
- Plating systems
- External fixator system

Reduction and stabilization methods

- Indirect reduction using traction table with axillary crutch support under limb
- Free leg positioning on radiolucent table over radiolucent bolster with the use of percutaneous half pins as joysticks for fracture reduction (**Figure 13.5a**)
- Open reduction and application of bone clamps for fracture reduction
- Stabilization can be undertaken as described by the various techniques outlined above

Rehabilitation

- Early physiotherapy input to maintain muscle strength and mobility
- Early appropriate weight bearing as necessary
- Serial postoperative X-rays to confirm no loss of reduction and progression of union
- Supervised progressive follow-up directed to patient needs

Avoiding postoperative complications

Infection

Infections occurring following closed fractures are less than 1% compared with 2.4–4.8% in open fractures. Features suggestive of infection include pain, pyrexia, swelling, erythema and purulent discharge. Management of infection includes debridement of all infected tissue and bone, implant removal and antibiotics. Further surgical stabilization of the fracture may be required if the fracture hasn't united.

Nonunion and delayed union

This can be as a result of significant bone loss, poor vascular supply, soft tissue interposition, inadequate reduction, excessive fracture site distraction, infection, or severity of high energy trauma.

Nerve injury

Iatrogenic nerve injury, in the form of neuropraxia is usually the result of traction or compression of the nerve. Sciatic nerve injury is seen with excessive traction and pudendal nerve injury can follow compression against the perineal post during intraoperative traction.

Heterotopic ossification

Heterotopic bone formation has been variably reported in 9–60% of patients.

Compartment syndrome

Although rare following femoral shaft fractures, there should be a high index of suspicion for compartment syndrome in patients with intense pain out of proportion to what is expected. Tense swelling of the thigh and pain on passive stretching of the muscles of the three compartments of

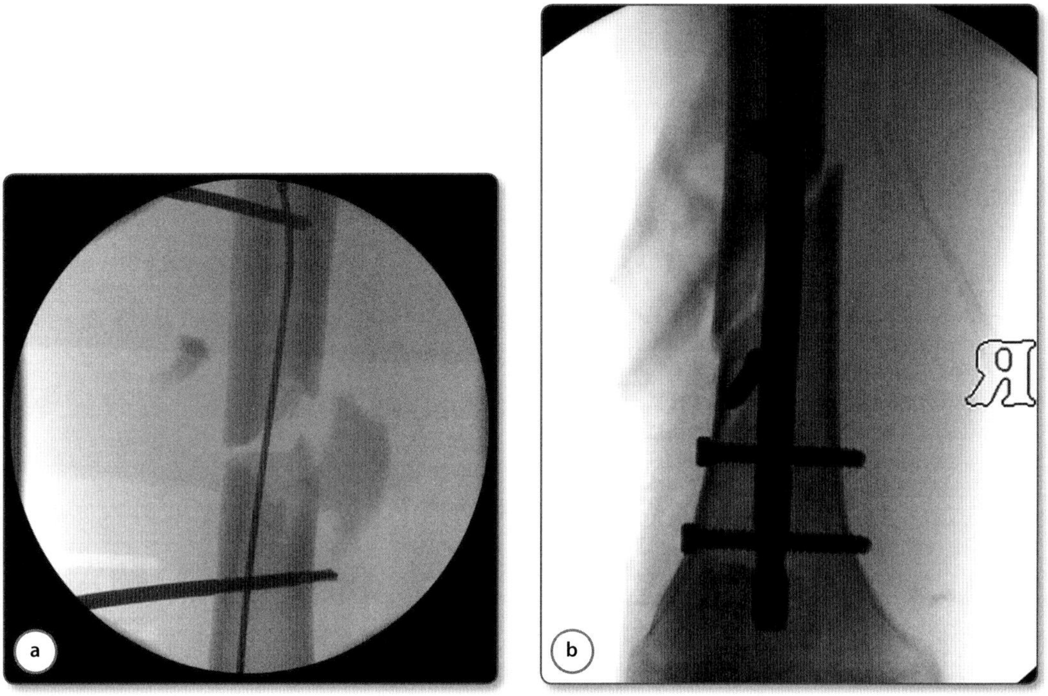

Figure 13.5 (a) Use of half pins to reduce and align fracture segments. (b) Poller blocking screws being used to maintain alignment of fragments around the narrower nail in the metaphyseal region.

the thigh are characteristic. Neurovascular compromise is a late finding. Treatment is emergency decompressive fasciotomy.

Malunion

Malrotation is a common complication of nailing, external fixation, traction and bridge plating compared to compression plating. Greater than 15° malunion occurs in up to 20–30% of patients and is symptomatic above this leading to functional limitations.

The incidence of axial mal-alignment is between 7–11% and can be defined as greater than 5–10° of angulation in the sagittal or coronal planes. This occurs more commonly in proximal and distal third shaft fractures due to the larger medullary canal diameter compared with middle third fractures which allow for a more intimate fit at the isthmus with the nail. Blocking screws/bolts can be used to maintain fracture alignment (**Figure 13.5b**).

Other complications include a femoral refracture and implant complications of broken nails, broken screws and bending of nails. Traumatic and iatrogenic damage to the surrounding muscles can lead to weakness. Knee stiffness can be as a result of damage to the muscles, disuse or immobilization. Ectopic bone formation can be as a result of a head injury which can largely affect the knee.

Summary of learning points

- Familiarity of traction table and patient setup obligatory for successful fracture screening and efficient operative surgical progression
- Appreciate femoral version on contralateral uninjured side in order to assess reduction/ rotational profile
- Choose correct nail entry point in relation to manufactures' operative technique (reduces risk of malreduction)
- Avoid prolonged closed reduction attempts
  - Flex the knee to eliminate deforming force of gastrocnemius e.g. retrograde nailing (**Figure 13.2b**)
  - Use a supporting crutch to correct femoral recurvatum
  - Half-pin 'joysticks' to aid reduction (**Figure 13.5a**)
  - Muscle interposition can prevent closed reduction despite reduction manoeuvers
- Avoid thermal necrosis in narrow canals, alternative methods of stabilization may be preferable
- Ream 1–2 mm greater than nail diameter

Further reading

De Campos J, Vangness CT Jr, Merritt PO, Sher J. Ipsilateral knee with femoral shaft fracture. Examination under anaesthesia and arthroscopic evaluation. Clin Orthop 1994:178–182.

Lefaivre KA, Starr AJ, Stahel PF, Elliott AC, Smith WR. Prediction of pulmonary morbidity and mortality in patients with femur fracture. J Trauma 2010; 69:1527–1535.

Nork SE. Femoral shaft fractures. In: Court-Brown CM, Heckman JD, McQueen MM, et al., (Eds). Rockwood and Green's Fractures in Adults, 8th edn (Vol. 2). Philadelphia: Wolters Kluwer Health/Lippincott Williams & Wilkins, 2015.

Ostrum RF, Marcantonio A, Marburger R. A critical analysis of the eccentric starting point for trochanteric intramedullary femoral nailing. J Orthop Trauma 2005; 19:681–686.

Stannard JP, Schmidt AH. Surgical Treatment of Orthopaedic Trauma: A Comprehensive Text and Video Guide, 2nd Edition. New York: Thieme, 2016.

Vangness CT Jr, De Campos J, Merritt PO, et al. Meniscal injury associated with femoral shaft fracture. J Bone and Joint Surg Br 1993; 75:207–209.

Yang KH, Han DY, Jahng JS, et al. Prevention of malrotation deformity in femoral shaft fracture. J Orthop Trauma 1998; 12:558–562.

14 Intra-articular knee fractures

Mike Kelly

Introduction

These injuries occur within both the high-energy injury spectrum and increasingly the osteoporotic low-energy spectrum. The needs of the differing populations vary and therefore the management strategy needs to be tailored appropriately. In the elderly, this will be the need to rehabilitate to weight-bearing as quickly as possible. In the young, the emphasis can be on achieving the best articular congruency and alignment where periods of protected weight bearing can be tolerated.

Incidence

The incidence of distal femoral fractures is approximately 1/100 000/year (0.5% of fractures) with a predominance in the elderly. The average age of a patient is 77 years and the incidence is higher in women. The demographic is similar to the hip fracture population, albeit slightly younger, and 30% will have a prosthesis in the femur, either hip, or a knee.

The incidence of tibial plateau fractures is 10–13/100 000/year (1.2% of fractures). It has a bimodal distribution in both men and women. In the younger population, there is a male predominance and the mechanism is high-energy trauma. In the older populations there is a female predominance and it results from low-energy trauma.

Mechanism of injury

In the younger population, the majority are high-energy injuries resulting from road traffic accidents, high-energy sports collisions or falls from height. In the elderly, it is most often a fall from standing height, usually with a twisting motion for the distal femur. For tibial plateau fractures, a valgus force to the knee is the most common mechanism. The most useful classification system is that proposed by Lao in 2010. This describes the injury to the bone in terms of the columns involved (lateral, posterior and medial) and can be used to plan a fixation strategy. The typical valgus injury produces a lateral column injury. As the energy of transfer rises, the posterior and medial columns then become involved.

Initial management/ prioritization

Advanced Trauma Life Support assessment takes priority, followed by splintage/soft tissue stabilization and appropriate radiological imaging, in conjunction with a directed neurovascular examination. If any wounds are present these should be appropriately toileted, photographed and covered with sterile dressings and BOAST 4 guidelines followed

If the patient remains physiologically compromised and the fractures are not controlled in a back slab then a spanning external fixator can be applied.

A CT scan is strongly recommended in fractures around the knee. In at least 30% of cases, a CT scan will alter the surgical strategy. This figure is likely to be an underestimate.

Considerations for surgery

The considerations for surgery and the goals will depend on the patient group. The elderly represent a similar cohort to those with hip fractures and the same principles should be applied. They respond very badly to nonoperative treatment and intervention is aimed at restoring weight-bearing as quickly as possible to facilitate the earliest possible return to functional independence. They do not tolerate restrictions

Case example: Bilateral intra-articular distal femoral fractures

A middle-aged driver of a car was involved in a head-on collision, sustaining bilateral deformed knees. Further imaging (**Figures 14.1** and **14.2**) demonstrated the complex comminuted intra-articular nature of the injuries. The soft tissue envelope was amiable to early surgery. She was taken to theater and positioned on a radiolucent table, with the aid of a radiolucent triangle under each thigh in-turn. A direct lateral approach to the distal femur allowed articular reduction and intra-fragmentary lag screw stabilization of the joint surface, before spanning plates were applied sub muscularly with the aid of an aiming guide (**Figure 14.3**).

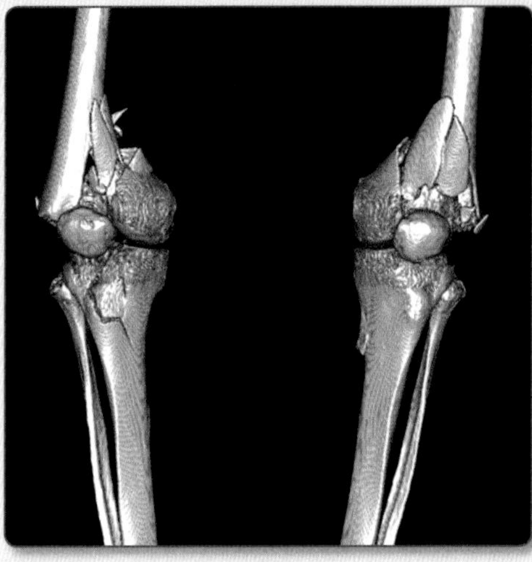

Figure 14.2 Rendered 3D CT images of the case illustrated in Figure 14.1, showing multiple bilateral distal femoral fracture fragments extending into joint and right proximal tibial fracture.

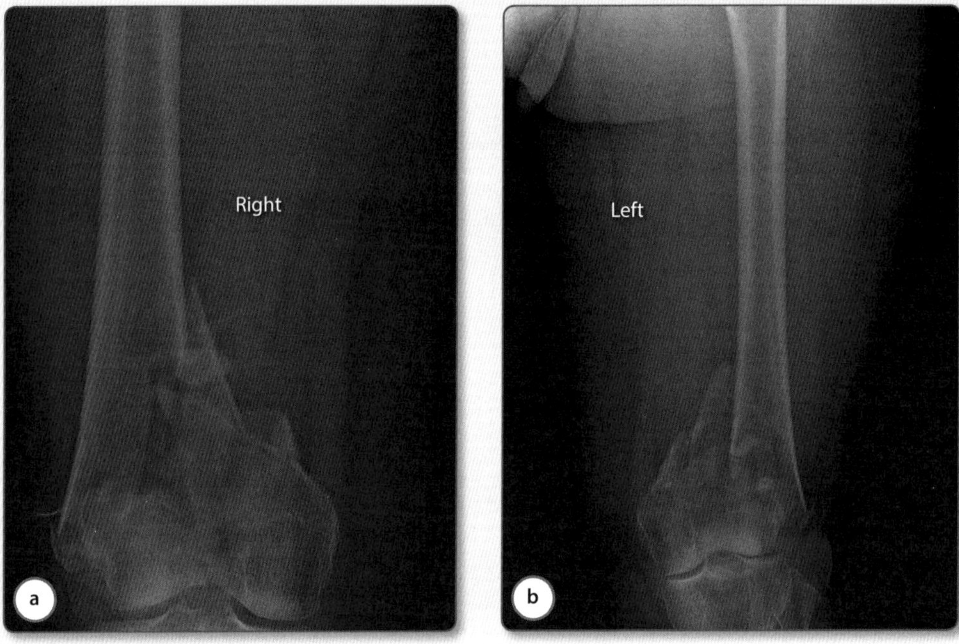

Figure 14.1 (a, b) Preoperative AP X-rays of bilateral inarticular distal femoral fractures.

Case example: *continued.*

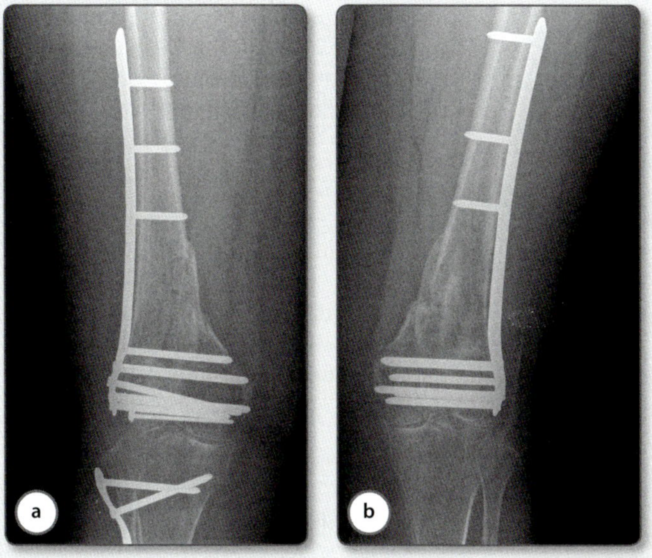

Figure 14.3 Postoperative AP X-rays of the case illustrated in Figure 14.1.

to weight bearing whether in the operative or nonoperative setting so any strategy has to allow for this. It is well documented that prolonged bed rest or hoisting bed-to-chair is disastrous in this patient group.

In the young, the primary aim of treatment is to maintain articular congruency and leg alignment with progression of rehabilitation.

Theater layout and patient positioning

The leg can be positioned over a radiolucent bolster, with flexion of the knee to reduce the pull of the hamstrings and gastrocnemius (**Figure 14.4**). This allows unrestricted access to both the femur and tibia for application of spanning external fixators and also for definitive surgical stabilization.

Initial management of injury

In high-energy injuries, the application of an external fixator allows stabilization of the fractures and protection of the soft tissue envelope, as well as being analgesic for the patient. Surgical planning in conjunction with CT scans can then be undertaken.

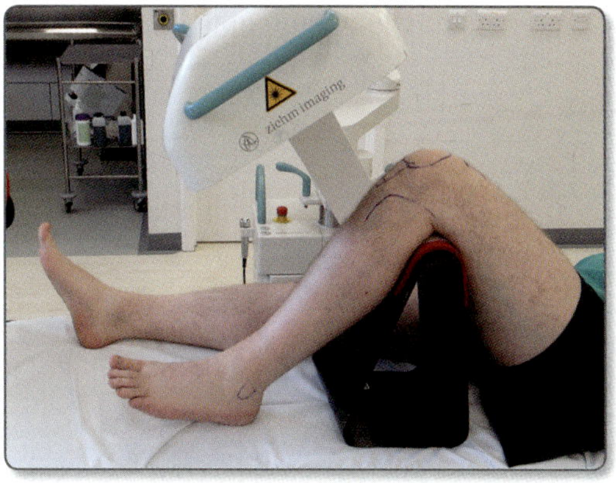

Figure 14.4 Proposed theatre set-up with patient on radiolucent table with knee over bolster. These radiolucent triangles come in varying sizes and can be rotated depending on whether operating on the distal femur (see Figure 22.3a for distal femur set-up) or proximal tibia (tibial plateau set-up shown).

Review of surgical approaches

Lateral distal femur

- Make an incision centered on lateral aspect of distal femur aiming toward tibial tuberosity

(**Figure 14.5a**) and incise the iliotibial band. Pay attention to the geniculate vessels and treat accordingly (**Figure 14.5b**)
- Perform a lateral joint arthrotomy as necessary to deal with inarticular fracture components (**Figure 14.5c**)
- For proximal access elevate vastus lateralis again paying attention to perforators
- Proximal screws can be inserted percutaneously if using a lateral plating system with aiming guide

Medial distal femur

- Make a medial incision in line with the femoral shaft (**Figure 14.6a**). The deep fascia of the thigh is then split in line with the skin incision, paying attention for the saphenous nerve
- Elevate the muscle fibers of vastus medialis anteriorly (**Figure 14.6b**), paying attention to perforating and geniculate vessels
- The distal interval is between vastus medialis anteriorly and adductor magnus posteriorly (**Figure 14.6c**)

Lateral tibial plateau

- Make a lazy-S incision with the horizontal component just at level of lateral meniscus (**Figure 14.7a**), opening the iliotibial tract
- Elevate tibialis anterior muscle off Gerdy's tubercle exposing fracture site
- Undertake a sub-meniscal arthrotomy and insert suture for joint inspection and later meniscal repair (**Figure 14.7b**)
- A varus stress on the knee with retraction of the stay suture gives good access to assess the lateral tibial plateau
- The distal limb of a lateral plate can be slid submuscularly down the anterior compartment for fracture stabilization

Medial tibial plateau

- Make an incision running from the medial epicondyle toward the posteromedial edge of the tibia (**Figure 14.8a**)
- Then, retract the pes anteriorly and the medial head of gastrocnemius posteriorly, giving

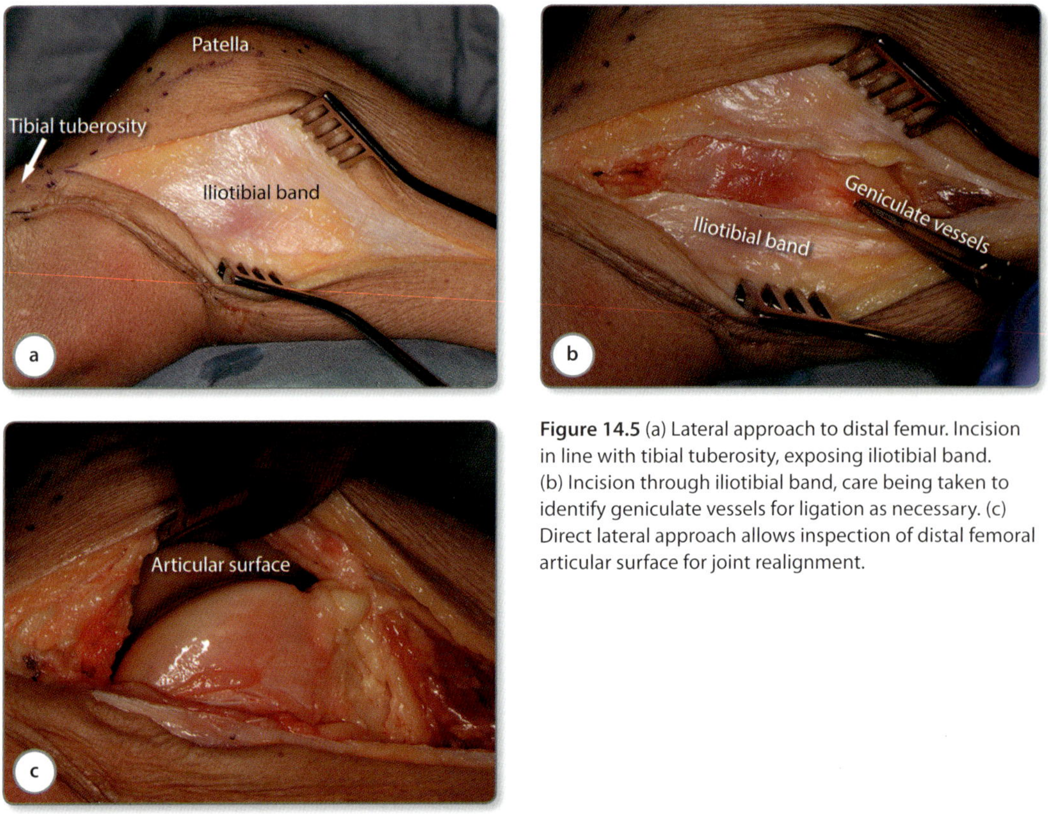

Figure 14.5 (a) Lateral approach to distal femur. Incision in line with tibial tuberosity, exposing iliotibial band. (b) Incision through iliotibial band, care being taken to identify geniculate vessels for ligation as necessary. (c) Direct lateral approach allows inspection of distal femoral articular surface for joint realignment.

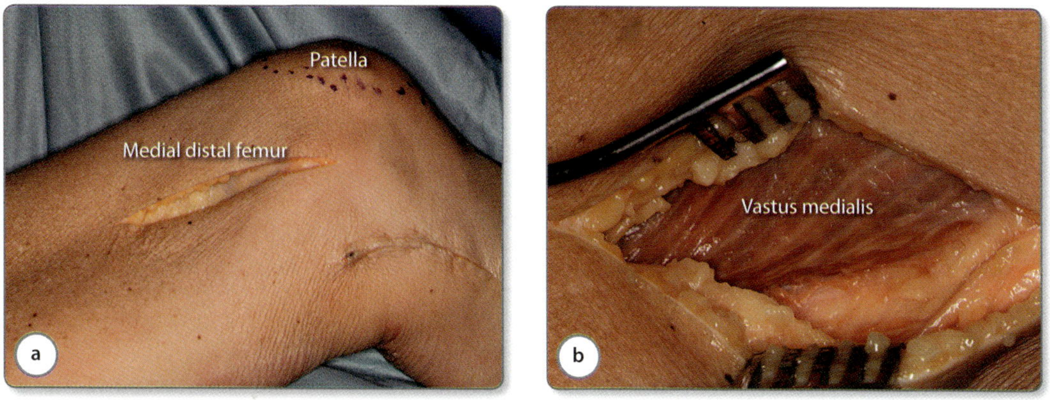

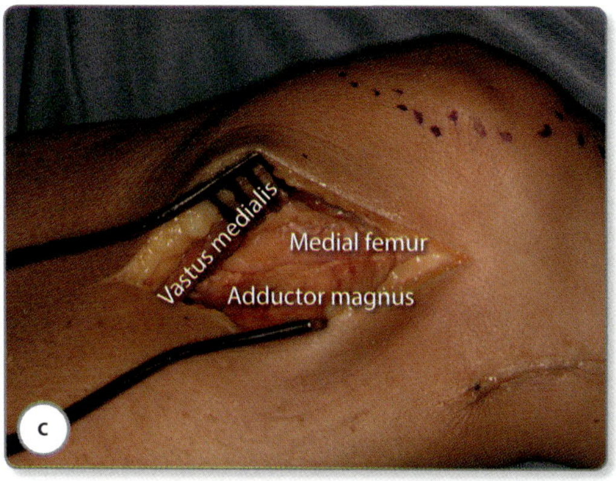

Figure 14.6 (a) Incision parallel to distal femur, equidistant from patella to posterior margin of medial femoral condyle. (b) The deep fascia over vastus medialis is split and the interval between vastus medialis and adductor magnus is identified. The saphenous nerve may be encountered. (c) Access to the medial femur is obtained by elevating vastus medialis anteriorly.

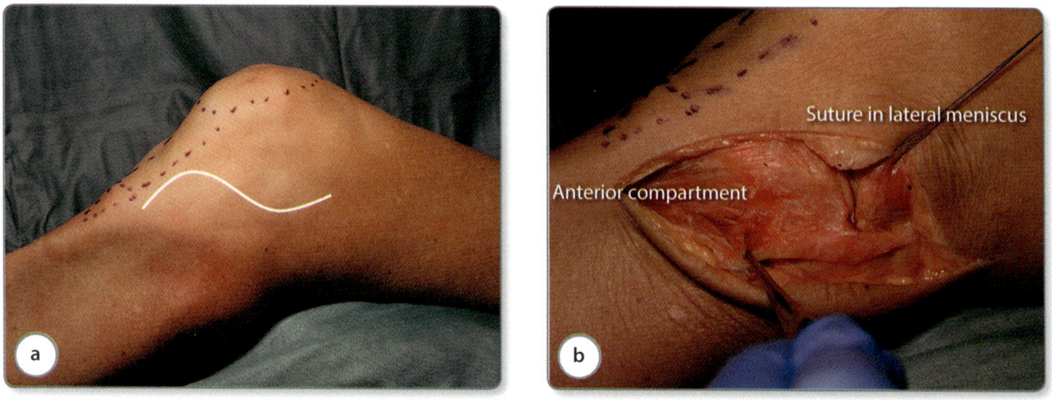

Figure 14.7 (a) Skin incision for lateral tibial plateau approach. (b) Iliotibial band incised and soft tissue elevated off anterior compartment. Stay sutures inserted in lateral meniscus and submeniscal arthrotomy performed in order to visualize lateral tibial plateau.

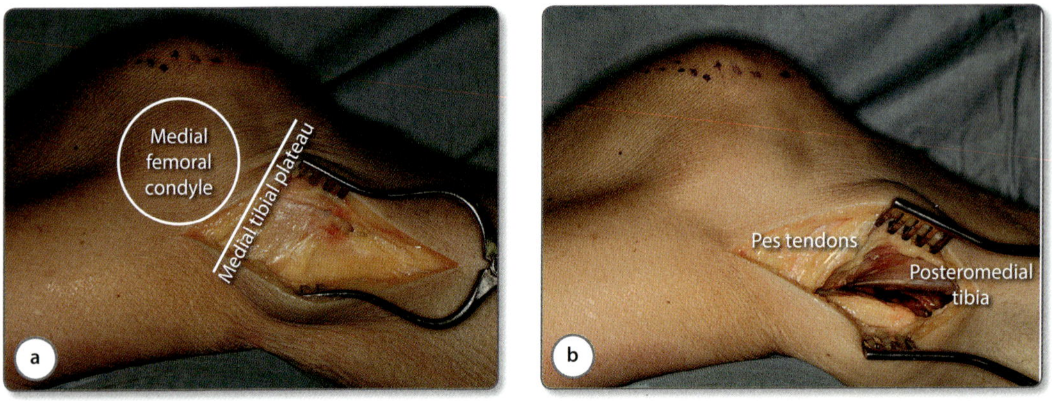

Figure 14.8 (a) Medial proximal tibial incision for application of buttress plate. Outline of tibial plateau and femoral condyle marked. (b) Medial head of gastrocnemius retracted posteriorly and pes retracted anteriorly giving access to the posteromedial proximal tibial surface.

access to the medial proximal tibia (**Figure 14.8b**). This allows application of a medial or posteromedial buttress plate

Posterior knee

- Position the patient prone with protection of pressure areas
- Make a lazy-S incision with horizontal component just at level of posterior skin flexion crease, and limbs suprolaterally and infromedially (**Figure 14.9a**)
- Identify the medial head of gastrocnemius and insert stay sutures and tenotomize (**Figure 14.9b**)
- Place a retractor under the medial head of gastrocnemius, while flexing the knee slightly. This will allow access in order to submuscularly elevate soleus and popliteus off the posterior tibia
- A Hohmann retractor can then be placed across to the lateral side of the tibia, but care being taken not to forceable retract due to the neurovascular structures
- Flexing the knee relieves pressure on the neurovascular structures while retracting. This gives access to posterior proximal tibia (**Figure 14.9c**) allowing the application of a posterior buttress plate

Equipment requirements

- Radiolucent table and positioning aids
- Radiolucent triangles
- External fixator set with appropriately sized Schanz pins
- External fixator removal set
- Battery drill and drill bits for pilot holes
- Periarticular plates/retrograde nails for distal femoral fractures
- Small fragment set
- K-wires
- Threaded K-wires/Schanz pins
- Osteotomes/laminar spreader
- Howarth elevator
- Specific reduction clamps – king tong, circular clamps

Method of external fixator application

- Position the patient safely as above, and confirm X-ray access
- Perform a pre-wash and scrub followed by routine preparation and draping
- Anterior or anterolateral bicortical femoral pilot holes are created with an appropriately sized drill, before 5/6 mm Schanz pins are inserted by hand
- A similar technique is applied to the medial face of the tibia, again positioning the Schanz screws out with the zone of injury
- An appropriately stable frame is then constructed under radiographic control with traction and reduction maneuvers as necessary (**Figure 14.10**)
- Elevate the limb to reduce soft tissue swelling
- Commence pin site and anti-deep vein thrombosis (DVT) care in accordance with unit policy

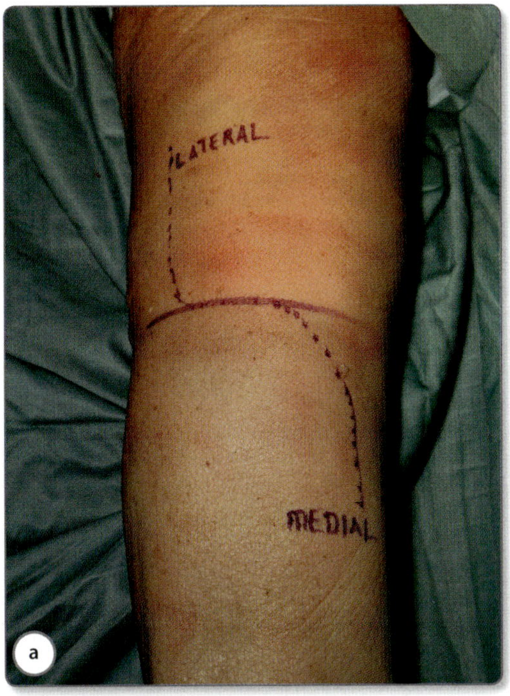

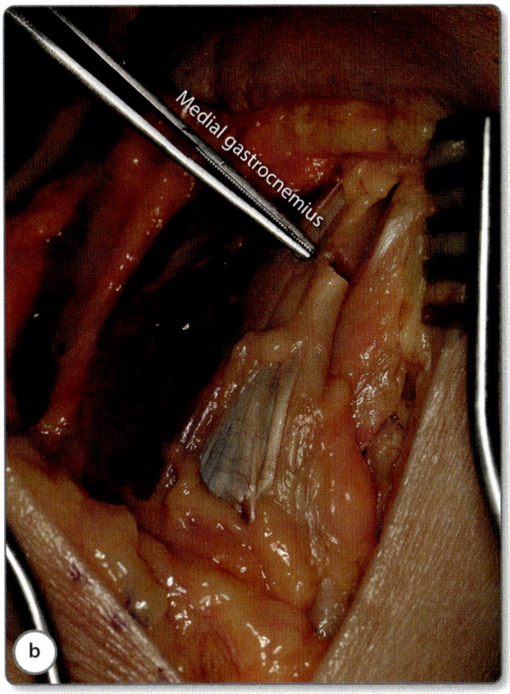

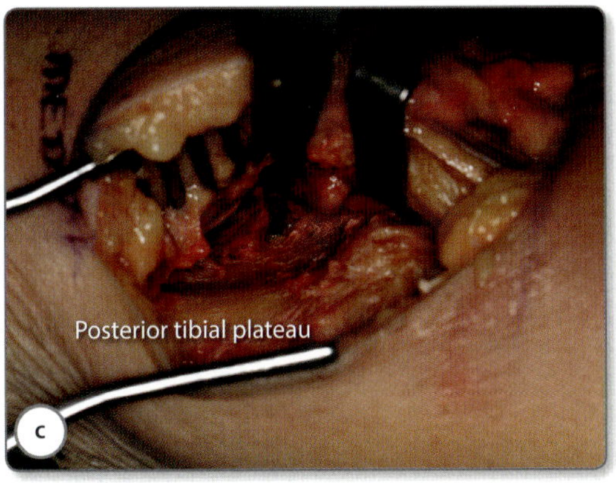

Figure 14.9 (a) Skin incision for posterior approach to tibial plateau. (b) Medial head of gastrocnemius can be tenotomized for easier access and later repaired. (c) Lateral retraction of the medial head of gastrocnemius and sub periosteal elevation of soleus and popliteus gives access to posterior tibial plateau.

- Arrange CT imaging to assess fracture configuration for definitive fracture fixation (**Figure 14.2**). Axial, coronal, sagittal as well as three-dimensional (3D) rendered views need to be carefully assessed for each clinical case

Reduction and stabilization methods

Definitive surgery is planned on a semi-elective basis once the soft tissue envelope is healthy. This can be 2–3 weeks post-index injury in high-energy trauma. Careful review of CT images is essential for operative planning and patient positioning.

Distal femur

Using a triangle with the knee at approximately 20° will facilitate the easy reduction and treatment of the majority of fractures. A detailed and accurate preoperative plan is the most essential part of the strategy and will predict and deal with most of the difficulties likely to be encountered. 3D imaging with fine cut CT scans facilitate this and are particularly useful

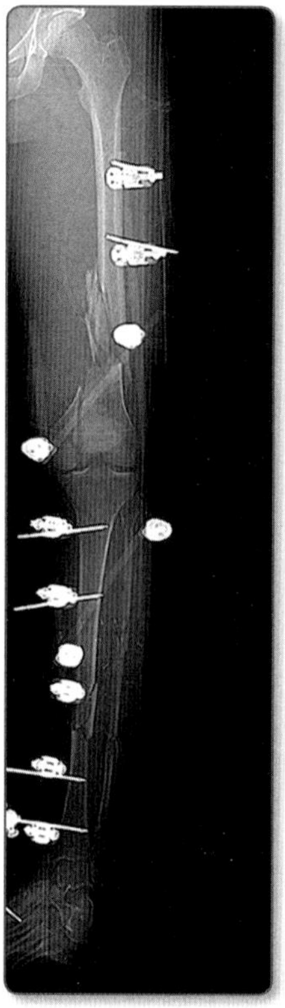

Figure 14.10 Example of multifragmentary lower leg injury with 'floating knee pattern' which has been temporarily stabilized with a spanning external fixator prior to definitive surgery.

in identifying coronal plane fracture lines, often missed in apparently extra-articular distal femoral fractures.

In the extra-articular fractures either a retrograde nail or plate can be used. The nail may require blocking wires/screws to maintain fracture reduction. The plate will allow easier direct/indirect reduction but at the expense of a much larger biological footprint.

With intra-articular fractures, the medial condyle is almost always in the correct position and therefore plan to build back on to this. The lateral incision is recommended for most fractures and by extending to Gerdy's tubercle and opening the joint, an anatomic reduction can be achieved.

Tibial plateau

If a staged approach is to be used then generally the posterior incision and stabilization is carried out first. This is mostly the application of a posterior buttress plate. Care should be taken to use only short screws (10–14 mm) in the metaphysis, as longer screws can interfere with the subsequent anterior approach and fixation. In addition, do not leave the diaphyseal screws proud anteriorly as these will affect subsequent plate positioning and can cause subcutaneous irritation to the patient.

If a dual approach is used then open both at the start and work through both. The advantage of this is that implant position can be readjusted without repositioning the patient. The disadvantage is that access and reduction are more difficult. For simple lateral column injuries, surgical access is through the split in the depressed fragment. If there is significant depression then the use of osteotomes and/or laminar spreaders to recruit and elevate the local (and usually crushed down) metaphyseal bone to form a subarticular layer, is a useful technique. Temporary fixation with K-wires then allows either a separate raft of subarticular screws to be inserted (**Figure 14.11a**) or they can be inserted through the proximal aspect of modern plating systems.

With higher energy injuries, it is important to deal with the medial and posterior column injuries first and build from there. There is usually considerable comminution and the lateral meniscus is often incarcerated in the lateral fragments and needs to be retrieved before addressing the joint surface. There are many circumstances where accurate articular reduction cannot be achieved but it is then essential to restore column height, particularly on the lateral side (**Figure 14.11b**), if salvage procedures are to be undertaken in the future.

Grafting materials

Local or synthetic/commercial products can be utilized at operating surgeon discretion as required, to fill structural voids.

Rehabilitation

- Request physiotherapy review and input when surgical wounds are satisfactory:
  - Range of motion exercises
  - Early appropriate weight bearing as necessary
  - Hinged knee braces as necessary
  - Serial postoperative X-rays to confirm no loss of reduction and progression of union over the following months
  - Supervised progressive follow-up

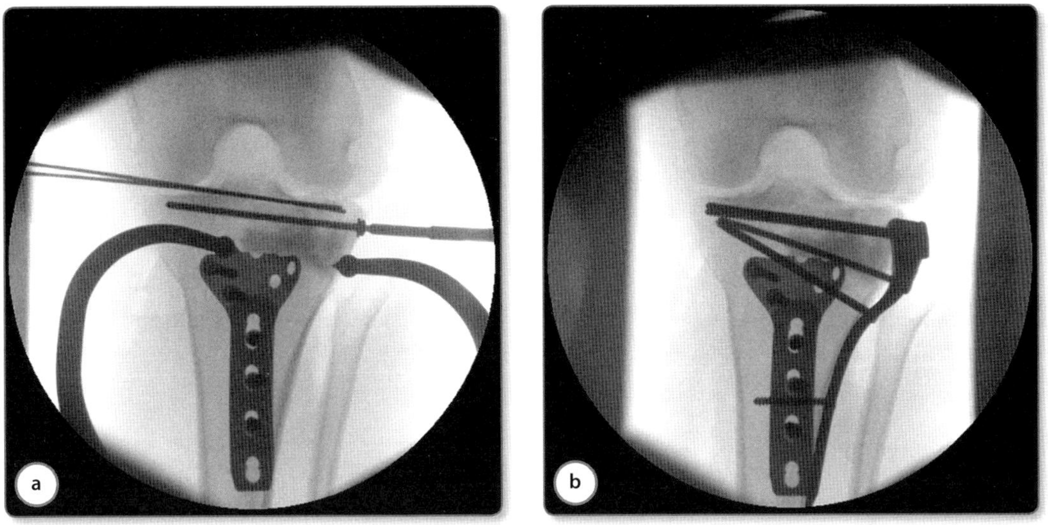

Figure 14.11 (a) Intraoperative image showing position of posterior buttress plate (2-stage procedure: patient positioned prone then supine) followed by elevation of joint line, temporary fixation with lateral to medial K-wires (driven out medially so not to interfere with metal work) followed by insertion of raft of screws. (b) Application of anatomical lateral plate following joint reduction and insertion of separate raft of supporting screws.

Avoiding postoperative complications

Infection/wound healing problems

- Staged protocol for fixation
- Careful soft tissue handling
- Tension-free wound closure
- Avoidance of hematoma formation
- Maintaining a well hydrated/warm patient
- Elevate limb to reduce soft tissue swelling
- Prescribe postoperative antibiotics and anti-DVT treatment in accordance with unit policy

Loss of reduction

- Thorough review of CT scans with accurate surgical planning and knowledge of specific surgical approaches
- Stable fixation of fracture specific components and grafting as necessary
- Protected weight-bearing with patient compliance +/– knee bracing

Post-traumatic degenerative change

- Often determined at time of original injury, but can be reduced by accurate joint reduction, stable fixation and early active joint motion

Salvage options

The overall percentage of conversion to total knee replacement following actively managed tibial plateau fractures is approximately 5–7%. This is a 3% increased risk over the noninjured population. The incidence for distal femoral fractures is very small because most of these occur in the elderly and other co-morbidities and patient tolerance often predicate against further surgical intervention. Increasingly for the severe distal femoral fractures in the elderly endoprosthetic replacement is being used in preference to fixation as a primary surgical option, allowing early unrestricted mobility.

Summary of learning points

- Have a strategy dependent on level of energy and patient phenotype
- Familiarity with approaches and complete gamut of approaches, following careful CT evaluation: may require multiple surgical approaches in same or separate sittings
- Familiarity with implants
- Attention to soft tissues: may require application of a spanning external fixator to allow soft tissues to settle
- Patient – specific rehabilitation regimens

Further reading

Arastu MH, Kokke MC, Duffy PJ, Korley RE, Buckley RE. Coronal plane partial articular fractures of the distal femoral condyle: current concepts in management. Bone Joint J 2013; 95:1165–1171.

Henderson CE, Lujan TJ, Kuhl LL, et al. 2010 mid-America Orthopaedic Association Physician in Training Award: healing complications are common after locked plating for distal femur fractures. Clin Orthop Relat Res 2011; 469:1757–1765.

Luo CF, Sun H, Zhang B, Zeng BF. Three-column fixation for complex tibial plateau fractures. J Orthop Trauma 2010; 24:683–692.

Nork SE, Segina DN, Aflatoon K, et al. The association between supracondylar-intercondylar distal femoral fractures and coronal plane fractures. J Bone Joint Surg Am 2005; 87:564–569.

Wähnert D, Hoffmeier K, Fröber R, Hofmann GO, Mückley T. Distal femur fractures of the elderly – different treatment options in a biomechanical comparison. Injury 2011; 42:655–659.

15 Periprosthetic fractures of the hip: pelvis and femur

James Holland, Clive Duncan

Introduction

Fractures around hip implants are a challenging problem bridging the increasing speciality divide between trauma and elective hip arthroplasty and, therefore, demand a team approach and careful multidisciplinary planning for a successful outcome. The United Kingdom National Joint Registry has reported a year on year increase in the number of primary hip replacements carried out from 69,000 in 2007 to 76,000 in 2013. The median age for hip replacement is 70 years and, thus one of the main challenges in periprosthetic fracture surgery is to restore a secure, stable reconstruction in deteriorating quantity and quality of bonestock, often in elderly patients.

Incidence

Periprosthetic fractures are the reported indication for surgery in 10% of the 8,000 hip replacement revisions performed every year in England and Wales, and are the fourth most common reason for revision after aseptic loosening, lysis, or unexplained pain and dislocation.

Mechanism of injury

As would be expected from the median age at total hip replacement (THR) and increasing life-expectancy, periprosthetic fractures are usually sustained after simple falls, but are occasionally the result of direct trauma. Risk factors for a fall are addressed, as with neck of femur fracture, but additional factors may predispose to periprosthetic fracture and compromise surgical management.

- Bone quality as influenced by:
  - Age
  - Steroid use
  - Rheumatoid arthritis
  - Stress-shielding and local osteolysis around well-fixed implants
- Biomechanics:
  - Varus THR stem
  - Stiff knee
- General conditions:
  - Poor balance, ataxia
  - Neuromuscular conditions; cerebrovascular accident, poliomyelitis, Parkinson's disease
- Implant:
  - Malalignment
  - Loosening

Initial management/ prioritization

Periprosthetic fractures require a multidisciplinary approach from initial admission onwards by the acute trauma team, the involvement (where appropriate) of elderly care specialists and the interaction of trauma surgeons and revision hip surgeons.

Management can be distilled down into treatment of:

- The patient
- The fracture
- The pre-existing implant

The patient

Treatment of the patient requires the usual rapid assessment and optimization of limb support, pain control, oxygenation and resuscitation. Early admission and anesthetic, together with geriatric/ elderly care assessment is ideal, followed by the establishment of a surgical plan based on the patient's fitness for surgery. There is no evidence that delays to optimize a patient's medical status compromise the final outcome.

Early communication between the trauma team and revision hip specialist is vital. Knowledge of the patient's history regarding the hip replacement is invaluable. Details of the prosthesis, and any recent follow-up clinical information, together with radiology, will help to classify the fracture and aid management. Pre-existing pain may indicate loosening or infection prior to fracture.

In general, treatment goals are:

- Pain relief, fracture healing
- A stable implant
- Preservation of bone and leg length
- Restoration of early mobilization and return to normal function

The fracture

Traditionally, these fractures have been classified according to the Vancouver system, which then provides a guide as to best management (**Table 15.1**; **Figure 15.1**). The reliability and validity of this approach has been established in separate studies from both Europe and North America. The system was developed with reference to the femur alone.

More recently, this has been superseded by the Unified Classification System (UCS). The purpose of the UCS is fourfold:

1. To unify the classification systems already in use relating to a number of joints
2. To include three types not previously included (D, E and F as outlined below)
3. To apply it to all periprosthetic fractures regardless of the bone broken and joint involved
4. To use a simple and common language in achieving those goals

Therefore, following hip replacement, it applies to the femur and pelvis.

To assist with its understanding and recall, the following UCS mnemonic has been proposed:

Type A: Apophyseal (greater and lesser trochanters, anterior inferior and superior spines, or ischium)

Type B: Bed of the implant or very close to it; stem or cup (therefore femoral shaft or acetabulum)

Type C: Clear of the implant (the remainder of the femur, or the ilium, superior and inferior rami)

Type D: Dividing one bone which supports two implants (fracture femur after hip and knee

Table 15.1 Vancouver classification

Type	Incidence	Level of fracture	Subtype
A	4%	Trochanteric	A (G): Greater trochanter A (L): Lesser trochanter
B	87%	Around stem	B (1): Prosthesis stable (18%) B (2): Prosthesis unstable (45%) B (3): Bone inadequate (37%)
C	9%	Distal to stem	No subtype

From Duncan CP, et al: Instr Course Lect 1995; 44:293–304.

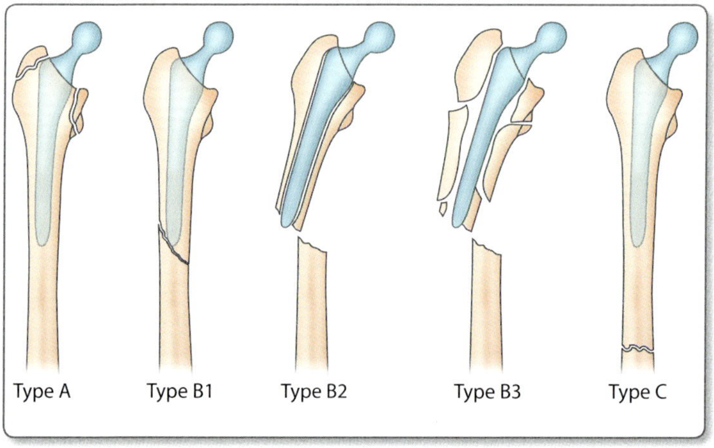

Figure 15.1 Vancouver classification.

replacement, or fracture pelvis after bilateral hip replacement

Type E: Each of two bones supporting one replacement (therefore both the femur and pelvis)

Type F: Facing or articulating with an implant (such as the acetabulum after hemiarthroplasty)

As with the Vancouver system, type B is subdivided into B1 (implant is well fixed), B2 (implant is loose), and B3 (implant is loose and bone support is poor). Again, after hip replacement, this subdivision applies to the stem and to the socket.

Pre-existing implant

Previous history of the implant is helpful. Pre-existing pain may suggest a loose prosthesis. History of infection will affect treatment. Previous radiographs will again highlight any previous problem or confirm a well-fixed device. Any incipient problem short of obvious loosening (e.g. lucent lines, focal osteolysis, polyethylene wear) that may influence revision over fracture fixation should be noted.

If femoral revision is to be considered, the acetabular component should be inspected to ensure that it is not worn, is securely fixed and of an appropriate head size and material compatible with the revision planned. Elective socket revision is often considered to allow the use of a large head size (36–40 mm) to reduce the risk of postoperative dislocation.

Knowledge regarding the characteristics of device in situ will aid extraction planning for revision. Cemented implant extraction is markedly aided by ultrasound cement removal tools (OSCAR: Orthosonics, Maidenhead, UK), high-speed burrs and traditional tools in the revision hip armamentarium. Cementless devices have differing fixation patterns and all have appropriate extraction tools supplied with forward plannning.

For either fixation or revision, it is important to establish the presence or absence of prostheses in the knee which may affect reconstruction (interprosthetic fracture).

Principles of treatment

The principles of treatment are based on the UCS classification type.

Type A (apophyseal)

Two questions need to be asked. Firstly, is the soft tissue attached to this apophysis important to the function of the arthroplasty? Secondly, if yes, is the fracture displaced? This divides the fractures into those that can be observed, and those that require intervention:

Observed: anterior superior iliac spine, anterior inferior spine, ischium, lesser trochanter, and some undisplaced greater trochanters.

Not usually observed: acutely displaced greater trochanter. Some judgement is required here, as nonacute trochanteric fractures with a small fracture fragment seldom improve with fixation alone.

Type B (bed of the stem or cup)

Again, two questions need to be asked. Is the implant stable (B1)? If not (B2), is there adequate bone to support a straightforward revision (B3 if not)?

The broad principles of management can be summarized as follows:

B1 femur: reduction and fixation, ideally with minimally invasive osteosynthesis (MIPO).

B1 acetabulum (usually an intraoperative event): add screws if recognized during operation (not needed if cemented cup): touch weight-bearing and crutches if recognized postoperatively.

B2 femur: revision and fracture fixation with a longer stem.

B2 acetabulum: fracture fixation and cup revision.

B3 femur: complex reconstruction and revision, sometimes requiring segmental replacement.

B3 acetabulum: commonly associated with pelvic discontinuity: complex reconstruction.

Type C (well clear of the implant)

C femur: reduction and fixation, with MIPO if feasible.

C pelvis: standard treatment of fracture pelvis.

Type D (dividing one bone which supports two implants)

D femur (dividing the femur between a hip and knee replacement): need to use the exercise of 'block out analysis.' In other words, if you block out the knee replacement, what fracture is this for the hip? It will be a type B or C. Next, block out the hip and ask what type is this for the knee? Again it will be a type B or C. A rational treatment plan will follow, requiring revision of one, both or neither of the arthroplasties.

D pelvis (dividing the pelvis between a bilateral hip replacement): again use block out analysis and ask if the fracture to the pelvis involves either hip replacement (socket), and if yes, is it a B1, B2, or B3? Usually, it involves neither socket.

Type E (each of two bones supporting one replacement)

E femur (pelvis and femur): block out analysis is again useful. If you block out the pelvis, what type of fracture is this for the femur? It can be an A, B or C. A rational treatment plan follows. Next block out the femur and ask the same question of the pelvis. Usually it will be a B2 or B3. Again a treatment plan follows.

E pelvis (both femur and pelvis): apply the same principles as above.

Type F (facing or articulating with an implant)

F femur (facing or articulating with an arthroplasty): the type F fracture cannot affect the femur.

F pelvis: the acetabulum can fracture following hemiarthroplasty for a fracture neck of femur. The principles of management depend on the degree of fracture displacement; observe and mobilize with protected weight-bearing if slight; consider intervention if substantial and if the health of the elderly patient justifies such an approach.

Specifics of treatment

Type A: fractures of greater trochanter

- Stable/undisplaced – conservative therapy
- Unstable/displaced > 5 mm – open reduction internal fixation (ORIF) with cable-plate system
- Any local osteolysis – consider THR revision

Failure to treat displaced fractures leads to a painful, weak Trendelenburg gait. Complications of surgery include nonunion which occurs with plate systems of 11%, but this is worse with cerclage wire (20–30%).

Type B1: fracture around stem with stable implant

Treatment is stable fixation of the fracture, leaving stem in situ.

Requirements

- Good quality AP and lateral views of the whole femur and hip
- Previous X-rays
- Arthroplasty opinion
- Diagnosis of a stable stem is imperative – failure of surgery is often due to undiagnosed B2 fracture (i.e. a loose prosthesis), or a poorly performed hip replacement
- Correct alignment of prosthesis and femur with no bone loss is needed. Varus stem alignment > 6° of stem is a contraindication for internal fixation
- Stable fracture fixation is required. Any comminution or bone loss due to osteoporosis will severely affect fracture healing as endosteal bone viability is already compromised
- Poor outcome is expected using fixation with screws or wires or a single conventional plate alone

Recommended technique

- Double plating with proximal screws and/or cerclage cables. Contoured plates should be applied at 90° to each other – lateral and anterior. At least four screws proximally and distally are required
- Single plate with strut graft. Attention must be paid to obtain an appropriately-sized and contoured strut graft. For effective fixation and incorporation, the graft must be burred and contoured for maximum bone-to-bone surface contact
- Standard femoral plates are usually inadequate for modern fixation. Large plates with cabling facilities (e.g. Dall-Miles; Stryker) are better. More advanced locking plates with polyaxial screw capabilities to avoid cement or implant are now available and may obviate the need for double plating, but they are still being evaluated

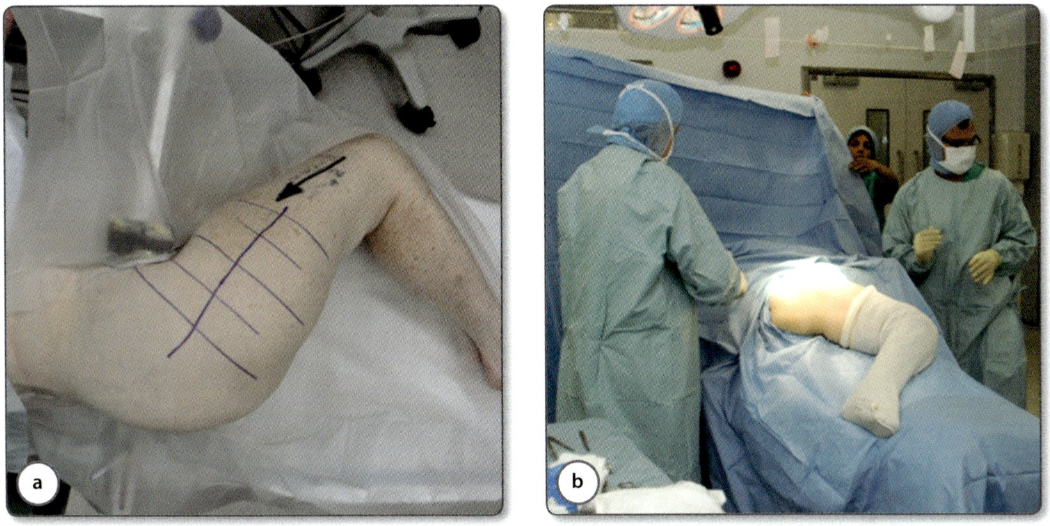

Figure 15.2 (a, b) Patient in the lateral position for fixation.

Theater layout and patient positioning

- Lateral position and lateral approach (**Figure 15.2**) to give access to anterior, lateral and posterior aspects of the femur
- Access remains for extended posterolateral approach and revision if necessary

Type B2: fracture around stem with unstable implant

Surgical treatment is the combined revision of the loose prosthesis with bypass of the fracture with intramedullary fixation (i.e. a long THR stem).

- The prosthesis of choice is a distal fixation device with modular taper fluted uncemented design; the modular body section adjusts for leg length, offset and anteversion
- Long-stem cemented devices are usually avoided due to the difficulties of cement extravasation through the fracture site, risking nonunions and loss of pressurization
- Consider the acetabulum and dislocation risk – this may also need revision if worn or loose. Cup revision will allow a full choice of bearing size and material options

Theater layout and patient positioning

Femoral revision surgery is not the remit of this chapter, but there are two basic approaches. Each utilizes the lateral patient position, with supports and padding suitable for up to 4 hours of surgery. Appropriate THR extraction equipment should be on-hand [e.g. cement removing set, ultrasound cement removal (OSCAR), uncemented component removal tools and full reconstruction capability].

Endosteal approach

The endosteal approach can be used when the bone quality is good, the fracture can be well-reduced and there is a straight femur (no proximal femoral remodelling). It is less traumatic than extended osteotomy, with less bleeding and a quicker recovery. This approach also allows for a cement-in-cement revision stem (but this is not favored by the author). The fracture is exposed through an extended posterior approach and can then be reduced and held with a plate and cables. The THR stem can then be dislocated and revised from above.

Transfemoral approach

The transfemoral approach is more commonly used as this has the dual advantage of speed of extraction and accuracy in revision stem placement. It is also the approach of choice for comminuted fractures in poor quality bone, which unfortunately are more common. The fracture is approached via an extended posterior approach (**Figure 15.9a**) which is then opened retaining as much soft tissue attachment as possible then used and adapted as a modified extended trochanteric osteotomy

Case example: B1 transverse fracture

A 65-year-old woman, 5 years after primary THR after a mechanical fall. X-rays show a well-fixed cemented THR (**Figure 15.3a**). Classification – Vancouver B1 transverse fracture at tip of well-fixed stem. Surgical treatment was with accurate reduction and an anterolateral plate with a posterolateral strut graft (**Figure 15.3b**). At 6 months, union of the fracture and full graft incorporation is seen **Figure 15.3c**)

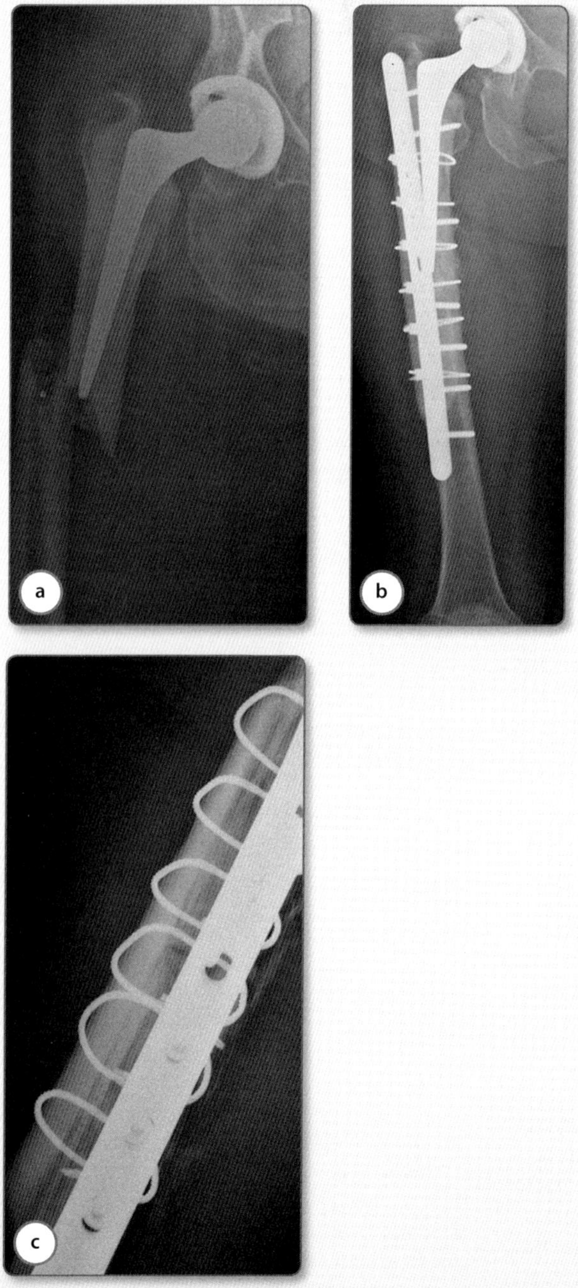

Figure 15.3 (a) A well-fixed cemented THR. (b) Surgical treatment with accurate reduction and anterolateral plate with posterolateral strut graft. (c) At 6 months, union of the fracture and full graft incorporation is seen.

Case example: B1 fracture

A 75-year-old woman suffered a B1 fracture around the tip of a well-fixed 20-year-old Charnley stem (**Figure 15.4a**). Long locking plate fixation was employed (**Figure 15.4b–d**).

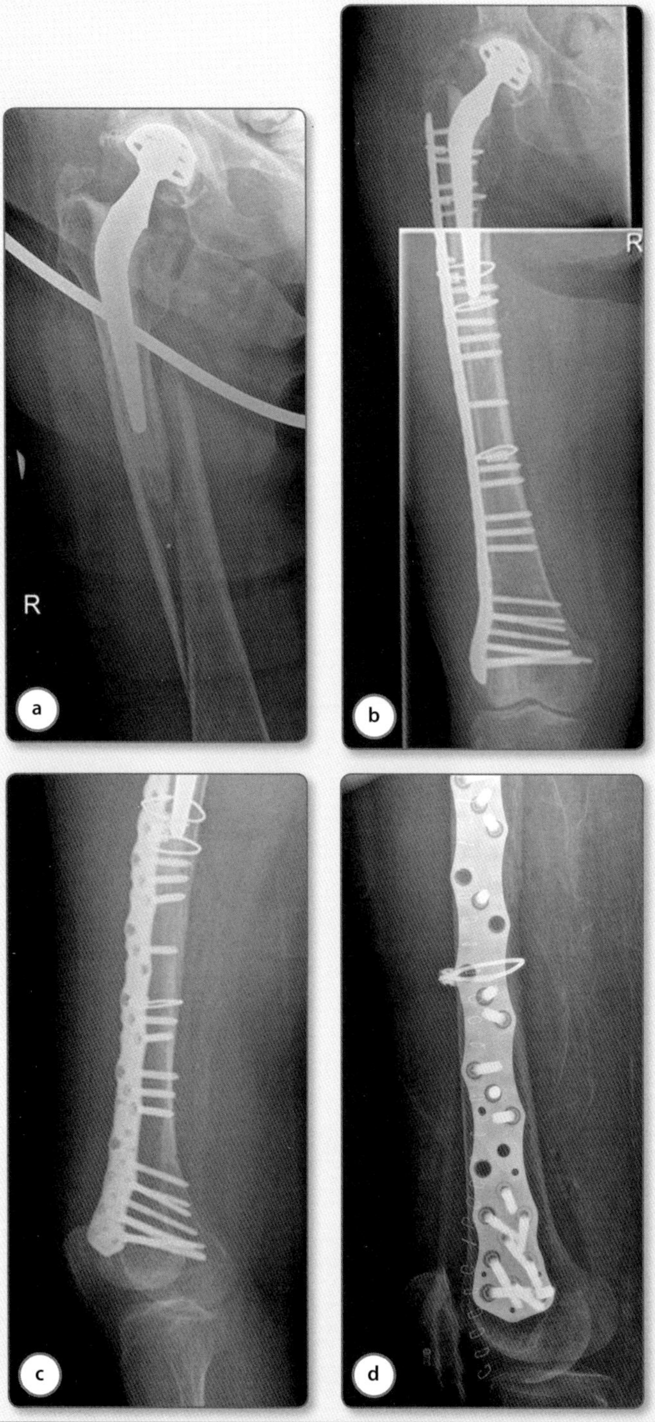

Figure 15.4 (a) B1 fracture around tip of well-fixed 20-year-old Charnley stem. (b–d) Long locking plate fixation.

Case example: B1 fracture fixation failures and salvage

Correct diagnosis and treatment plan for B1 fracture (**Figure 15.5a**) was implemented, but poorly performed. There is poor fracture reduction and inadequate proximal fixation (**Figure 15.5b, c**). Displacement occurred requiring full revision (**Figure 15.5d**).

Failed double-plate fixation of B1 fracture due to poor bone healing (**Figure 15.6a**). Extremely poor proximal femoral bone after component removal resulted in a B3 situation and required an uncemented bypass stem and supplementary strut graft to augment proximal femoral bone stock (**Figure 15.6 b, c**).

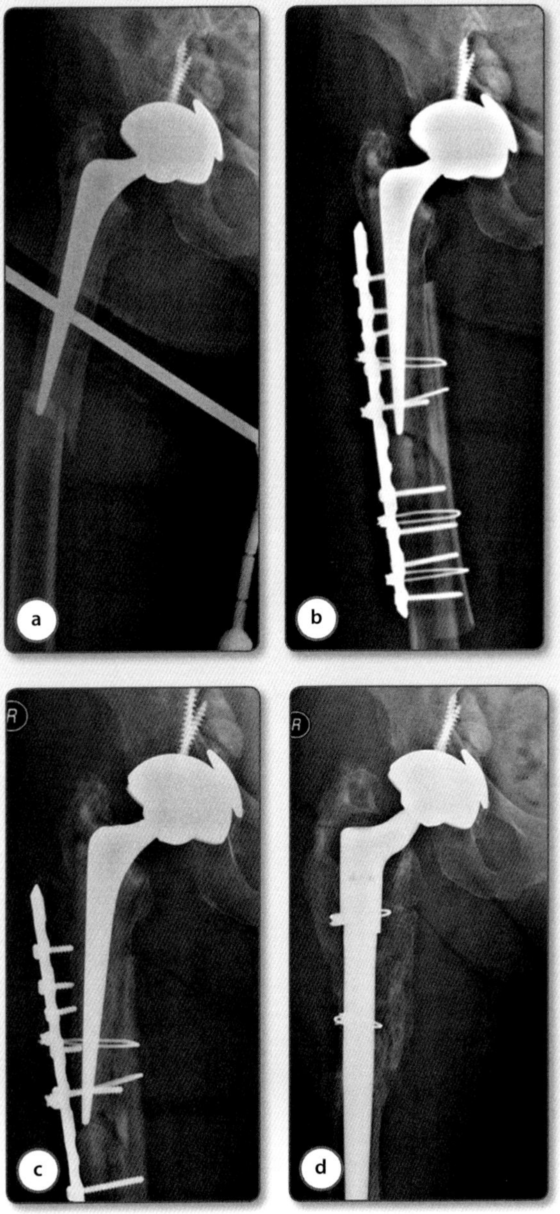

Figure 15.5 (a) Correct diagnosis and treatment plan for B1 fracture. (b, c) There is poor fracture reduction and inadequate proximal fixation. (d) Displacement occurred, requiring full revision.

Case example: *continued.*

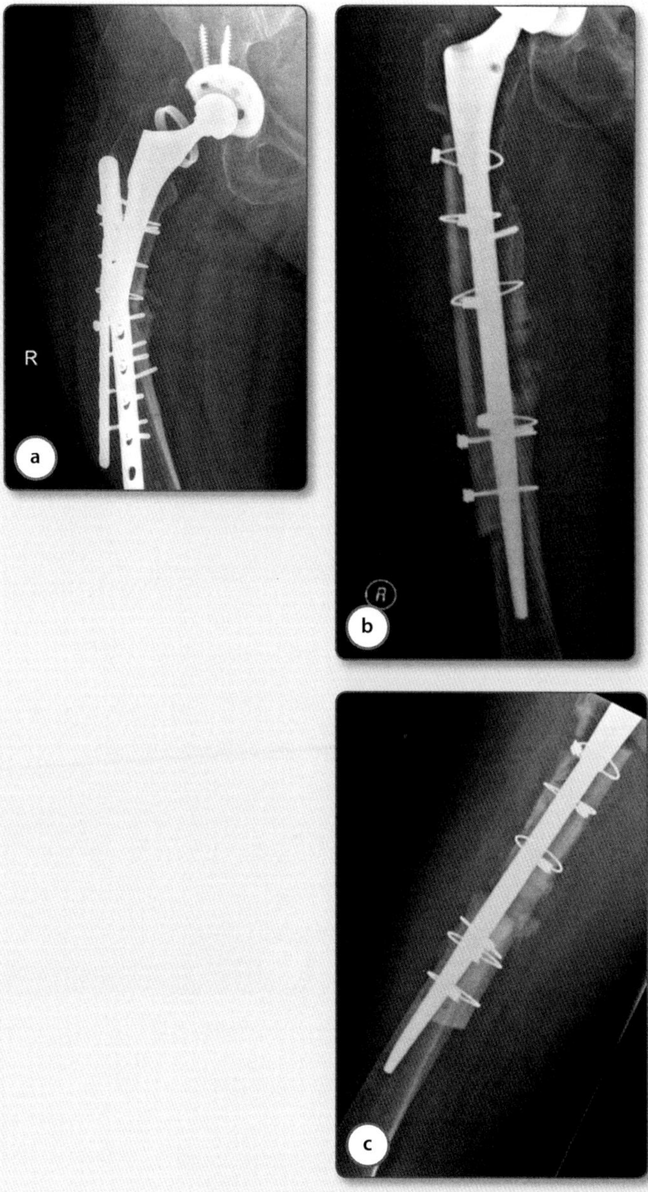

Figure 15.6 (a) Failed double plate fixation of B1 fracture due to poor bone healing. (b, c) Revision surgery requiring uncemented bypass stem and supplementary strut graft to augment proximal femoral bonestock.

Case example: Clinical B2 case (endosteal approach)

A 62-year-old woman presented with a B2 fracture below femoral stem (**Figure 15.7a**). Although the stem was not technically loose, there were lucent lines seen on recent X-rays (**Figure 15.7b**) and it was therefore likely to be unstable and fail in the near future. Surgical treatment was to reduce the fracture and hold it in place with a plate and cables, thus allowing dislocation and revision from above in the usual way (**Figure 15.7c**).

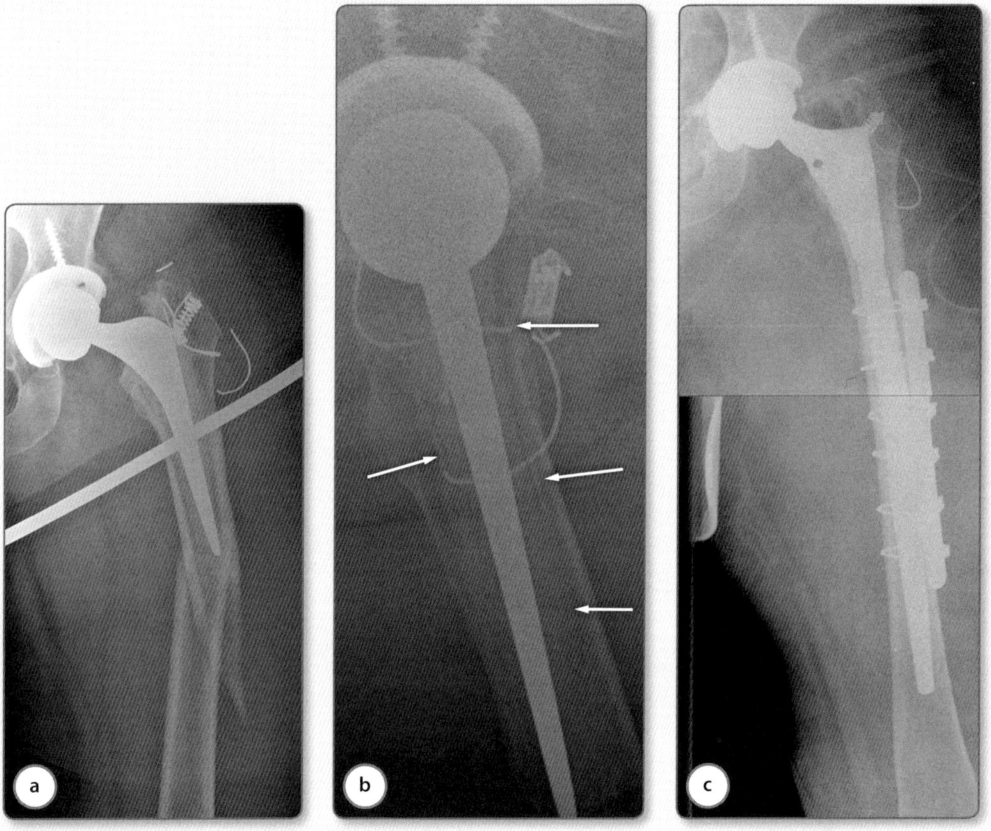

Figure 15.7 (a) B2 fracture below femoral stem. (b) Lucent lines (marked with arrows) seen on recent X-rays, indicating high risk of future failure. (c) Plate and cables system applied to allow dislocation followed by revision long stem bypass procedure.

Case example: Clinical B2 case (transfemoral approach)

A 54-year-old man with a previous large head-metal-on metal THR suffered a traumatic fall down stairs (**Figure 15.8 a–c**). Revision was via a modified ETO. The cup and bearing were revised due to a poor prognosis of the bearing surfaces (**Figure 15.8d**).

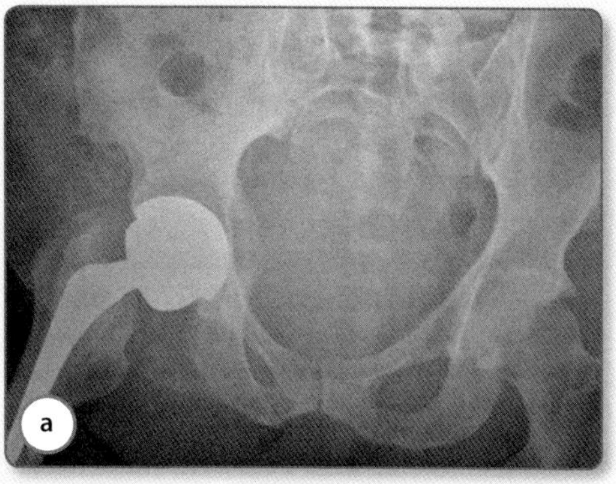

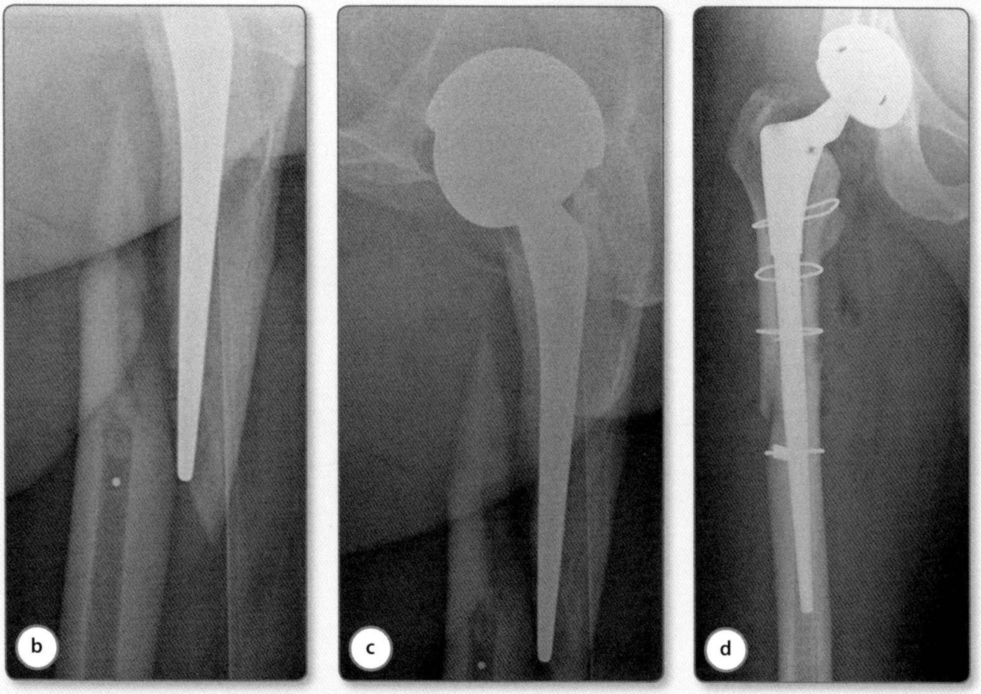

Figure 15.8 (a–c) B2 fracture of large metal-on-metal head components. (d) Revision via transfemoral osteotomy and long stem bypass.

(ETO). The prosthesis can then be rapidly removed, together with the cement (**Figure 15.9b**). One 'prophylactic' safety cable at the zone of fixation at the opening of the distal femur is recommended in case of occult fracture extension. Direct distal reaming can then allow accurate distal stem insertion, followed by modular body trials and definitive reconstruction (**Figure 15.9c**). The proximal femoral bone is then restored around a proximal implant, ideally with only two cables for maximum vascularity (**Figure 15.9d**). Comminution of trochanteric bone may necessitate the use of a cable-plate system to prevent trochanteric escape.

Type B3: fracture around stem with un-stable implant and inadequate bone

Similar to B2, but distal fixation is much more tenuous due to poor bone stock (Paprosky grade 3–4). An additional strut graft augmentation may be needed to restore proximal bone above the fracture. Additional distal fixation may also be needed as a conventional modular taper fluted stem may not be sufficient. Cemented or distal locking prostheses, endoprostheses are preferred.

Type C: fracture distal to prosthesis (similar to B1)

Options

- Locking plate fixation +/– strut graft for added biological stability and long-term bone supplementation
- Specialist plates with polyaxial locking options and cable systems
- Combinations of both of the above

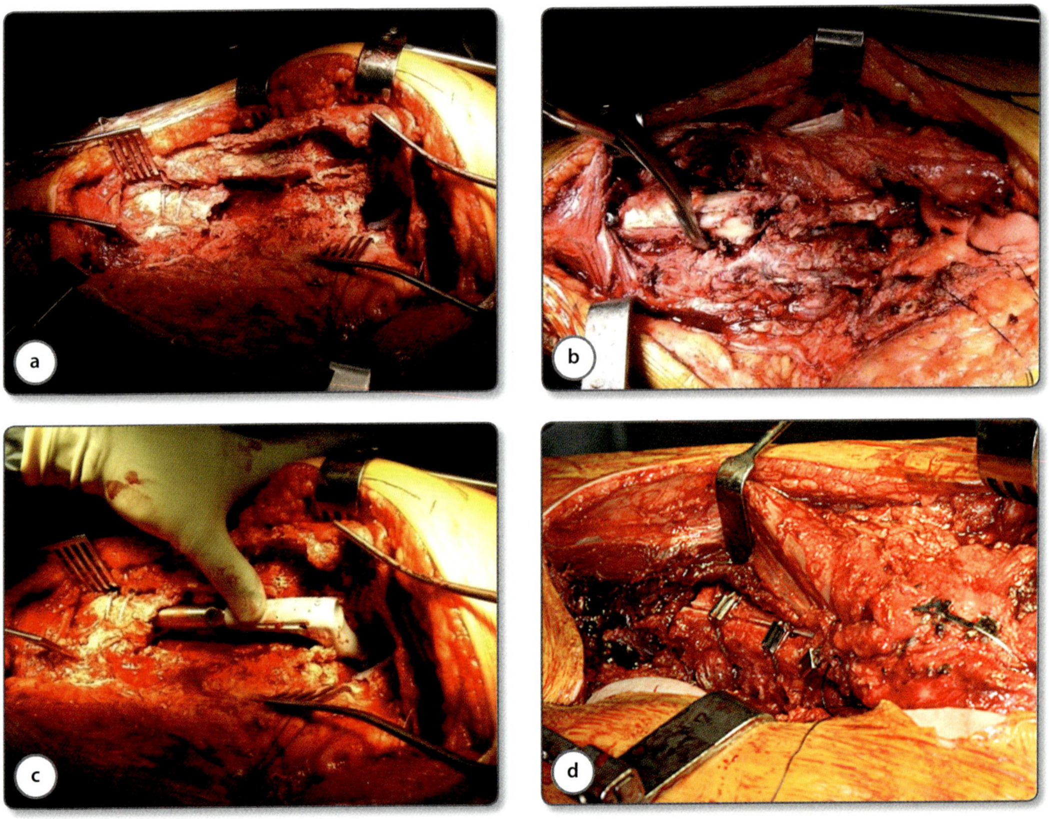

Figure 15.9 (a) Proximal osteotomy through fracture site. (b) Access for direct cement removal. (c) Insertion of prosthesis through osteotomy site. (d) Repair of osteotomy site using cables.

Summary of learning points

- Periprosthetic fractures present a multidisciplinary challenge requiring careful planning to obtain the most appropriate treatment for:
  - The patient
  - The fracture
  - The existing implant
- Classification systems can provide guidelines, but each case needs to be carefully assessed. Patients are often elderly with poor biology which must be optimized for what may be lengthy and physiologically compromising surgery
- An early specialist arthroplasty opinion is ideal. If the patient's surgery must be delayed for the most appropriate and best intervention in the most appropriate environment, there is no evidence to suggest that this is in any way detrimental

Case example: B3 type fracture

An 85-year-old man fell at home resulting in a B3 type fracture at the tip of a loose Charnley stem with poor bone (**Figure 15.10a**). Preoperative planning and templating with modular taper fluted stem was undertaken (**Figure 15.10b**). The previous stem was removed via a modified ETO, with cables to protect the distal femur while the stem is inserted. The rest of the stem is constructed and the proximal femur closed over (**Figure 15.10c**). In this case, the cup was electively revised to allow a larger head to reduce the risk of dislocation. Leaving the cup would have mandated a 22 mm head size.

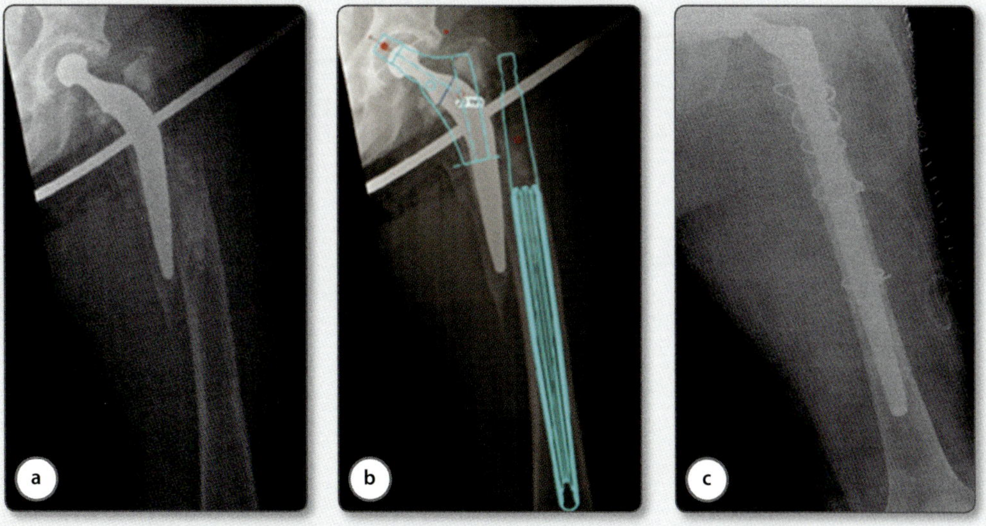

Figure 15.10 (a) B3 type fracture at tip of loose Charnley stem with poor bone quality. (b) Preoperative planning and template with modular taper fluted stem. (c) Stem removed via modified extended trochanteric osteotomy, cables were utilized to protect the distal femur while the stem was inserted before the rest of the stem is constructed and the proximal femur closed over the implant.

Case example: B3 type fracture

A 90-year-old woman fell onto an uncemented hemiarthroplasty (**Figure 15.11a**) resulting in a B3 fracture – Paprosky grade 4 femur – distal locking prosthesis (**Figure 15.11b**).

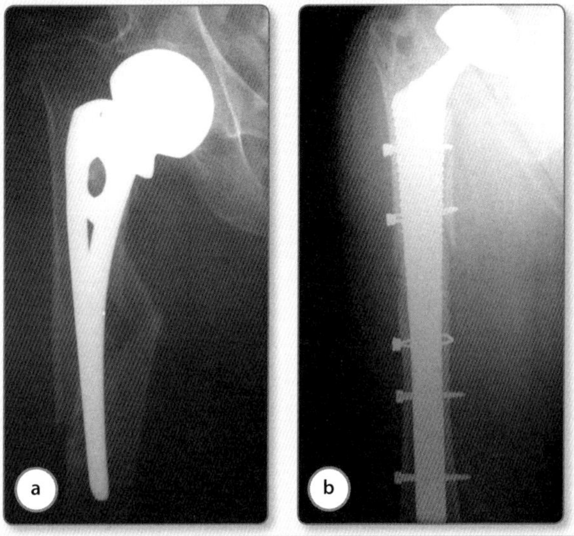

Figure 15.11 (a) B3 fracture around uncemented hemiarthroplasty. (b) Revision surgery with distal locking prosthesis, and bipolar cup.

Case example: B3 type fracture

A 58-year-old juvenile rheumatoid patient with three previous THRs suffered a fracture at the tip of unstable long-stem cemented THR (**Figure 15.12 a, b**). Grade 4 femur: a distal locking device was required (**Figure 15.12c**).

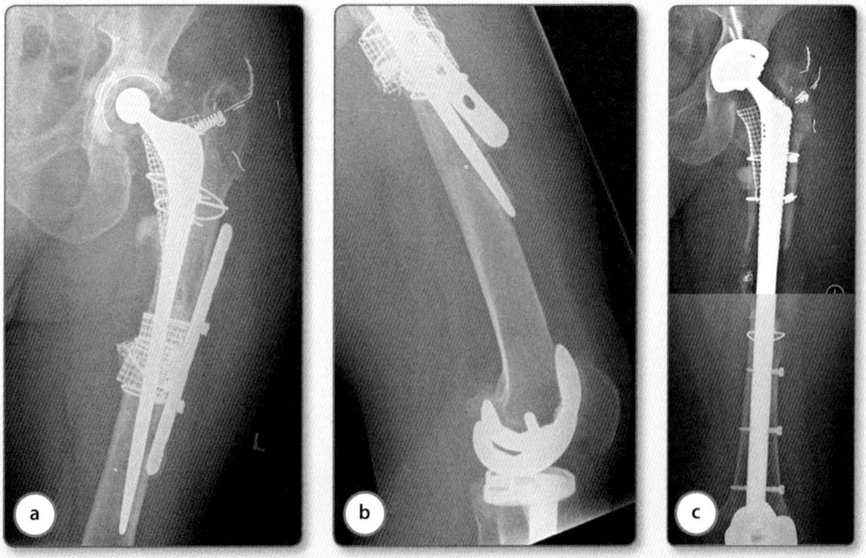

Figure 15.12 (a, b) X-rays of B3 case example with fracture at the tip of unstable long-stem cemented THR. (c) Distal locking device required.

Case example: B3 type fracture

A 79-year-old woman after femoral 'explosion' type B3 typical of polished taper stems. The resulted in a 'log-splitter' effect with direct trauma. She was stable prior to the fall (**Figure 15.13a**), B3 after impact (**Figure 15.13b**), with revision to both the femur and bipolar acetabular component (**Figure 15.13c**).

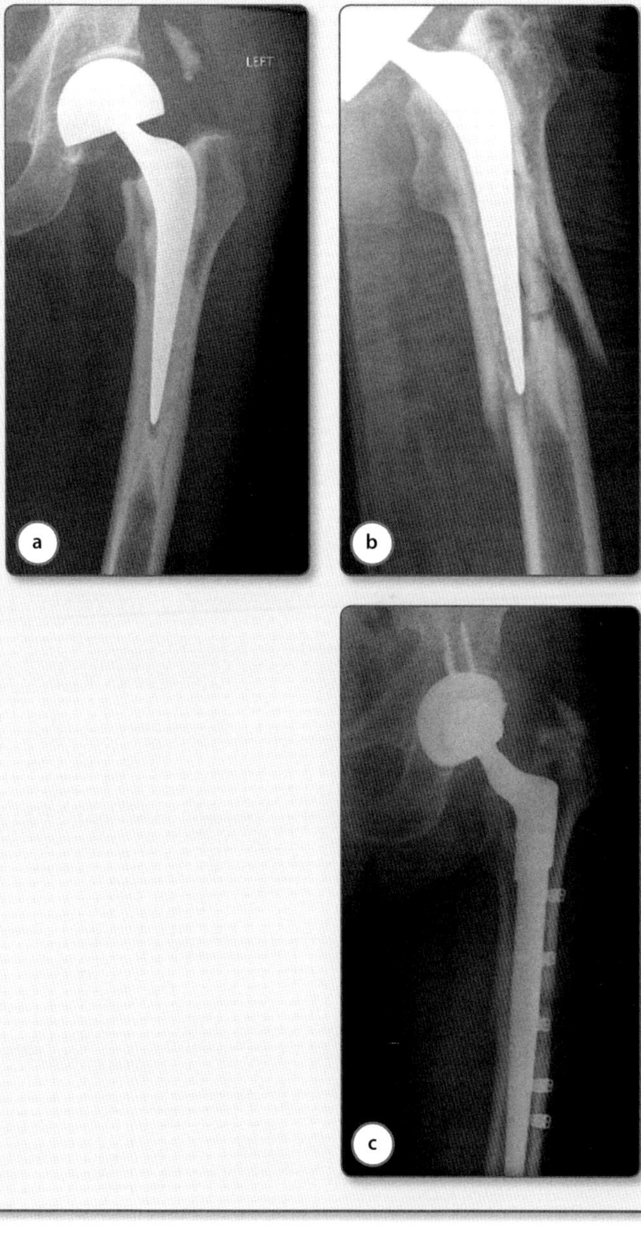

Figure 15.13 (a) Stable well-fixed cemented bipolar hemiarthroplasty. (b) B3 pattern in polished taper stem. (c) Revision of femoral component and insertion of uncemented acetabulum.

Case example: Type C fracture

A 74-year-old woman 1 year after total hip replacement fell on ice (**Figure 15.14a, b**).

She was treated with a direct lateral approach, elevation of vastus lateralus and double-plating with supplementary cables (**Figure 15.14c**).

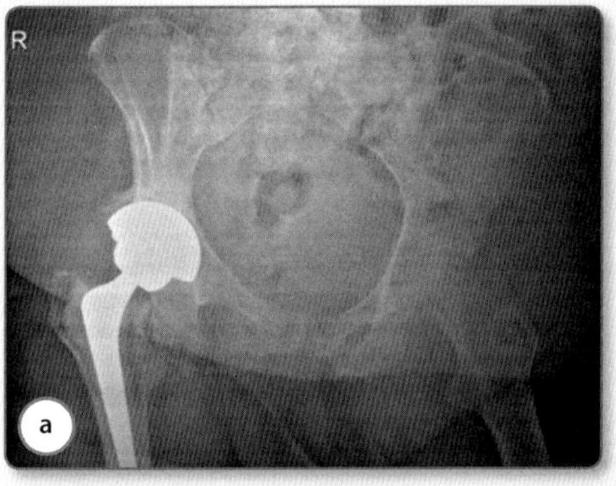

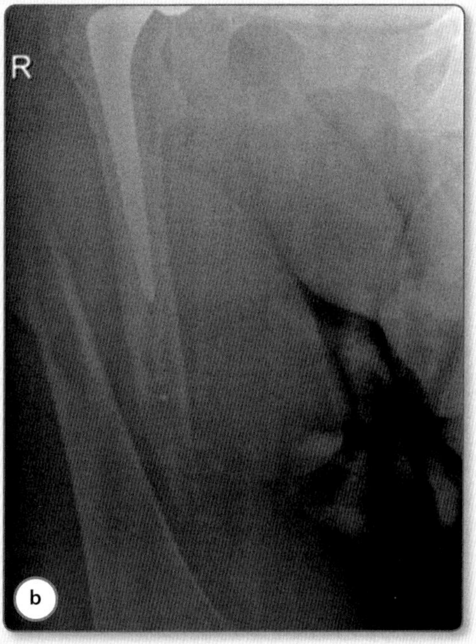

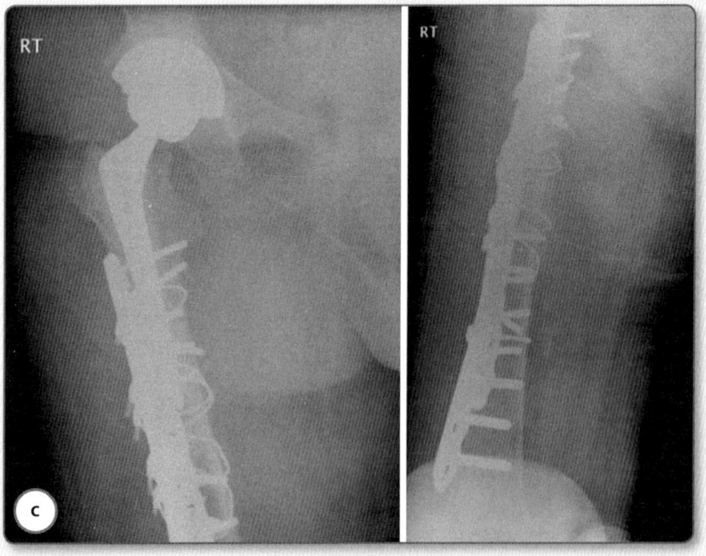

Figure 15.14 (a, b) Stable right total hip replacement with fracture distal to cement plug. (c) Stabilization with double plating.

Case example: Type C fracture

An 87-year-old man was confused and fell 6 weeks following displaced intracaspular femoral neck fracture (**Figures 15.15a–c**), suffering a long spiral fracture distal to a well-fixed stem. He was treated with a single polyaxial locking plate and cabling system.

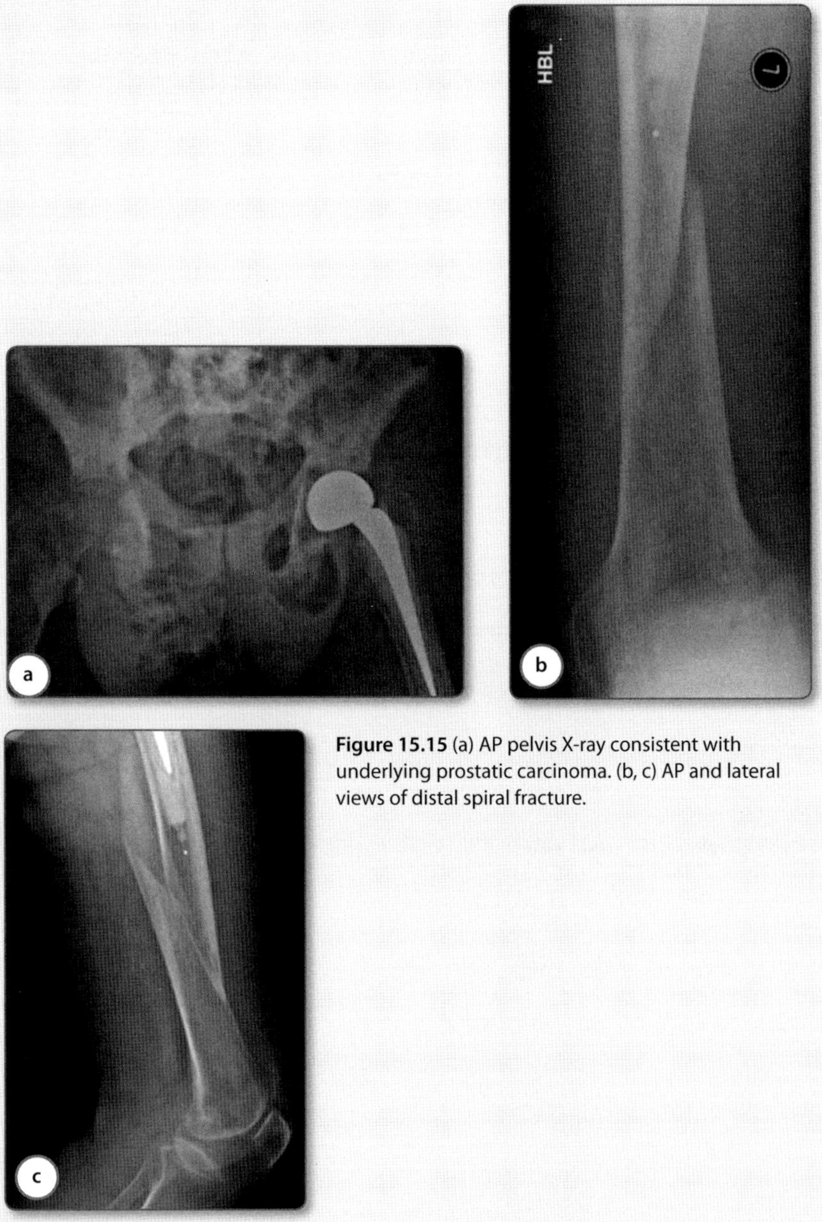

Figure 15.15 (a) AP pelvis X-ray consistent with underlying prostatic carcinoma. (b, c) AP and lateral views of distal spiral fracture.

Further reading

Duncan CP, Haddad FS. The Unified Classification System (UCS): improving our understanding of periprosthetic fractures. Bone Joint J 2014; 96-B:713–716.

Haddad FS, Duncan CP, Berry DJ, et al. Periprosthetic femoral fractures around well-fixed implants: use of cortical onlay allografts with or without a plate. J Bone Joint Surg Am 2002; 84-A:945–950.

Lindahl H, Malchau H, Oden A, Garellick G. Risk factors for failure after treatment of a periprosthetic fracture of the femur J Bone Joint Surg Br 2006; 88:26–30.

Tadross TSF, Nanu AM, Buchanan MJ, Checketts RG. Dall-Miles plating for periprosthetic B1 fractures of the femur. J Arthroplasty 2000; 15:49–51.

Vioreanu MH, Parry MC, Haddad FS, Duncan CP. Field testing the Unified Classification System for periprosthetic fractures of the pelvis and femur around a total hip replacement: an international collaboration. Bone Joint J 2014; 96-B:1472–1477.

16 Acute knee dislocation

Kanishka Milton Ghosh, David Deehan

Introduction

Knee dislocations are defined as complete tears of both cruciate and collateral ligaments. In addition to ligament damage, the energy required for traumatic knee dislocation can damage neurovascular structures with the popliteal artery and common perineal nerve being particularly at risk. The long-term morbidity from multiligament knee injuries is substantial and includes pain, instability, and stiffness of the affected joint.

Incidence

Multiligament injuries to the knee are rare injuries accounting for less than 0.02% of all orthopaedic injuries. They are defined as disruption of two of the four major stabilizers of the knee; the anterior cruciate ligament (ACL), the posterior cruciate ligament (PCL), the medial collateral ligament (MCL), and the lateral (fibular) collateral ligament (LCL). In a prospective cohort of 2,265 patients with knee injuries presenting to five tertiary referral centers over a 10-year period, only 11% involved patients with multiligament knee injuries. Of these patients, 70.5% involved the ACL and MCL (making it the most common presenting pattern) and 11.9% involved the ACL and LCL. Dislocation of the tibiofemoral joint is a more serious injury with adverse long term consequences.

Mechanism of injury

Multiligament knee injuries vary from high-velocity injuries from motor vehicle crashes to more common low-velocity sports related injuries. But both injury patterns are associated with neurovascular damage.

Initial management/ prioritization

A full history and examination of the patient must be undertaken following Advanced Trauma Life Support protocol. Examination usually reveals gross joint instability. The condition of the soft tissues should be assessed, with any wounds dressed appropriately and the leg temporarily splinted. Peripheral nerve function should be documented with the motor and sensory function of the tibial and common peroneal nerves assessed. The incidence of common peroneal nerve (CPN) injury is approximately 20% after knee dislocation with a higher incidence after posterolateral patterns of injury. Complete nerve transection is rare but severe stretching often produces a neurotmesis and a guarded prognosis.

Palpable pedal pulses with comparisons to the contralateral limb for symmetry is of the highest priority especially if a knee dislocation is suspected. The popliteal artery is tethered at the adductor hiatus proximally and soleal arch distally. This results in the vessel having little tolerance to stretching. The vascular damage can range from intimal tears to complete disruption.

Measurement of ankle brachial index (ABI) is a useful tool to rule out gross arterial compromise. An ABI of 0.8 or higher is reassuring but a CT angiogram is the most sensitive test to rule out intimal tears and vascular compromise. A senior vascular opinion is mandatory in such clinical cases.

The 'dimple' sign is often pathognomonic of an irreducible posterolateral knee dislocation. This occurs when the medial femoral condyle buttonholes through the anteromedial joint capsule.

The immediate priority is joint reduction. Simple traction, counter-traction under sedation and analgesia in the emergency room can reduce most acute dislocations. Failed reduction in the emergency department results in urgent expedition to the operating theater.

Temporary stabilization can be achieved using a simple extension splint or in more unstable injury patterns – a spanning external fixator can be applied. This has the advantage of improved stability, protection of the soft tissues and allowing vascular surgical access as necessary.

In the absence of a limb 'at risk', a simple 'look, feel and move' method of evaluation can be used. Swelling and its location can indicate the degree of injury and the likely structures involved. Capsular rupture allows blood to extravasate into the surrounding soft tissues and can lead the examiner to underestimate the extent of the injury. Knee examination is often more useful and more accurately performed under a general anesthetic.

Imaging is essential to corroborate clinical findings and plan surgery. Concomitant fractures, especially of the tibial plateau and distal femoral condyle are reported in at least 10–20% of patients presenting with multi-ligament knee injuries and dislocations. Associated fractures are generally associated with poorer outcome and must be addressed when restoring mechanical joint alignment and stability. Plain radiographs may demonstrate bony avulsions pathognomic of ligamentous injury (e.g. Segond fractures, Pellegrini–Stieda lesions, tibial spine avulsion). Stress X-rays are seldom required before surgery with the advent of magnetic resonance imaging (MRI), but may be useful under image intensifier screening in theater to assess the degree of instability.

MRI is highly sensitive and specific for soft tissue injuries but provides poor visualization of bony injuries. The major role of MRI is to gather an inventory of injured ligamentous structures (as well as associated meniscal and chondral injury) which will allow surgical planning. Unfortunately, this may not be available in the acute setting.

An algorithm for the initial management of multiligament knee injuries and dislocations is demonstrated in **Figure 16.1**.

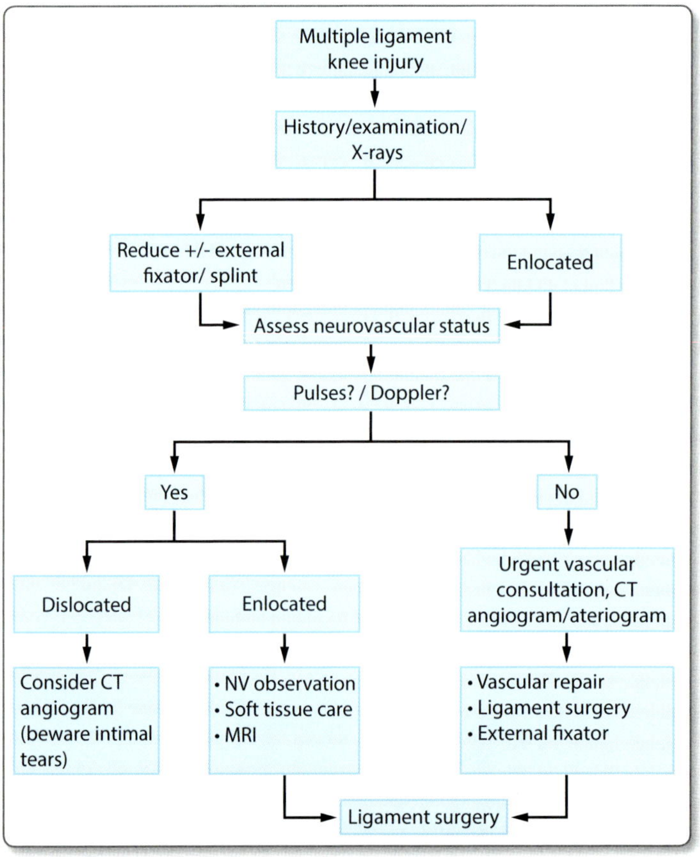

Figure 16.1 Algorithm for initial management of suspected knee dislocation or severe multiligament knee injury.

Case example: Knee dislocation with neurovascular compromise

A 42-year-old previously-well man was a front seat passenger in a van involved in a high-energy collision, which resulted in him being trapped in the cab of the vehicle for more than 2 hours. His right knee was hyperextended during the extraction process. He was transferred directly to the resuscitation suite of the emergency department, where examination confirmed a pulseless partially insensate leg, below a clinically deformed knee. He was taken to theater as a matter of urgency.

On-table mobile X-ray screening confirmed an absence of periarticular fractures but an anterior dislocation of the knee (**Figure 16.2a**). This was reduced closed on the operating table after intubation and an external spanning frame applied to stabilise the knee region (**Figure 16.2b**). Combined vascular and plastic surgery teams then used medial and lateral approaches respectively for vascular repair (**Figure 16.2c**) and exploration of the common peroneal nerve (**Figure 16.2d**). Prophylactic fasciotomies of all four lower leg compartments were undertaken intra-operatively.

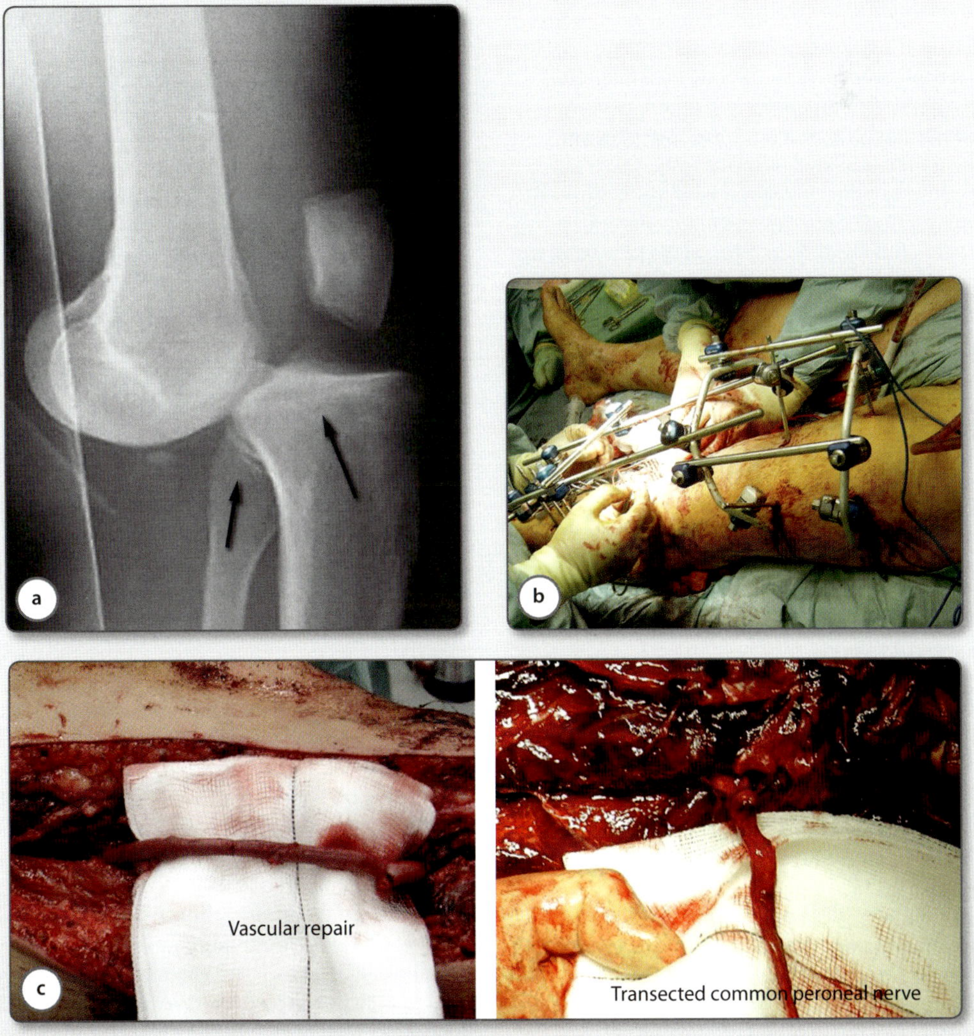

Figure 16.2 (a) Lateral X-ray of dislocated knee joint. (b) Reduction and stabilization of dislocated knee joint with spanning external fixator, allowing vascular reconstruction. (c) Left-hand image: reverse vein graft used as vascular repair. Right-hand image: transected CPN.

Considerations for surgery

A methodical approach to evaluation and treatment is required. Operative methods include repair, repair plus augmentation, or reconstruction of injured structures combined with bracing and rehabilitation in the short term.

Recent studies suggest that early surgical reconstruction of disrupted knee ligamentous structures is associated with better functional outcomes and a lower risk of residual joint stiffness. Caution must be exercised with any form of limited (endoscopic) approach in the acute setting where the capsule could be incomplete, leading to fluid extravasation and early compartment syndrome.

In the absence of neurovascular injury, early reconstruction should only be considered when the soft tissues allow and where essential resources (e.g. allograft tendons) and surgical expertise are available. Alternatively, a two-stage procedure can be considered with initial limited reconstruction of the capsule and collateral ligaments followed by an interval (6–12 weeks) to allow capsular healing with combined cruciate ligament reconstruction being performed as a staged procedure.

Theater layout and patient positioning

The patient is supine, with a high-thigh tourniquet and side support (**Figure16.3**).

Review of tendon harvesting

Arthroscopic soft tissue knee reconstruction is outwith the remit of this chapter, but the technique of hamstring harvesting is as follows:

- Make an anteromedial vertical incision over pes anserinus, care being taken not to damage the saphenous nerve. Open the tendon sheath (**Figure 16.4a**)
- Separate semitendinosus from gracilis and break down any vincula using a gemini artery forceps (**Figure 16.4b**)
- Insert tendon stripper to harvest graft, excess muscle can be scrapped off the tendon as necessary to give a clean graft (**Figure 16.4c**)

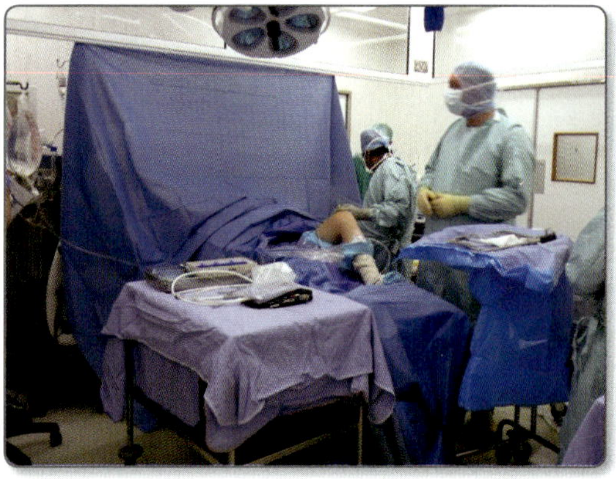

Figure 16.3 Theater layout and patient positioning.

Equipment requirements

- Tendon harvesting equipment: Linvatec tendon stripper/micro deSoutter saw
- Arthroscopic equipment including dyonic 4.5 mm and 5 mm shavers
- Interference screws/endobutton/other means of fixation
- Access to allograft/synthetic graft material
- Image intensifier

Reduction and stabilization methods

Sustaining a twisting and hyperextension injury while playing football resulted in a hospital attendance for one unlucky student. MRI was arranged and confirmed complete disruption of the ACL, PCL and posterolateral corner. He was referred for physiotherapy and to a specialist knee surgeon. There was no neurovascular deficit and normal distal pulses and active motor function of the CPN. Repeat assessment confirmed a positive Lachman, soft end point to anterior and posterior drawer, positive dial test, normal neurovascular deficit, LCL 3 laxity. He was counselled for reconstruction, brace support postoperative requirement for chemical DVT prophylaxis and risk of graft failure. He underwent ACL (central third patellar tendon autograft), PCL – contralateral semi T and gracilis autograft, LCL/PLC (Larsen type) using ipsilateral semi T. Fixation was by means of round cannulated interference (RCI) screws and proximal

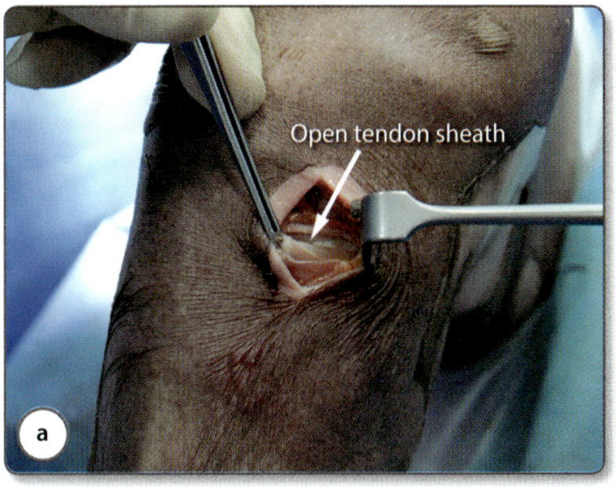

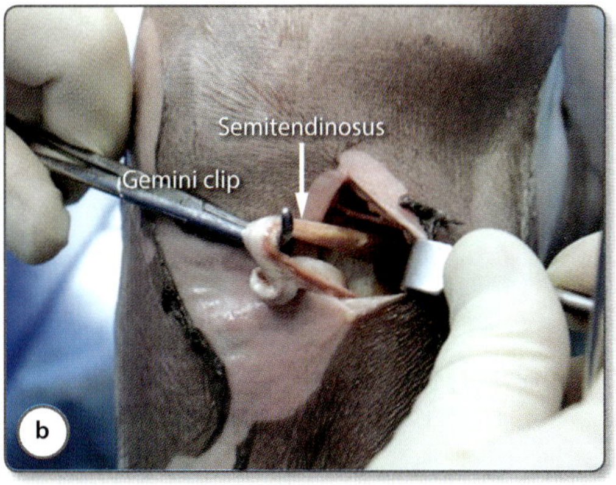

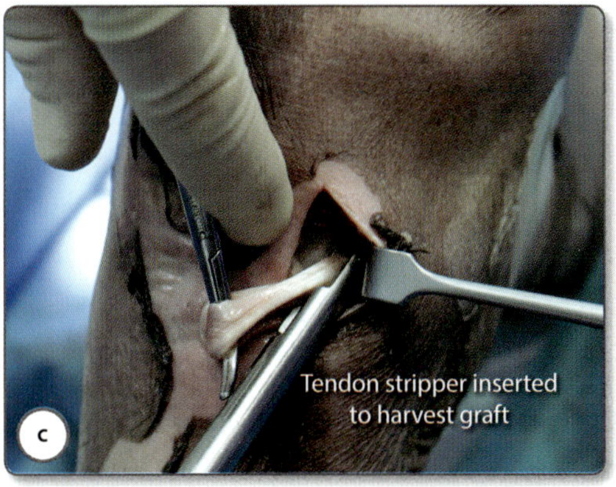

Figure 16.4 (a) Anteromedial vertical incision over pes anserinus. (b) Isolation of semitendinosus. (c) Insertion of insert tendon stripper to harvest graft.

endobutton for the PCL graft (**Figure 16.5**). He was treated in a brace 0–30° for 4 weeks and then 0–90° for a further 4 weeks. At 4 months, there was full movement and a stable knee without pain.

Posterolateral corner reconstruction (Figure 16.6)

- Make a lateral vertical incision, curved posteriorly and centered between Gerdy's tubercle and the fibular head inferiorly and the lateral femoral epicondyle proximally
- Locate, dissect out and protect the CPN as it winds around fibular head. This is best located proximally in the surgical field where it lies posterior to short head of biceps
- Divide the iliotibial band (ITB) in the line of its fibers: anterior two-thirds and posterior one-third
- Peel back the ITB anteriorly and posteriorly to expose the lateral femoral condyle, the insertion of the popliteus tendon (more anterior structure) and the fibular collateral ligament (more posterior structure)

Grafting materials – autograft versus allograft

Autografts can be harvested from the ipsilateral or contralateral extremity and include hamstring tendon, bone-patellar tendon-bone or quadriceps tendon. Allografts allow for a far greater selection of tissues to include the aforementioned tissues as well as Achilles tendon with calcaneal bone plug, anterior tibialis tendon, or posterior tibialis tendon. Use of allografts eliminates donor site morbidity, decreases dissection time, can reduce the number of surgical incisions, and has the potential to reduce postoperative pain and stiffness. However, possible disadvantages include greater cost, the potential for disease transmission, and a delay in incorporation.

Rehabilitation

Early active motion in a brace with close supervision by experienced physiotherapists is essential to achieving good long-term outcomes and avoiding joint stiffness. Multiligament knee

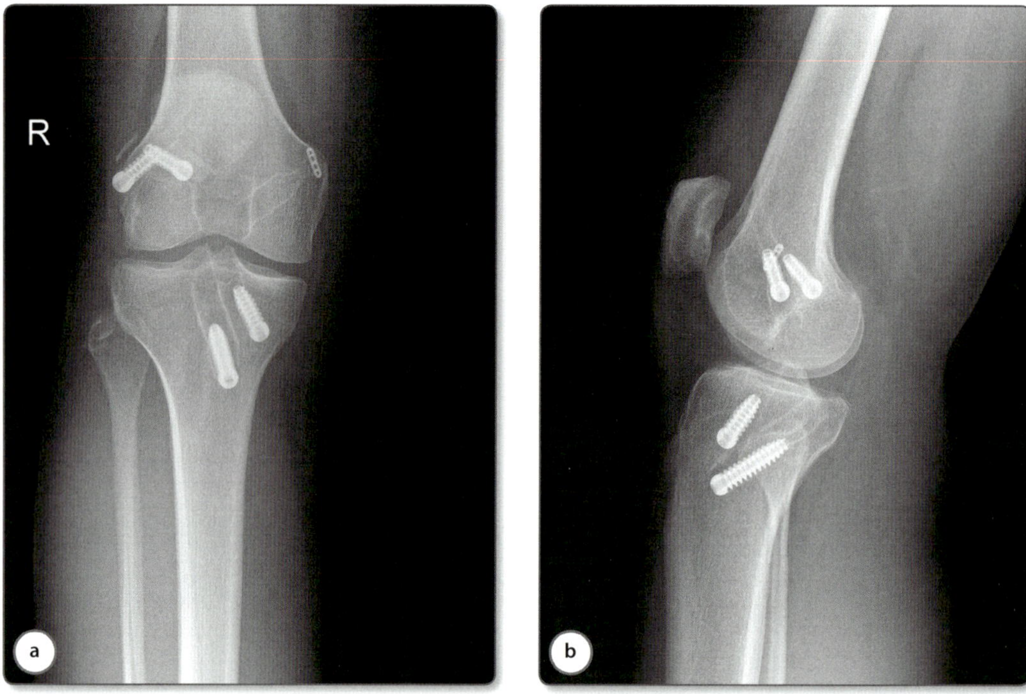

Figure 16.5 (a) AP and (b) lateral postoperative X-rays of reconstructed multi-ligament knee injury.

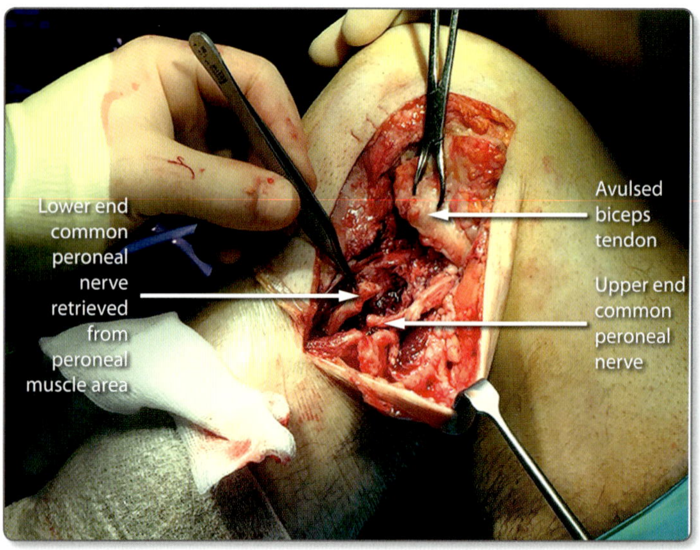

Figure 16.6 Lateral knee anatomy in severe posterolateral injury.

injuries or dislocations must be managed more cautiously than their counterparts with single ligament injuries. In the first phase, a hinged knee brace should be retained for at least 6 weeks after which full weight bearing can be commenced. From 6–12 weeks the brace can be discarded or replaced with a sports brace. During this phase the patient focuses on regaining range of motion, joint proprioception and quadriceps strengthen using closed chain exercises. Hamstring resistance exercises are avoided to protect the PCL repair. The third phase, from 12–18 weeks involves return to light exercises and running. After 18 weeks the patient can return to light sports, improve quadriceps and hamstring strength and start plyometric training. At 8–9 months, patients can return to competitive sporting activities. It is important to stress that the surgeon should be involved regularly in the management of the postoperative rehabilitation. Each case is unique and often needs tailoring to the individual. Chemical thromboprophylaxis (allowing and being cognizant of the risk of bleeding) is being increasingly considered relevant due to the early immobilization. Ready access to ultrasound scanning to exclude above-knee thrombosis is useful.

Summary of learning points

- A thorough examination is essential for the correct diagnosis to assess neuromuscular integrity and the pattern of ligament injury
- Early joint reduction and application of a spanning external fixator stabilizes the knee joint should vascular intervention be necessary in the acute setting
- Surgery should be carried out by a specialist with the appropriate skills set and where resources (e.g. allograft) are readily available
- The goals of treatment are restoration of knee stability and early range of motion
- Staged procedures often yield the best results in terms of functional outcome
- Rehabilitation should be performed by specialist physiotherapists and need to more cautious than single ligament injuries

Further reading

Cook S, Ridley TJ, McCarthy MA, et al. Surgical treatment of multiligament knee injuries. Knee Surg Sports Traumatol Arthrosc 2015; 23:2983–2991.

Dedmond BT, Almekinders LC. Operative versus nonoperative treatment of knee dislocations: a meta-analysis. Am J Knee Surg 2001; 14:33–38.

Fanelli GC, Orcutt DR, Edson CJ. The multiple-ligament injured knee: evaluation, treatment, and results. Arthroscopy 2005; 21:471–486.

Mook WR, Miller MD, Diduch DR, et al. Multiple-ligament knee injuries: a systematic review of the timing of operative intervention and postoperative rehabilitation. J Bone Joint Surg Am 2009; 91:2946–2957.

Robertson A, Nutton RW, Keating JF. Dislocation of the knee. J Bone Joint Surgery 2006; 88:706–711.

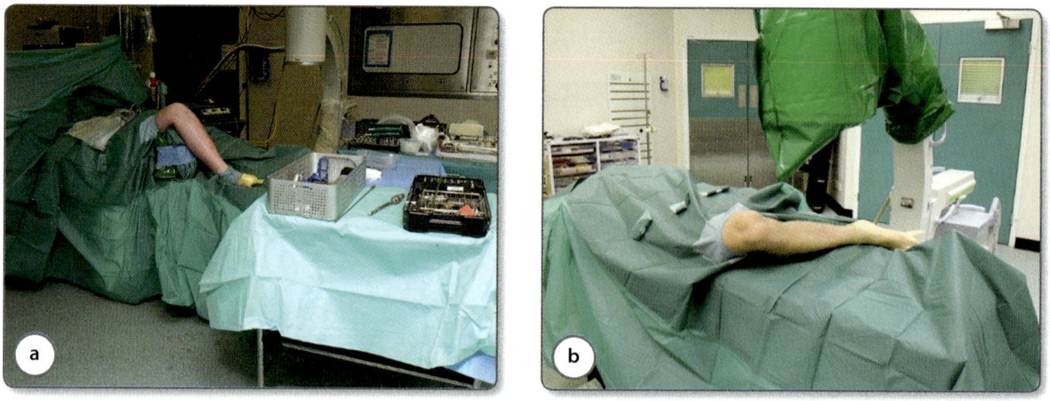

Figure 17.3 (a) Theater setup using a bolster under the injured leg. (b) Injured leg in 'figure of four' position.

operating table. A sandbag is placed under the contralateral buttock to avoid external rotation of the injured leg (**Figure 17.3b**). The fluoroscopic C-arm remains in the vertical position and does not need to rotate to obtain the lateral view. An anteroposterior (AP) view can be obtained by flexing the hip and knee. A tourniquet is not used with this setup.

Review of surgical approaches

Nail entry

Skin incision

- Make a longitudinal midline incision centered over the distal pole of the patella to the tibial tubercle
- The patella tendon can be split or an incision made either side of tendon. For more proximal fractures, a suprapatellar entry point can also be used

AP view

- The fibula head should be superimposed by the lateral tibial plateau by 50%.
- The entry point is commonly in line with the medial aspect of the lateral tibial spine, in line with the medullary canal (**Figure 17.4a**)

Lateral view

- The posterior aspects of both femoral condyles should be superimposed
- On the lateral view, the entry point is on the anterior edge of the tibial plateau (**Figure 17.4b**)

Plating

Plating is used generally where the fracture extends more into the proximal and distal thirds of the tibia. The anteromedial side of the tibia has limited soft tissues coverage and often may be injured. The anterolateral approach can therefore be used for plating.

Anterolateral approach

- Make a longitudinal incision 1 cm lateral to the tibial crest (**Figure 17.5a**)
- Release the muscles of the anterior compartment to expose the tibia. Proximally, tibialis anterior is released (**Figure 17.5b**). More distally, the interval between peroneus brevis and extensor digitorum longus is used (see Chapter 18)

Fasciotomies

A four-compartment decompression of the lower leg can be achieved via two incisions: anterolateral and posteromedial.

Anterolateral incision

- The landmarks are the lateral tibial crest and fibula. Position the incision half-way between the two (**Figure 17.6a**)
- The anterior compartment fascia is incised longitudinally. A further transverse incision across the intermuscular septum gains access to the lateral compartment (**Figure 17.6b**)
- At the distal end of the fasciotomy, take care to identify and protect the superficial peroneal nerve which pierces the crural fascia at around 10–12 cm above the lateral malleolus

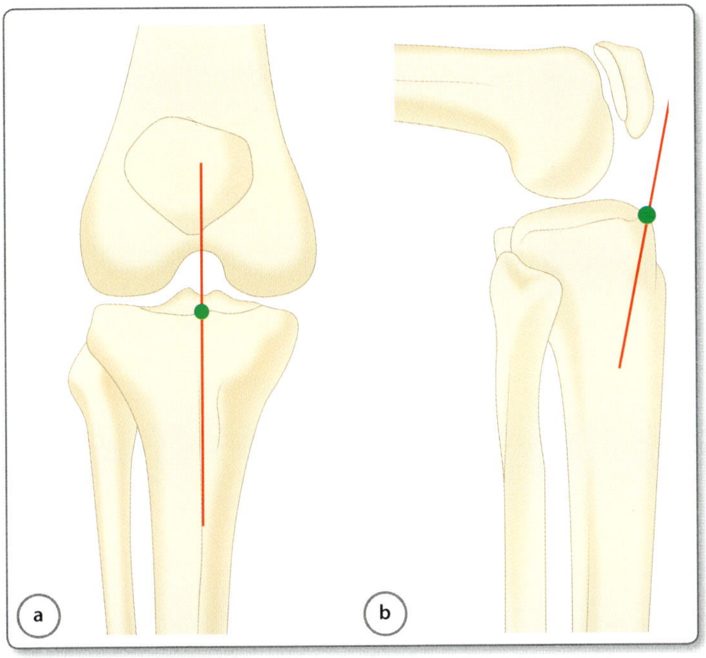

Figure 17.4 (a) Anteroposterior and (b) lateral view of nail entry site.

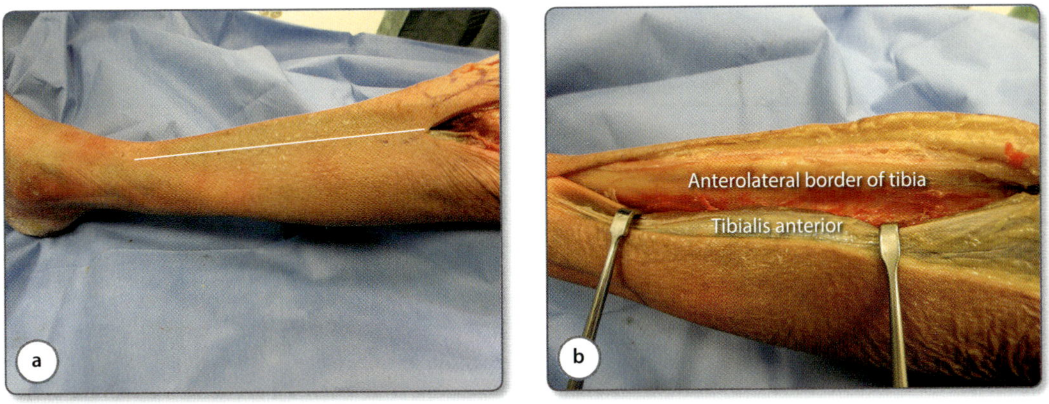

Figure 17.5 (a) Proposed skin incision for anterolateral incision. (b) Release of tibialis anterior to expose anterolateral aspect of tibia.

Posteromedial incision

- The landmark is the medial tibial crest. Make a longitudinal incision 2 cm posterior to the medial tibial crest (**Figure 17.6c**)
- Split the fascia longitudinally along the whole length of the compartments. Both the superficial and deep posterior compartments can be accessed through this one incision
- Be aware the long saphenous vein and saphenous nerve which should be protected
- At the proximal end, ensure the soleal bridge is released in order to achieve full decompression of the deep posterior compartment (**Figure 17.6d**)

Equipment requirements

- Radiolucent table
- Thigh tourniquet (for the approach only, not to be used whilst reaming)
- Intramedullary nailing set

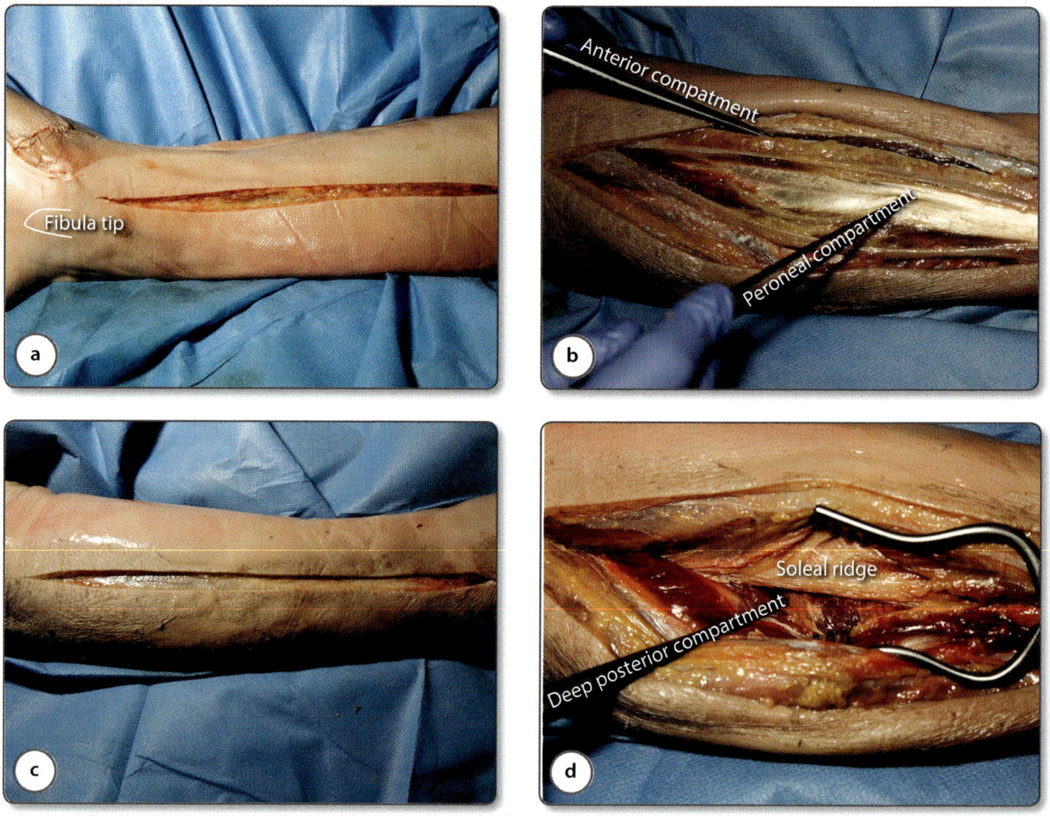

Figure 17.6 (a) Proposed skin incision for decompression of anterior and lateral/peroneal compartments. (b) Fascial incisions are then created in the anterior and lateral/peroneal compartments to release the pressure. (c) Proposed medial based incision for decompression of superficial and deep posterior compartments. (d) Posterior deep compartment entered by releasing soleus from the tibial surface.

Reduction and stabilization methods

- Reduction and stabilization may be achieved by various methods.
- Manual traction and manipulation
- Poller/blocking screws direct the intramedullary nail and aid fracture reduction in oblique fractures. It is placed in the acute angle formed at the intersection between a longitudinal line drawn along the shaft of the tibia and along the fracture line (**Figure 17.7**)
- The main fracture fragments can be manipulated using reduction forceps, application of Schanz pins or in the case of open fractures where the fracture is exposed, a plate with unicortical screws can provide temporary stability

In more proximal fractures, due to deforming forces by the quadriceps, an apex anterior deformity occurs when the knee is hyperflexed during intramedullary nailing. To avoid this, the leg can be semi-extended and a suprapatellar entry point used.

If there is distraction at the fracture site on nail entry, the distal locking screws can be inserted first. The nail can then be 'back-slapped' to gain cortical contact between the distal and proximal fragments or some nails allow compression. The nail needs to be adequately sunk to allow room for it to be knocked back proximally.

The final position of the intramedullary nail with the use of Poller screws is shown in **Figure 17.2**.

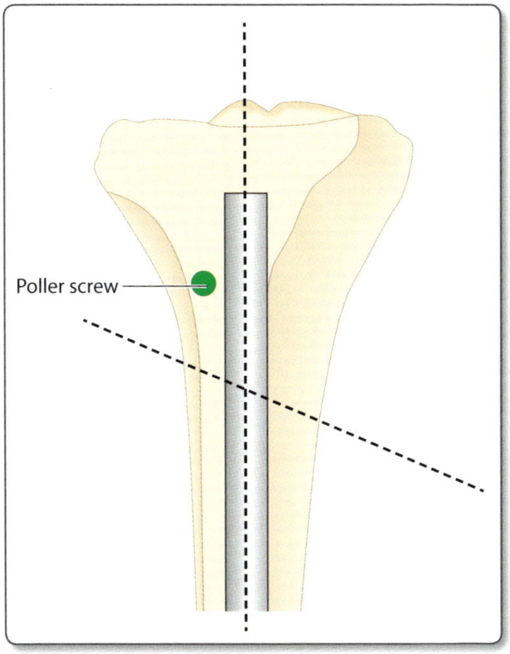

Figure 17.7 Placement of Poller/blocking screw.

Rehabilitation

Request physiotherapy review and input when surgical wounds are satisfactory:

- Weight bearing status is dependent on fracture pattern and stability. Those with transverse fractures anatomically fixed may fully weight bear immediately postoperatively
- There may be limitations to mobilization determined by the plastic surgeon if a flap was necessary for soft tissue coverage
- Active assisted knee and ankle range of motion exercises
- Serial postoperative X-rays to confirm no loss of reduction and progression of union over the following months
- Supervised progressive weight-bearing exercises in conjunction with X-rays and clinical symptom monitoring

Avoiding postoperative complications

Infection/wound healing

- Careful soft tissue handling
- Prophylactic antibiotic administration
- In open fractures, aggressive early debridement and soft tissue coverage following BOAST 4 guidelines

Malunion

- Rotation should be checked with the contralateral leg if uninjured
- The tibial tuberosity should be in line with the middle of the ankle joint, usually along the second ray
- One fluoroscopic way of assessing rotation is to take a true lateral of the knee, rotate the fluoroscopic C-arm 100–105° and center at the ankle. This should give a true mortice view of the ankle if normal tibial torsion is restored
- Protected weight-bearing

Nonunion

- Avoidance of excessive soft tissue stripping
- Patient factors:
  - Smoking
  - Steroids
  - Excessive alcoholic consumption
  - Diabetes mellitus
  - Non-steroidal anti-inflammatory drugs
  - Poor nutrition
  - Noncompliance with postoperative instructions
- Particularly for open fractures, where infection risk is much greater than in closed injuries, aggressive debridement and timely soft tissue cover should be achieved

Compartment syndrome

- Prophylactic fasciotomies may be necessary in those where compartment syndrome risk is high

Neurovascular injury

- With the oblique proximal locking screw, take care that it is not too long as it can cause damage to the common peroneal nerve as it runs around the fibular head
- With distal lateral plating, the superficial peroneal nerve is a risk during the approach so care should be taken to protect it

Salvage options for nonunion

Exchange nailing

The old intramedullary nail is removed. The tibial canal is then reamed so that a new larger diameter and therefore stiffer intramedullary nail can be inserted. In cases of infection, the reamer aspiration irrigation (RIA) system can be used to debride the medullary canal and can also be used to harvest intramedullary, cancellous bone graft, often from the femur.

Fine wire frame

For bone loss, bone transport can be used with a circular frame. This may be achieved with compression-distraction at the fracture site, shortening with lengthening at a separate corticortomy site or use of a free bone graft.

Masquelat technique

With bone loss, initially a cement spacer is used to fill the dead space, which aids to form a bio active membrane as a reaction to the foreign material. The space is then filled with bone graft at a later date.

Posterolateral bone grafting

This technique can be used in infected nonunions of the middle and distal third of the tibia. In more proximal fractures this technique is not used as it presents a high risk to neurovascular structures. Previously traumatized soft tissue which is commonly in the anteromedial aspect is avoided using this approach. A large amount of graft can be used and stability is obtained by creating tibiofibular synostosis spanning the fracture site.

Summary of learning points

- Recognize that tibial fractures have the greatest risk of compartment syndrome and therefore monitor closely, particularly in the unconscious/obtruded patient. Consider prophylactic fasciotomies
- In open fractures, particularly of the tibia, early aggressive debridement and soft tissue coverage markedly reduces complications of infection
- In intramedullary nailing, obtaining the correct entry point is key to successful placement of the nail

Further reading

BAPRAS/BOA. Standards for the management of open fractures of the lower limb (online). www.bapras.org.uk. London: BOA/BAPRAS, 1991.

Hak DJ. Getting the Rotation Right: techniques for assessing rotation in intramedullary tibial and femoral nailing. Orthopaedics 2011; 34:33.

McQueen MM, Gaston P, Court-Brown CM. Acute compartment syndrome. Who is at risk? J Bone Joint Surg Br 2000; 82:200–203.

Bhandari M, Guyatt G, Tornetta P 3rd, et al. Randomized trial of reamed and unreamed intramedullary nailing of tibial shaft fractures. J Bone Joint Surg Am 2008; 90:2567–2578.

Toivanen JA, Väistö O, Kannus P, et al. Anterior knee pain after intramedullary nailing of fractures of the tibial shaft. A prospective, randomized study comparing two different nail-insertion techniques. J Bone Joint Surg Am 2002; 84-A:580–585.

18 Pilon fractures

Paul V Fearon

Introduction

A Pilon fracture is a high-energy inarticulate distal tibial fracture. These are difficult and challenging injuries and can be associated with long-term complications resulting in pain, functional impairment and disability.

Incidence

Although Pilon fractures account for only about 5% of tibial fractures. Approximately 10–20% of Pilon fractures occur in poly trauma patients and 10–30% are open fractures. As a result, they are often complex and difficult fractures to manage.

Mechanism of injury

The majority of patients have a history of a high-energy axial injury, such as falling from a height. Patients often have concomitant injuries, such as trauma to the calcaneum, knee, hip or spine. Compartment syndrome of the foot and lower leg can result and must be excluded.

Case example: Closed pilon fracture

A man in his thirties fell off a ladder sustaining an isolated injury to his right ankle region. He underwent ATLS assessment before being referred to the receiving orthopaedic team. Initial AP and lateral X-rays (**Figure 18.1**) demonstrate the high energy injury associated with articular involvement.

He underwent a staged protocol management pathway: application of a spanning external fixator prior to CT scanning (**Figure 18.2**). Definitive stabilization utilizing the tibialis anterior approach for articular reconstruction (**Figure 18.3**), grafting and plate stabilization (**Figure 18.4**), once the soft tissues were amenable.

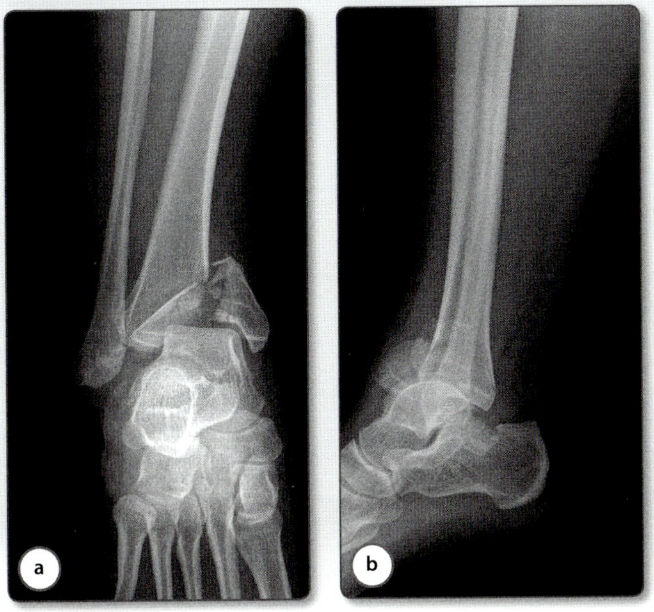

Figure 18.1 (a) Anteroposterior and (b) lateral radiographs of a pilon fracture.

Case example: *continued.*

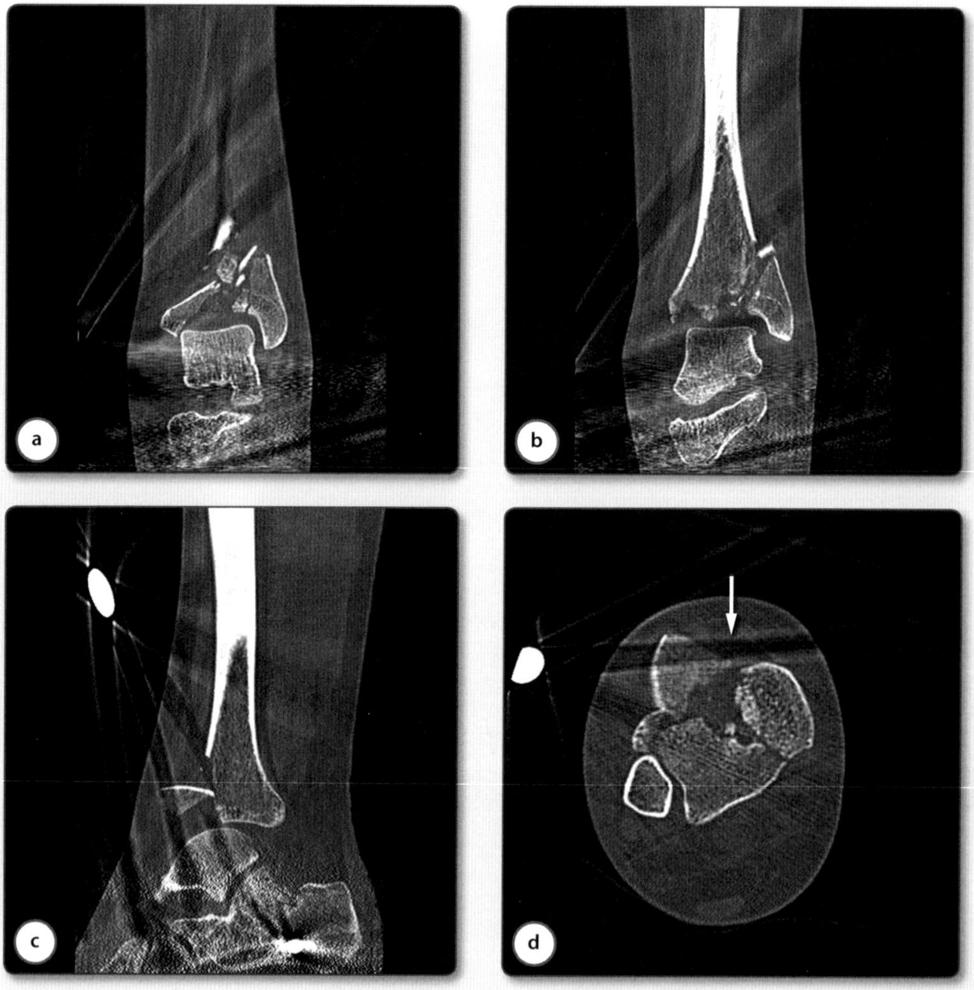

Figure 18.2 Pilon fracture. (a,b) Coronal views showing disruption of joint surface. (c) Sagittal view showing rotation of anterior fragment. (d) Axial image showing distribution of fracture lines.

Initial management/prioritization

Advanced Trauma Life Support (ATLS) assessment takes priority, followed by splintage/soft tissue stabilization and appropriate radiological imaging, in conjunction with a directed neurovascular examination.

Case example: *continued.*

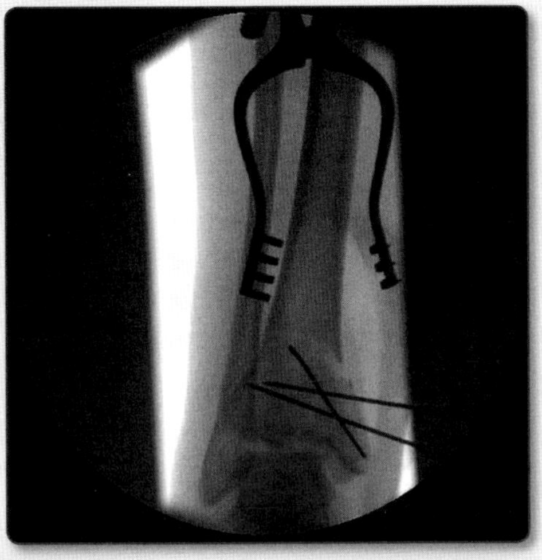

Figure 18.3 Tibialis anterior surgical approach for reduction of the depressed articular fragments and stabilization with K-wires. Voids were back filled with grafting materials.

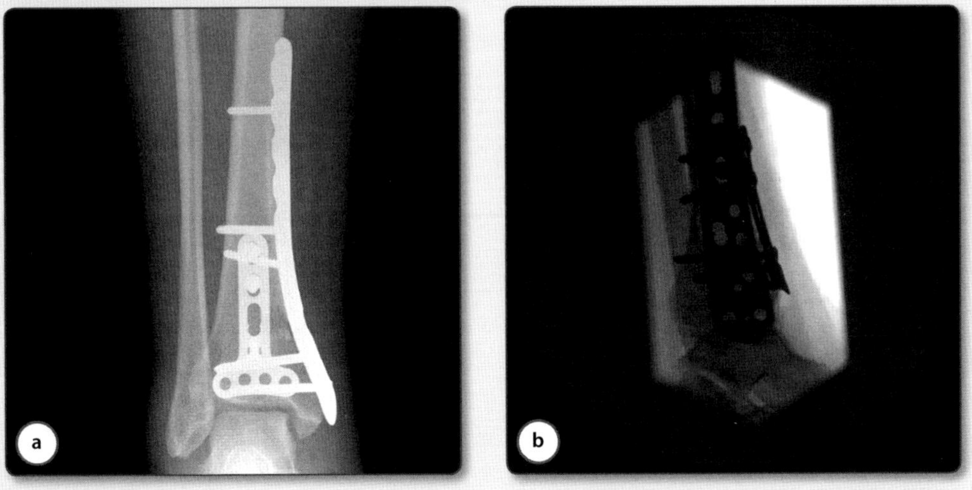

Figure 18.4 (a) Anteroposterior and (b) lateral radiographs showing final position of plates inserted via tibialis anterior approach.

Considerations for surgery

It is important to determine the patient's functional level, medical and social history, to reduce potential complications. The status of the soft tissue envelope needs to be carefully assessed and protected from further damage. The optimal management for Pilon fractures remains controversial, but a staged protocol is an acceptable method of treatment, allowing the soft tissues to recover from the initial trauma of the accident prior to planned surgical intervention. Operating through swollen, blistered, damaged skin is associated with an increased risk of infection and subsequent complications.

Theater layout and patient positioning

- A proposed theater set up and layout is illustrated in **Figure 18.5**
- Position the patient as for spanning fixator application (**Figure 18.6**). Positioning the patient in such a manner allows unrestricted access to the medial surface of the tibia and also the insertion of a medial to lateral os calcis transfixation pin
- Place the tourniquet with patient supine, before moving the patient into the desired position for definitive surgery
- Position the leg on a radiolucent block [allowing anteroposterior (AP) and lateral X-rays without moving the leg]
- Place a sandbag under the ipsilateral buttock, with the patient supine to prevent the limb from falling into external rotation
- Remove the majority of external fixator but leave one bar for stability whilst setting up the patient

Review of surgical approaches

Options will depend upon fracture configuration.

Tibialis anterior approach

- Identify the tibial crest and make an incision 5–10 mm lateral to this. Distally, curve the incision medially toward (but staying anterior to) the medial malleolus (**Figure 18.7a**)
- Keep the initial incision superficial and be aware of the neurovascular structures, particularly the saphenous bundle at the medial malleolus (**Figure 18.7b**)

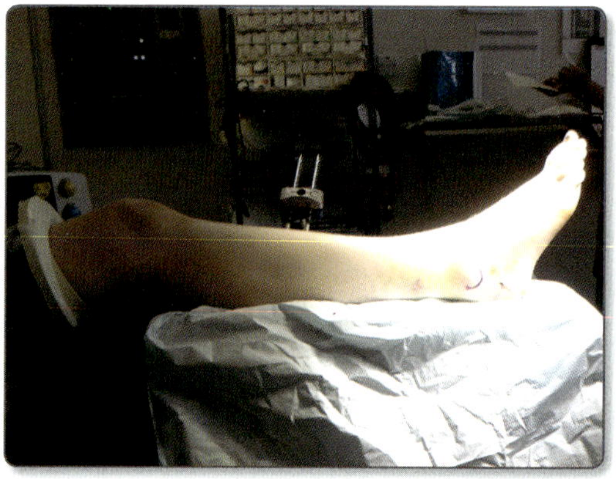

Figure 18.6 Limb elevated on radiolucent block. Patient pre-washed and scrubbed to reduce number of skin organisms prior to prep and draping.

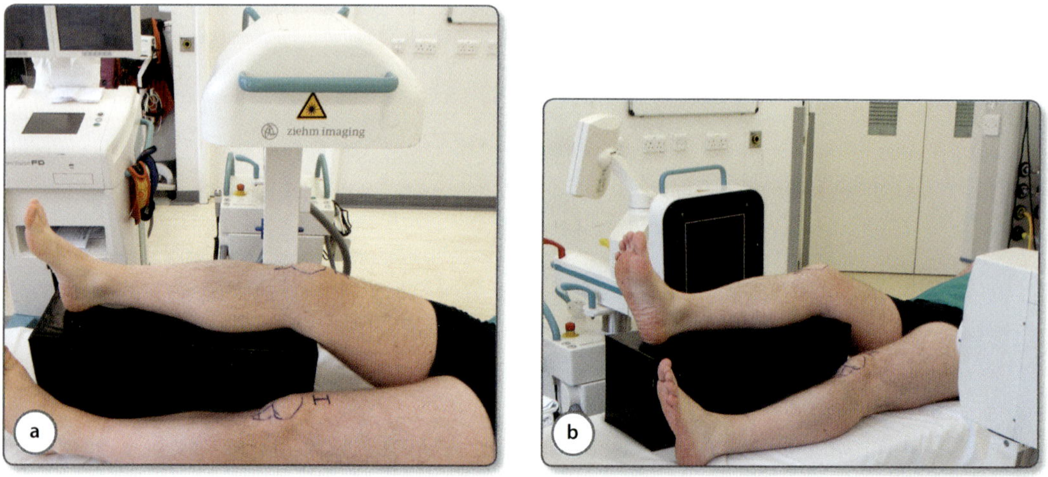

Figure 18.5 (a) Theater set up with radiolucent table and block. (b) Image intensifier and tourniquet on ipsilateral injured limb side. This gives the surgeon free access while positioned facing the medial tibial surface.

- Expose the tibialis anterior tendon (TAT) but do not open its sheath (**Figure 18.7c**). Develop a flap medially, exposing the anteromedial tibial surface. Keep the dissection extraperiostial
- Gain access to the anterior tibial surface by retracting the tibialis anterior laterally (**Figure 18.7d**). The fracture can be opened through the anterior window, allowing for reduction of the displaced joint fragments
- A medially based plate can be applied extraperiosteally, with the proximal screws inserted through percutaneous incisions, avoiding unnecessary soft tissue dissection (**Figure 18.7e**), as in the illustrated case example

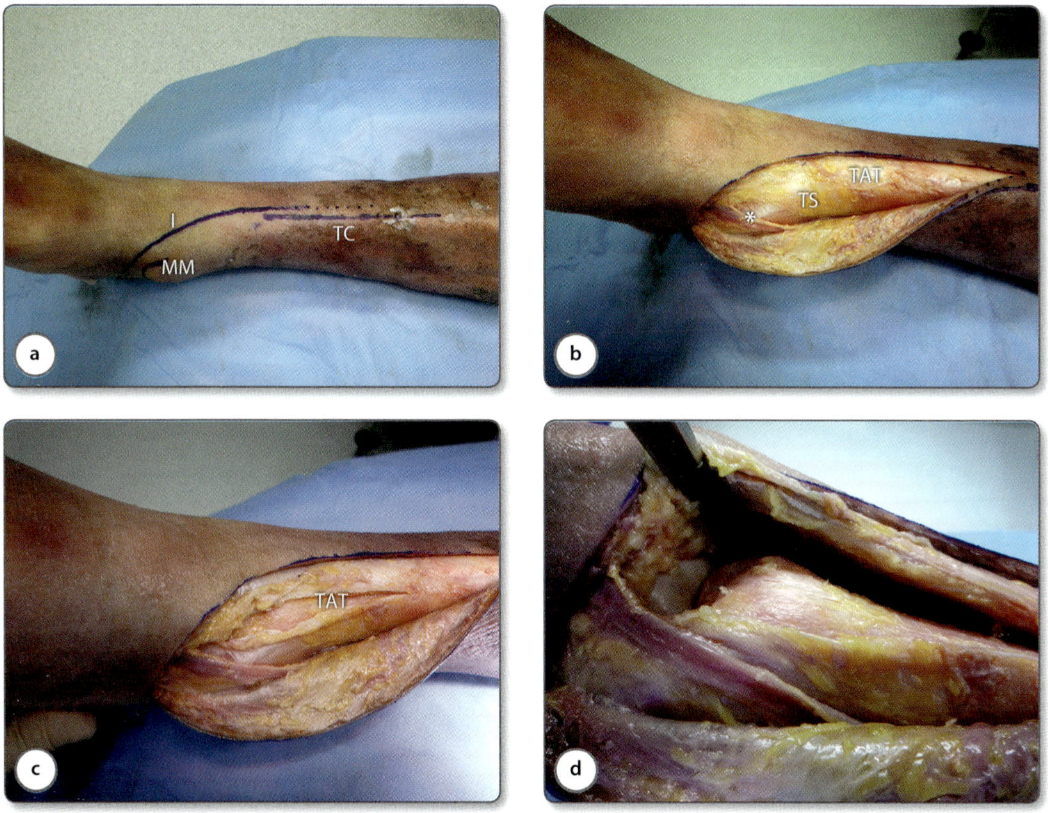

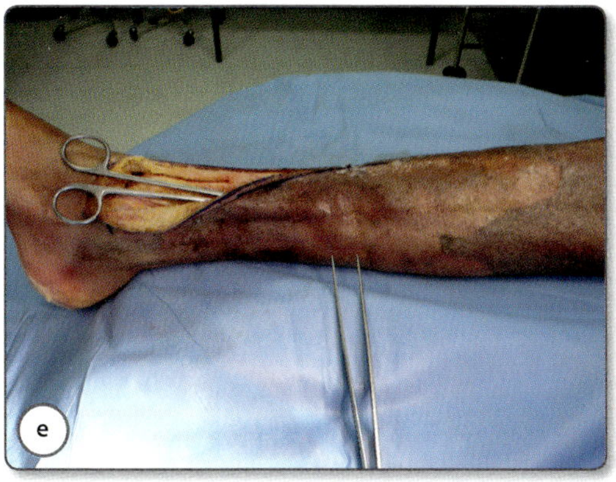

Figure 18.7 Tibialis anterior surgical approach. (a) Medial malleolus (MM), tibial crest (TC) and planned incision (I) marked. (b) Full thickness flaps created exposing anteromedial tibial shaft (TS). Saphenous neurovascular structures visible* and protected. (c) Anterior aspect to the distal tibia is gained by retracting TAT laterally. (d) Anterior and medial surfaces of the tibia are easily accessible, allowing for reduction, grafting and appropriate plating. (e) The incision does not need to be extended proximally as proximal screw insertion can be performed percutaneously.

Limited anterolateral approach

This approach can be used separately or in conjunction with the tibialis anterior approach to aid reduction, but care needs to be taken with the resulting skin bridge, which is at risk of necrosis.

- Perform an incision in line with the fourth metatarsal centered on the ankle joint. The superficial peroneal nerves needs to be identified and protected (**Figure 18.8a**)
- Divide the extensor retinaculum in line with the skin incision. Retract extensor digitorum longus (EDL) medially and peroneus tertius (PT) laterally. The anterior distal tibia and superior talar done are then visible (**Figure 18.8b**)

Medial posteromedial approach

- Plan the position of the incision in relation to the fragments to be reduced
- For the posteromedial approach make the incision between the Achilles tendon (AT) and medial malleolus (**Figure 18.9a**), avoiding the saphenous structures (**Figure 18.9b**)
- The flexor retinaculum is encountered and is divided carefully as later repair is required to avoid tendon subluxation (**Figure 18.9c**)
- Approach between the flexor digitorum longus and neurovascular structures (tibial nerve and posterior tibial artery), or the neurovascular structures and the flexor hallucis longus. The tendons can be subluxed from their bed to improve access (**Figure 18.9d**). This approach only allows indirect reduction of the posteromedial tibia for buttress plating. But it can also allow access to the posteromedial talus and medial calcaneum when the incision is enlarged distally

Posterolateral approach

- Apply a high-thigh tourniquet with patient supine prior to positioning in a lateral or prone position on a radiolucent table
- Utilize appropriate supportive blocks, allowing radiographs to be obtained, without interference from the opposite limb or the need to move the fractured limb
- Perform an incision between the fibula (F) and AT (**Figure 18.10a**)
- Identify and protect the sural nerve (**Figure 18.10b**)
- Dissect medial to peroneal muscles, with their lateral retraction
- Retract flexor hallucis longus medially to expose the posterior tibial surface (**Figure 18.10c**)

Timing of surgery

Definitive surgery is planned on a semi-elective basis once the soft tissue envelope is healthy and wrinkling. This can be as much as 2–3 weeks post index injury in high-energy trauma.

Equipment requirements

- Radiolucent table and bolster (**Figure 18.5**). This allows AP and lateral X-ray views to be obtained without moving the limb and potentially displacing fractures and further damaging soft tissues

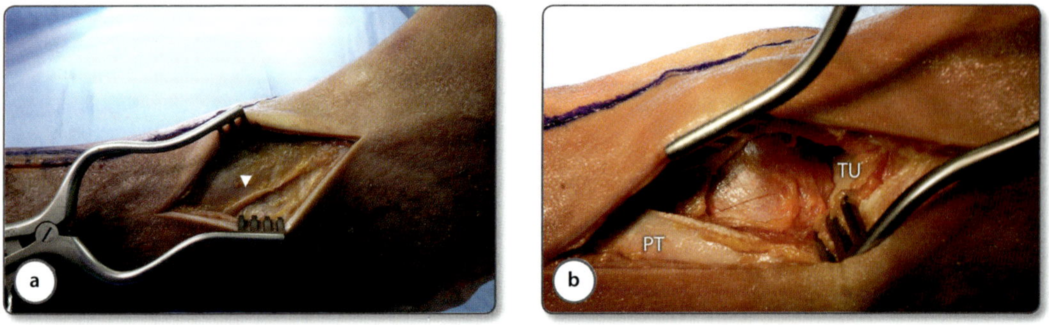

Figure 18.8 Anterolateral approach. (a) Identification and protection of superficial peroneal nerve (▼). (b) Following incision of the extensor retinaculum, EDL is retracted medially and PT laterally. This then gives intra-articular access to the anterolateral distal tibia and superior surface of talus (TU)

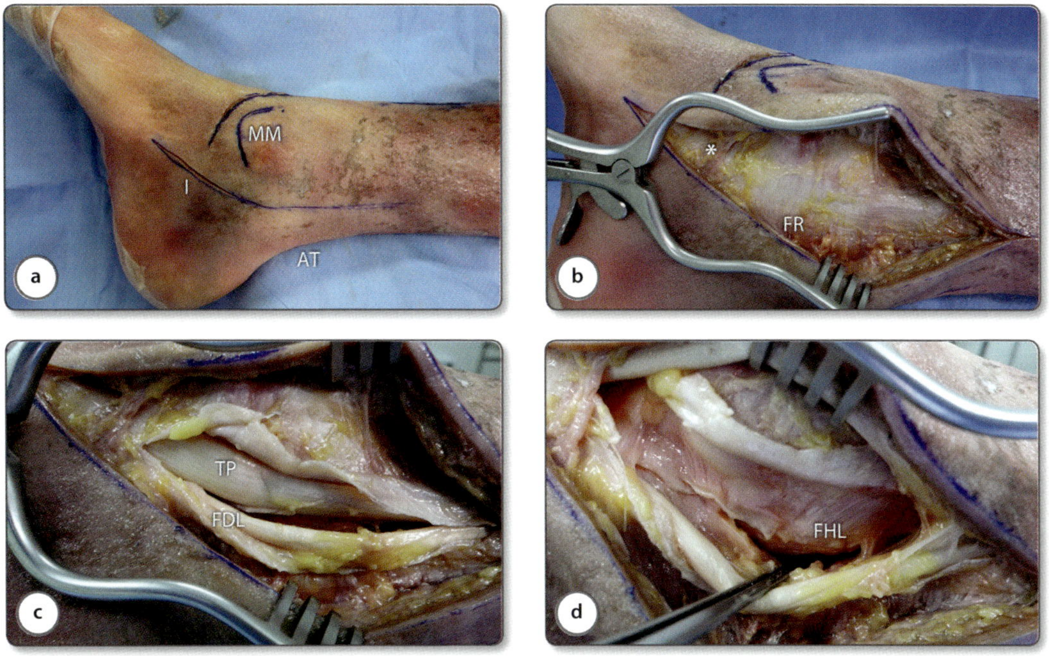

Figure 18.9 Medial/posteromedial surgical approach. (a) Planned surgical incision (I) centered between medial malleolus (MM) and Achilles tendon (AT). (b) The flexor retinaculum (FR) is encountered. At the inferior aspect of the incision the saphenous neurovascular structures are at risk (*). (c) The flexor retinaculum is carefully incised for later repair. This allows the tendons of tibialis posterior (TP), Flexor digitorum longus (FDL), and flexor hallucus longus (FHL) to be identified. (d) FHL in depth of approach. Forceps protecting FDL and neurovascular structures (TP displaced anteriorly from its bed).

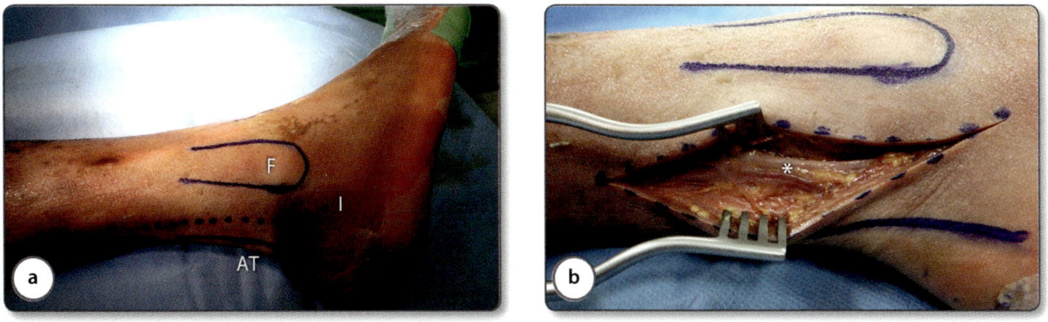

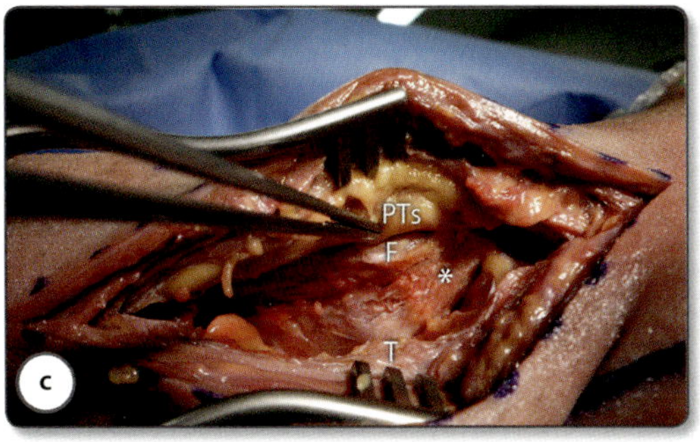

Figure 18.10 Posterior-lateral surgical approach. (a) Planned surgical incision (I) between fibula (F) and Achilles tendon (AT) for posterolateral approach to tibia. (b) Identification of sural neurovascular structures (*). (c) Peroneal tendons (PTs) retraced laterally with FHL retracted medially. Posterior surface of tibia (T) and fibula (F) accessed. Posterior syndesmotic (*) ligament complex should not be divided or it will destabilize ankle joint.

- Thigh tourniquet (not necessary for application of external fixator)
- External fixator set with appropriately sized Schanz and Denham pins
- Battery drill and drill bits for pilot holes
- In the majority of instances, small fragment sets are utilized, including:
  - Anatomical plates with locking options
  - Fine wires
  - Fixators-distractors
  - Reduction clamps
  - Grafting material

Reduction and stabilization methods

Method of external fixator application

- Position the patient's leg appropriately on the radiolucent block to allow free access to medial tibial surface and ankle region (**Figure 18.6**)
- Preform a prewash and scrub followed by routine preparation and draping
- Perform stab incision in Langer's lines on the medial face of the tibia, outside the zone of injury
- Predrill both near and far cortices (2.5 mm drill appropriate). This allows better fix of Schanz pins and avoids the 'crown necrosis' that occurs when pins are inserted by drill power
- Insert an appropriately sized Schanz pin (usually 5 mm or 6 mm) by hand, feeling for far cortex purchase - a stable frame protects soft tissues better, and is less likely to have issues with pin loosening. An image intensifier can be utilized to confirm adequate far cortex pin capture
- Drill a second parallel pilot hole (located appropriately, depending on the system used)
- Perform a medial os calcis stab incision, avoiding the neurovascular bundle. Then insert a Denham pin by hand, transfixing the os calcis in a medial to lateral direction
- Insert an optional mid-foot pin as necessary into the first metatarsal or tarsal bones, to prevent equinus positioning of foot
- Assemble a delta frame under radiographic control with traction and reduction maneuvers
- Lock the frame components and reinforce the structure as necessary
- Elevate the limb to reduce soft tissue swelling
- Commence pin site care in accordance with unit policy
- Arrange appropriate CT imaging to assess fracture configuration (**Figure 18.2**)

Definitive fracture fixation

From the CT slices in **Figure 18.2**, the axial image demonstrates anteromedial, and anterolateral fragments with a depressed intra-articular component. The sagittal split between the anteromedial and anterolateral fragments can be opened to access the intra-articular fragment (**Figure 18.2d**, white arrow). This can then be reduced, stabilized and grafted and the articular block attached to the shaft. In order to achieve this, a working knowledge of the appropriate surgical approaches is essential. The approach or approaches utilized will depend upon the fracture configurations identified from CT evaluation.

Reduction methods

Utilizing open exposures the joint surface needs to be recreated and held temporarily before backfilling any voids with graft material. Laminar spreaders, periosteal elevators and clamps/K-wires are useful to aid and hold reduction (**Figure 18.3**).

Grafting materials

Currently the use of artificial/biological material is gaining popularity due to the avoidance of donor site issues and increased availability of suitable grafting compounds. Commercial materials have structural as well as biological properties, suitable for use in reconstruction of displaced intra-articular fragments.

Stabilization methods

Using the tibialis anterior approach:

- Select an appropriate length of contoured distal tibia plate (distal tip often requires bending to avoid prominence)
- Place the plate extraperiostally on the anteromedial surface of the tibia (**Figure 18.7e**)
- Insert nonlocking screws initially to secure the position of the plate and pull it down against the bone

- Insert any further nonlocking screws as necessary, before locking screws
- The proximal screws in the anteromedial plate can be inserted percutaneously, avoiding the need to extend the surgical incision (**Figure 18.7e**)
- In order to buttress the anterolateral fragment joint fragment, a standard T-plate is utilized (**Figure 18.4**)
- Close tissue layers without tension
- Insert drain as necessary to avoid hematoma formation
- Apply bulky dressing and dorsiwedge type splint, to prevent equinus contracture at the ankle
- Elevate the limb to reduce soft tissue swelling
- Prescribe postoperative antibiotics and DVT prevention in accordance with unit policy

Rehabilitation

Request physiotherapy review and input when surgical wounds are satisfactory:

- Non weight-bearing exercises on injured limb
- Active assisted ankle and subtalar range of motion exercises with the limb iced to reduce swelling and aid in mobilization
- Serial postoperative X-rays to confirm no loss of reduction and progression of union over the following months
- Supervised progressive weight-bearing exercises in conjunction with X-rays and clinical symptom monitoring

Avoiding postoperative complications

- Infection/wound healing problems
  - Staged protocol for fixation
  - Careful soft tissue handling
  - Prescription of antibiotics
  - Tension-free wound closure
  - Avoidance of hematoma formation
- Loss of reduction
  - Thorough review of CT scans with accurate surgical planning and approach
  - Stable fixation of fracture components and grafting of voids as necessary
  - Protected weight-bearing with patient compliance
- Nonunion
  - Avoidance of excessive soft tissue stripping
  - Patient factors:
    - Smoking
    - Steroids
    - Excessive alcoholic consumption
    - Noncompliance with postoperative instructions
- Post-traumatic degenerative change
  - Often determined at the time of original injury, but can be reduced by accurate joint reduction, stable fixation and early active joint motion

Salvage options after failed fracture fixation

Options following the development of post-traumatic arthritic changes include:

- Removal of metal work combined with debridement of osteophytes and distraction with a spanning external fixator
- Total ankle replacement
- Ankle fusion (**Figure 18.11**)

Any such surgery post pilon fixation requires identification of previously used skin incisions, and careful planning of further incisions. This is to limit the increased risks associated with compromised wound healing and infection.

Summary of learning points

- Careful review of CT scans allows further understanding of the fracture configuration and accurate surgical planning
- Checking theater set up and equipment preoperatively allows time saving intraoperatively
- The tibialis anterior approach, respecting the soft tissues, can be used as an utilitarian approach for anterior joint reduction and fracture stabilization
- With fracture comminution and joint depression grafting of voids is advisable to maintain joint reduction

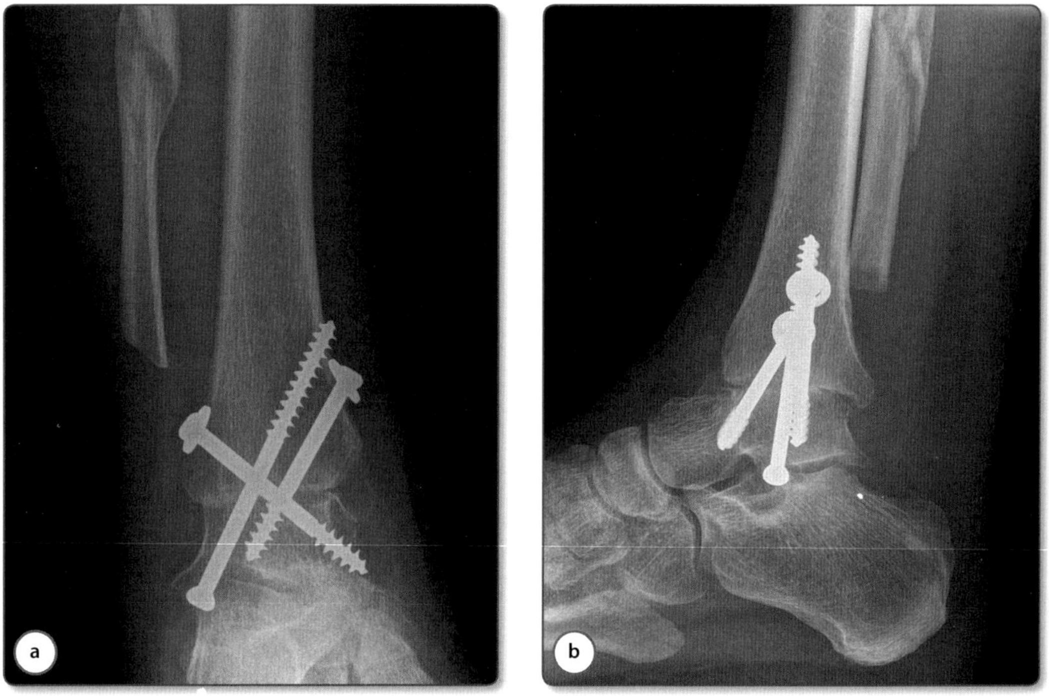

Figure 18.11 (a) Anteroposterior and (b) lateral views of one method of ankle fusion using large fragment partially threaded cancellous screws.

Further reading

Fearon PV, O'Brien PJ. What is the best treatment for pilon fractures? In: Wright JG (Ed). Evidence-based orthopaedics: the best answers to clinical questions. Philadelphia: Saunder/Elsevier, 2009.

Pollack AN, McCarthy ML, Bess RS, Agel J, Swiontkowski MF. Outcomes after treatment of high-energy tibial plafond fractures. J Bone Joint Surg Am 2003; 85-A:1893–1900.

Rüedi TP, Allgöwer M. The operative treatment of intra-articular fractures of the lower end of the tibia. Clin Orthop Relat Res 1979; 138:105–110.

Tarkin IS, Clare MP, Marcantonio A, Pape HC. An update on the management of high-energy pilon fractures. Injury 2008; 39:142–154.

Topliss CJ, Jackson M, Atkins RM. Anatomy of pilon fractures of the distal tibia. J Bone Joint Surg Br 2005; 87:692–697.

Tornetta P III, Gorup J. Axial computed tomography of pilon fractures. Clin Orthop Relat Res 1996; 323:273–276.

19 Ankle fractures

Charlotte Lewis

Introduction

Ankle injuries are among the most common of the bone and joint injuries encountered. The spectrum of injuries ranges from simple stable malleolus injuries to complex fracture dislocations with associated ligamentous involvement.

Incidence

Ankle injuries are common with an estimated incidence of 125/100000/year. Only 1–2% are open injuries. They occur equally in both sexes, affect a wide range of ages but are commoner in young men and old women. The elderly person's osteoporotic fracture is becoming more common. There is increasing concern regarding the failure of fixation in many ankles that are surgically fixed.

Mechanism of injury

The majority of ankle fractures are isolated low energy injuries often as a consequence of a fall. The Lauge-Hansen classification is commonly used as it is based on the mechanism of injury and can help with reduction maneuvers. The initial position of the foot is either supinated or pronated. Supination of the foot places tension on lateral structures of ankle, whereas pronation places tension on medial structures. The deforming force is then either rotational (internal or external) or translational (abduction or adduction)

Initial management/ prioritization

Assuming an isolated injury, the priority is to prevent further injury to the soft tissues and joint and give pain relief. A significantly displaced fracture needs urgent reduction to reduce any compromise to the overlying soft tissue envelope. This can be done in the emergency department using sedation and application of a splint. Ideally radiographs should be taken prior to the reduction to obtain good quality images without artefact from the splint; however, an ankle fracture-dislocation should not be left unreduced or unsupported. Any potential delay for imaging should be avoided and the ankle reduction performed expeditiously. A neurovascular assessment should be performed both before and after reduction, in accordance with BOAST 12 guidelines.

Considerations for surgery

The decision to operate on an ankle fracture rests on whether the ankle fracture is stable or not. Around 75% of ankle fractures at presentation are undisplaced, implying the talus is congruent in the mortice, despite small amounts of displacement of malleolar fragments. Weight bearing stress radiographs (mortise and lateral) are the most useful way of identifying the small number of undisplaced, unstable fractures. Manual or gravity external rotation stress radiographs are also useful in evaluation of deltoid ligament insufficiency. A medial clear space of ≥ 5 mm is compatible with a rupture of the deep deltoid ligament.

The goal of surgical treatment is to restore tibiotalar congruity, hold the fracture reduced till union avoiding potential complications and rehabilitate early.

Even with the increased risk of complications in the elderly or diabetic group, surgical fixation of an unstable ankle still has superior outcomes compared to nonoperative treatment. The advent of minimally invasive techniques such as percutaneous plating or the fibular nail has reduced the need for large wounds and potential wound complications.

Case example: Fracture dislocation of ankle with posterio-medial malleolar involvement

A middle-aged man fell while walking his dog. AP and lateral X-rays on presentation, prior to early reduction in ED, are shown in **Figure 19.1**. The ankle was reduced and placed in a back slab within 30 minutes. The results of a CT scan performed to confirm size and orientation of the medial and posterior malleolar fragments are shown in **Figure 19.2**. Surgical fixation was planned for the next suitable theater list. The patient was positioned supine on a radiolucent table and underwent inter fragmentary compression of the fibula using 2.7 mm screws followed by a third tubular neutralization plate. Medial fixation was undertaken via a posteromedial approach (**Figure 19.3**).

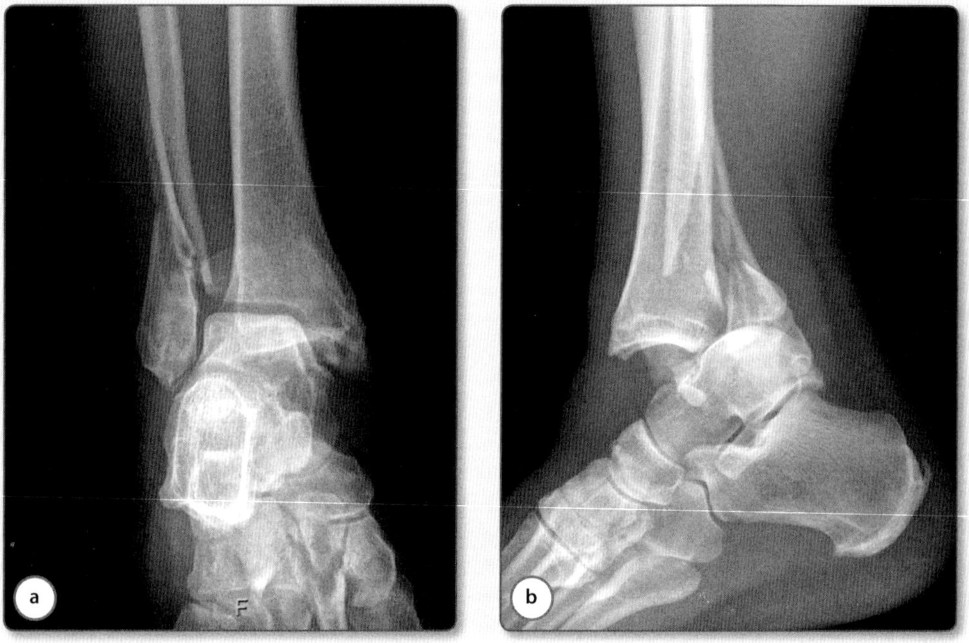

Figure 19.1 (a) Anteroposterior and (b) lateral X-rays of fracture dislocation of ankle.

Theater layout and patient positioning

- Theater setup is shown in **Figure 19.4**
- The patient is placed on a radiolucent table on a block to allow imaging of the ankle in the lateral position without moving the ankle
- A sandbag is placed under the ipsilateral buttock
- A tourniquet is placed on the thigh if utilized
- The limb has a 'social wash' with chlorhexidine and a sterile split sheet is applied above the knee to minimize contamination prior to standard preparation and draping

Review of surgical approaches

Lateral approach

- Identify the distal fibula tip and make an incision at the mid-lateral or posterolateral aspect of fibula, progressing proximally as necessary (**Figure 19.5a**)

Case example: *continued.*

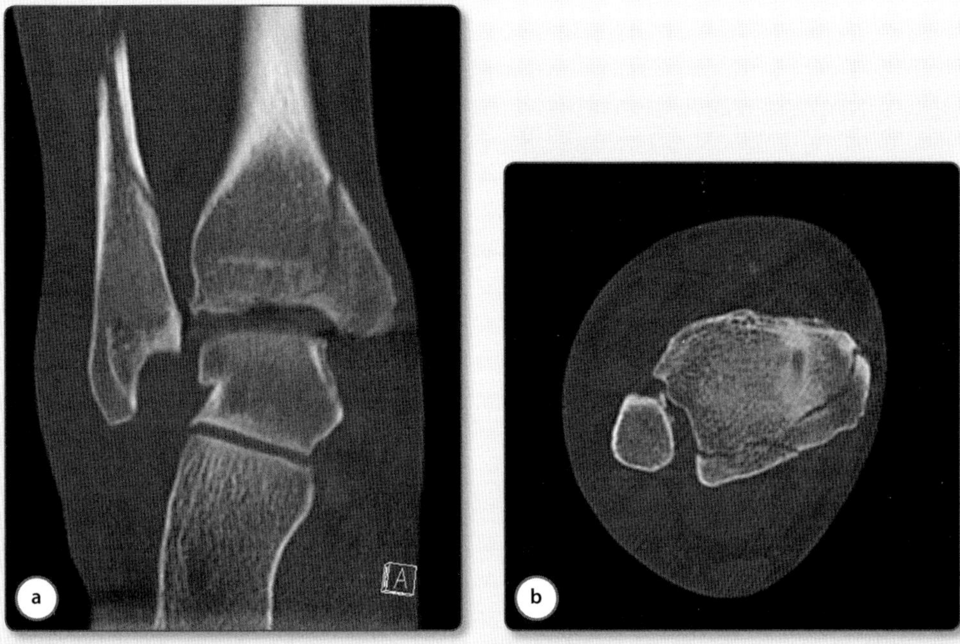

Figure 19.2 (a, b) CT images following reduction of ankle fractures, showing the position of a posterior fragment.

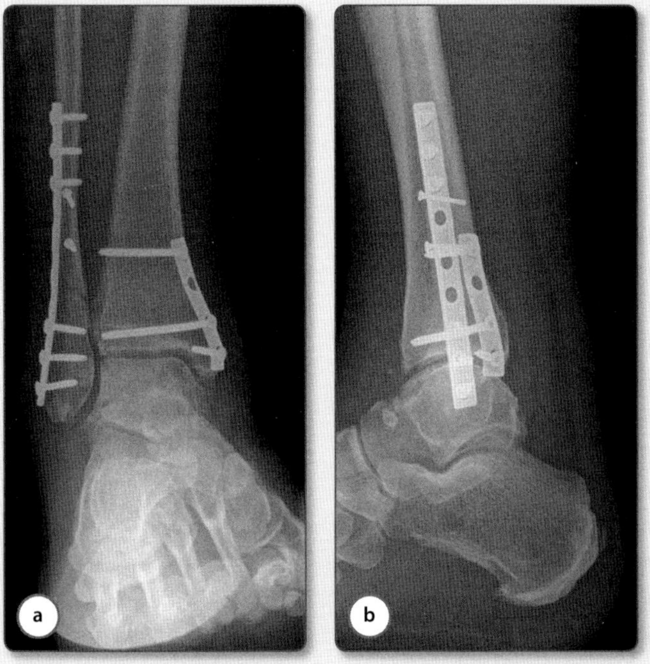

Figure 19.3 (a, b) Postoperative images of the case illustrated in Figure 19.1.

- Pay attention to peroneal tendons posteriorly and the superficial peroneal nerve entering surgical area from a proximal direction. Expose the fibula for surgical stabilization (**Figure 19.5b**)

Medial/anteromedial approach

- A direct medial or anteromedial incision just medial to tibialis anterior is performed (**Figure 19.6a**)
- The saphenous neurovascular structures are identified, protected, and retracted as necessary to allow visualization of the medial malleolar fracture and subsequent reduction and stabilization (**Figure 19.6b**)

Posteromedial approach

- See Chapter 18 (**Figure 18.9**)

Posterolateral approach

- See Chapter 18 (**Figure 18.10**)

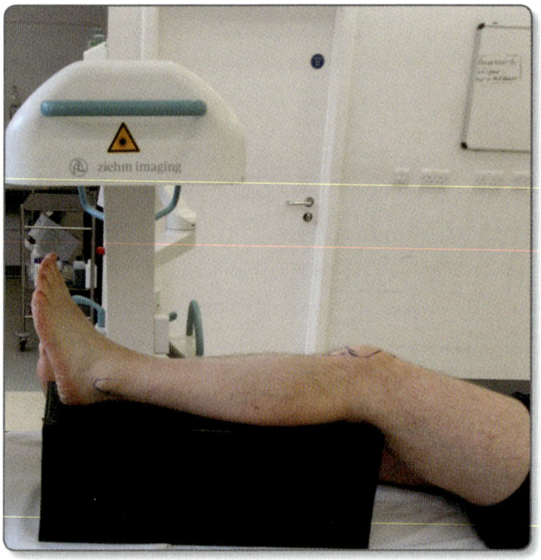

Figure 19.4 (a, b) Theatre setup with image intensifer coming in from opposite direction. Lateral image obtained by rotating C-arm through 90°, avoiding the need to rotate the fractured ankle.

Equipment requirements

- Radiolucent table and block or a theater pack of drapes if the patient is prone
- Thigh tourniquet applied but not inflated
- Small fragment set
- Anatomical locking plates if there are any concerns regarding bone quality
- 2.7 mm/2.4 mm screw set
- Large reduction clamp if syndesmotic injury is suspected, to avoid damage to soft tissues
- Battery drill able to oscillate, a selection of drill bits and a spare battery pack
- Suture anchors

Reduction and stabilization methods

Reduction

- The ankle is reduced, reversing the mechanism of injury

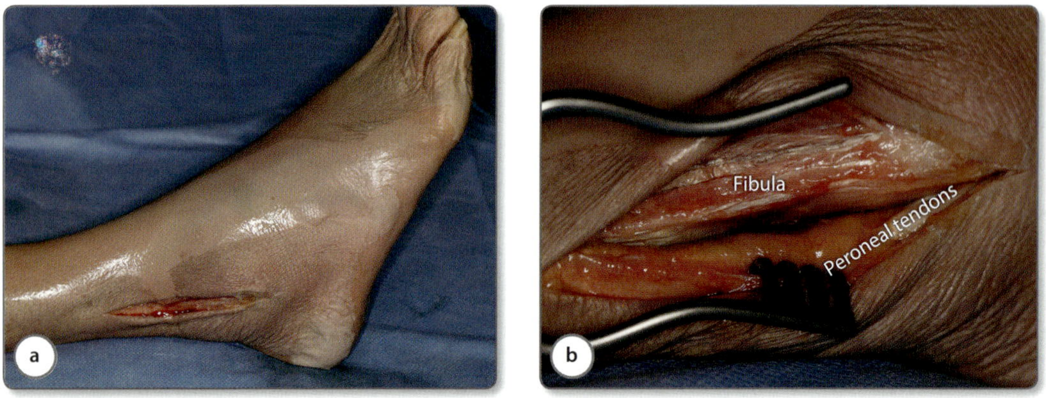

Figure 19.5 (a) Skin incision for lateral approach to distal fibula. (b) Exposure of lateral and posterolateral distal fibula.

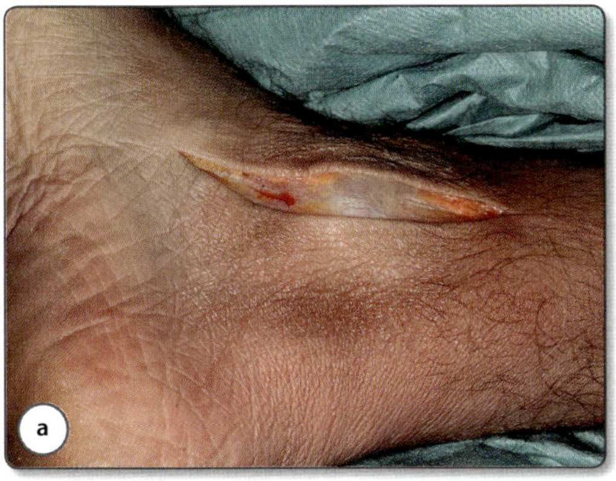
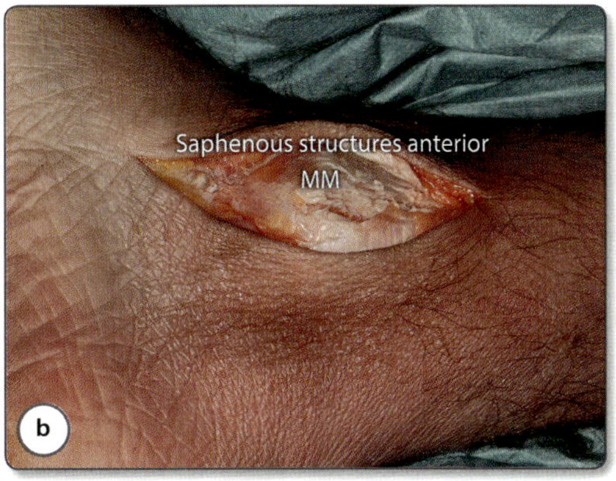

Figure 19.6 (a) Skin incision for medial approach to medial malleolus. (b) Saphenous structures retracted anteriorly for protection prior to exposing medial malleolus.

- Time should be taken using sharp dissection to clear the fracture ends without damaging critical small fragments, allowing interdigitation and confirming anatomical reduction
- Crocodile/pointed clamps either side of the fracture give traction and restore the length of fibula
- Care is required in patients with osteoporotic bone

Stabilization

- Lateral fixation is achieved using lag screws and a neutralization plate if possible
- If small fragments prevent the use of a standard 3.5 mm lag screw, dropping down a size to 2.7 mm or 2.4 mm screws can allow lag screw fixation
- If comminution is present, preventing the use of smaller lag screws, a plate may be used in bridging mode, leaving the fracture undisturbed
- Osteoporotic bones present a further challenge and may require the use of antiglide plates or locking plates
- Fibula nails can be used successfully in both the elderly and younger age group allowing surgical fixation in swollen, blistered ankles, leaving the fracture undisturbed
- In the illustrated case mentioned previously, 2.4 mm lag screws, a neutralization plate to the fibula fracture and a medial buttress plate to the posteromedial fragment were used. A small posterior malleolar fragment less than 25% of the articular surface was reduced and allowed to heal without fixation (**Figure 19.3**)
- Surgical closure
- Ideally deep soft tissue structures should cover the metalwork interrupted deep dermal sutures without tension followed by a continuous nylon to skin is favored by the author. Sterile dressing followed by a supportive back slab, holding the ankle in a neutral position is applied
- The limb is elevated postoperatively and instructions to monitor neurovascular status recorded. Additionally, a standard antibiotic regime and thromboprophylaxis pathway is prescribed

Rehabilitation

- The patient can be sent home the day after surgery on crutches if it is safe to do so
- Review the patient for removal of the backslab and sutures, perform a wound check and take follow-up radiographs 10–14 days post-surgery
- Full weight-bearing in a boot or suitable cast can be allowed if the surgeon is confident with fixation: the use of a boot allows early mobilization of the ankle

20 Os calcis fractures

Nicholas M Desy, Richard E Buckley

Introduction

Fractures of the calcaneus are often challenging and typically require a specialized skill set to manage optimally. The ideal treatment of displaced, intra-articular fractures remains a source of controversy, however several randomized control trials have been performed to help improve treatment algorithms. Minimally invasive techniques are also becoming increasingly common to avoid the soft tissue complications seen with the extensile lateral approach. Foot shape is very important for long-term best outcome.

Incidence

Calcaneus fractures represent 1–2% of all fractures in the human body and the calcaneus is the most common tarsal bone fractured (60% of all tarsal bone fractures). Approximately 75% of calcaneus fractures are intra-articular and 17% are open injuries.

Mechanism of injury

Calcaneus fractures usually occur from a high-energy axial load, often a fall from a height such as in construction workers. Motor vehicle crashes can also lead to fractures of the calcaneus. Associated injuries that also occur from an axial load can present concomitantly, such as pilon, hip and spine fractures. Lower-energy injuries can also occur in elderly patients with osteoporotic bone. Compartment syndrome of the foot is of concern and must be considered with calcaneus fractures.

Initial management/ prioritization

The initial management begins with Advanced Trauma Life Support (ATLS) followed by splinting of the affected extremity and appropriate radiographic assessment. Open fractures require tetanus investigation and urgent antibiotic administration.

Once the patient has been medically stabilized, calcaneus fracture management is planned based on patient characteristics, the soft tissue status and fracture pattern.

Considerations for surgery

Several factors are important to consider when treating calcaneus fractures.

Poor prognostic factors include:

- Older age (> 50 years old)
- Male gender
- Obesity
- Manual laborer
- Patients on worker's compensation
- A history of smoking
- Bilateral calcaneus fractures and patients with vascular disease

Nondisplaced fractures are treated nonoperatively. Displaced extra-articular fractures, such as tongue-type fractures can be treated well with surgery to reduce and stabilize the displaced fragment(s). Displaced intra-articular fractures are also usually treated with surgery (either with full open reduction and internal fixation or minimally invasive reduction with percutaneous fixation). The best outcomes are seen in young, female patients with sedentary jobs. The degree of comminution of the posterior facet is also prognostic and is used to guide treatment.

Initial management of injury

The patient's injured foot is immobilized in a below knee splint for pain control and soft tissue stabilization. Minimally invasive procedures are ideally performed within the first few days from the injury while the fracture fragments haven't commenced healing to allow for ease of fracture mobilization and reduction. This is in contrast to more extensive dissections, such as the extensile lateral approach where it is encouraged to wait for surgery until swelling subsides (usually at least 1–2 weeks) to prevent soft tissue complications.

Case example: Minimally invasive Os calcus treatment

A 53-year-old man presented to the emergency room following a fall from a ladder. The patient was cleared with an ATLS assessment and underwent X-ray examination of his left foot (**Figure 20.1**). A calcaneus fracture was identified and a CT scan was obtained for further characterization of the fracture (**Figure 20.2**). He was positioned lateral on a radiolucent table and, using a minimally invasive approach (**Figure 20.3**), the fracture was reduced and then stabilized with percutaneous fixation (**Figure 20.4**).

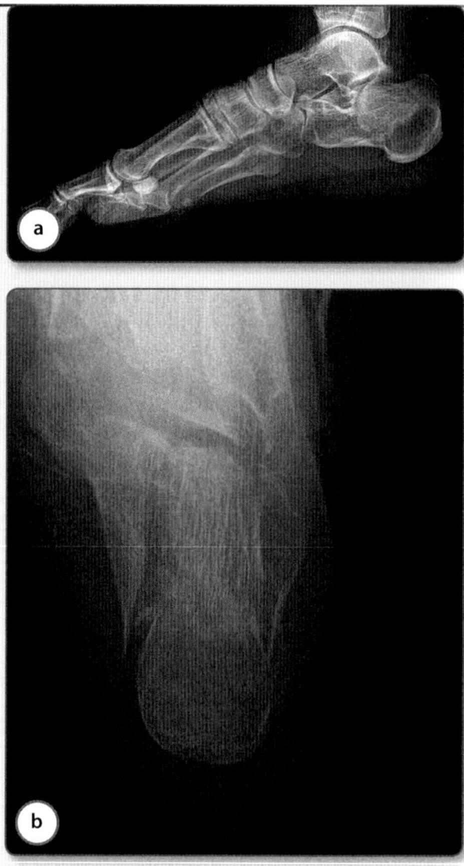

Figure 20.1 (a) Lateral and (b) Harris X-ray views of a calcaneus fracture.

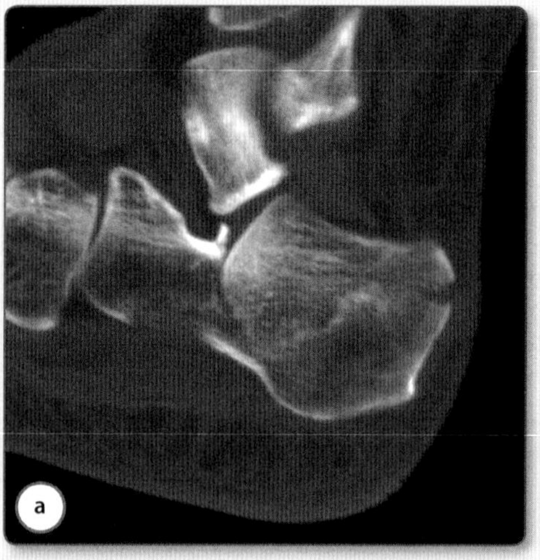

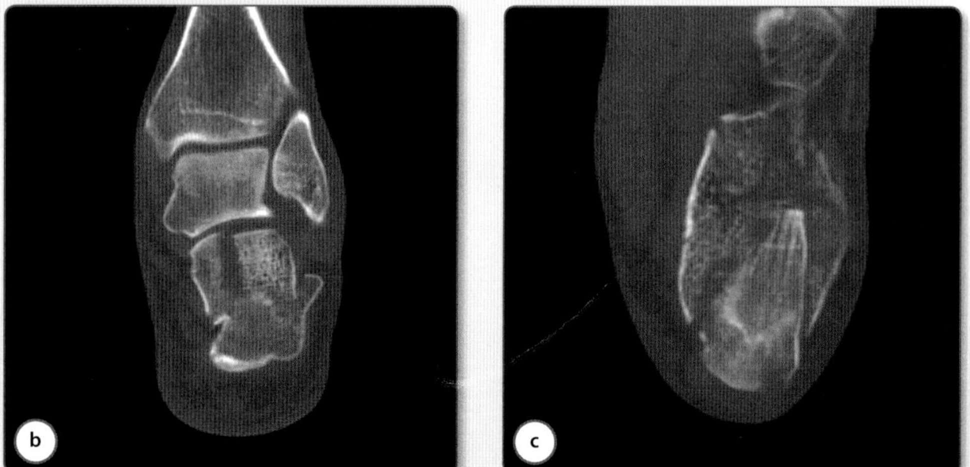

Figure 20.2 Calcaneus fracture. (a) Sagittal view demonstrating a displaced calcaneus fracture with a decreased Bohler's angle and angle of Gissane. (b) Coronal view showing the posterior subtalar joint with a gap along the joint surface. The primary fracture line is also visualized. (c) Axial view indicating widening of the calcaneus.

Case example: *continued.*

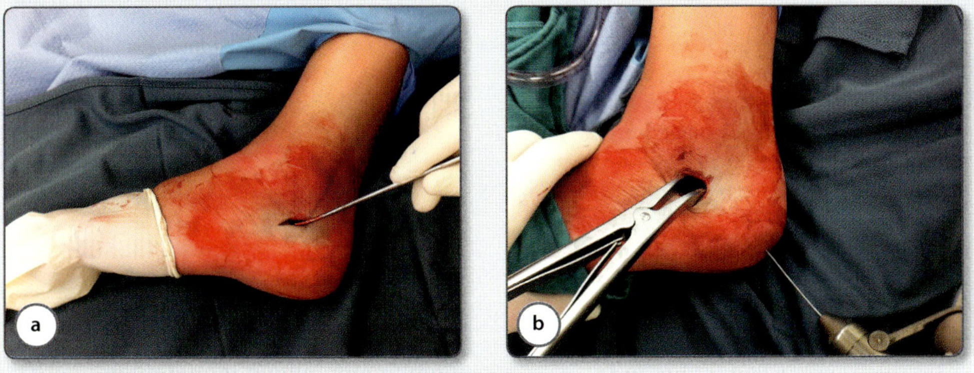

Figure 20.3 Surgical approach for minimally invasive fracture reduction. (a) A small incision is made over the fracture site near the angle of Gissane, and a Howarth or periosteal elevator is used to mobilize the fracture site. (b) A laminar spreader is then placed into the fracture site all the way toward the medial side of the calcaneus. The laminar spreader is spread apart perpendicular to the fracture site for fracture reduction.

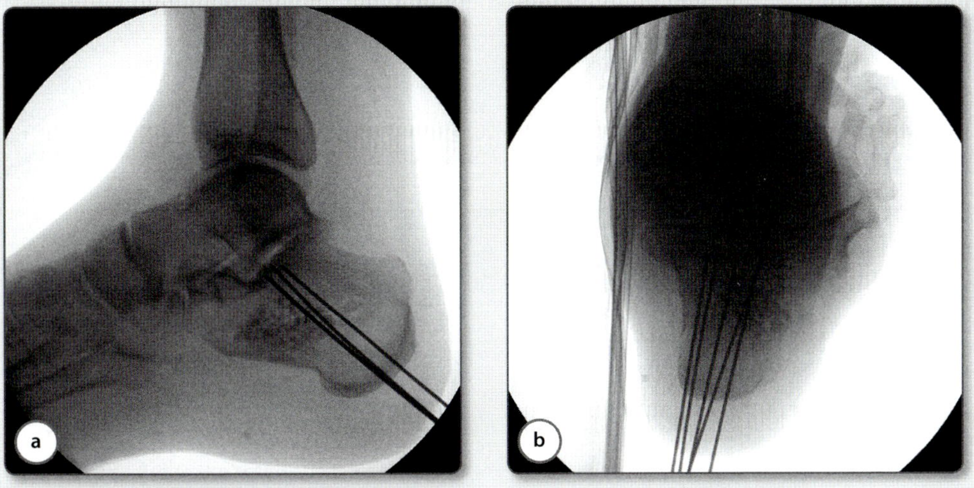

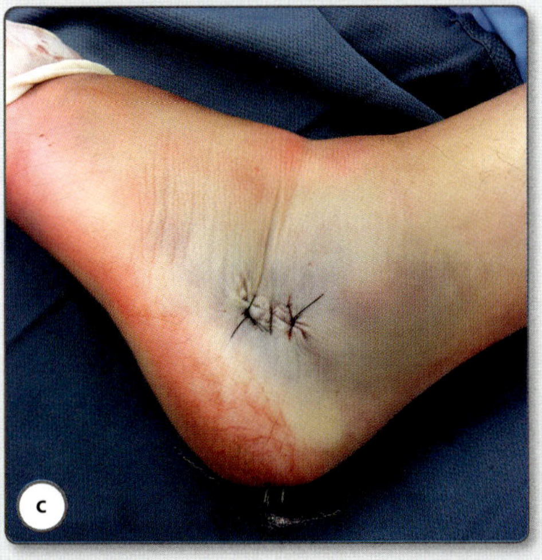

Figure 20.4 (a) Lateral and (b) Harris X-ray views demonstrating final minimally invasive reduction and percutaneous fixation using fully threaded Kirschner wires as well as bone void grafting material. (c) Intraoperative picture showing final wound closure with a 3-0 nylon suture. The Kirschner wires are cut near the skin.

Theater layout and patient positioning

The patient is positioned in the lateral decubitus position on a radiolucent table with a bean bag (**Figure 20.5a**). Placing the patient in slight over-rotation toward the prone position can help internally rotate the leg to allow for easier access to the lateral aspect of the operative foot. A raft/radiolucent block is placed under the affected extremity and a tourniquet is placed around the thigh of the injured leg. Lateral X-rays and Broden views can be taken (**Figure 20.5a, b**).

The image intensifier is positioned to enter at a 45° angle from the patient's front and the leg externally rotated to obtain a Harris view (**Figure 20.5c**).

Review of surgical approaches

The choice of surgical approach will depend on patient factors, soft tissue quality and fracture pattern.

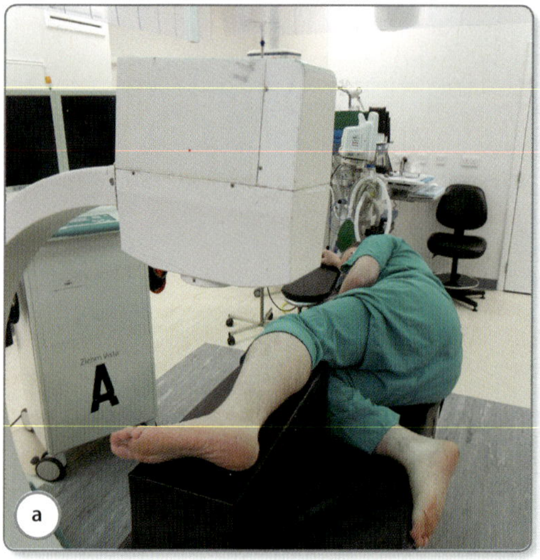

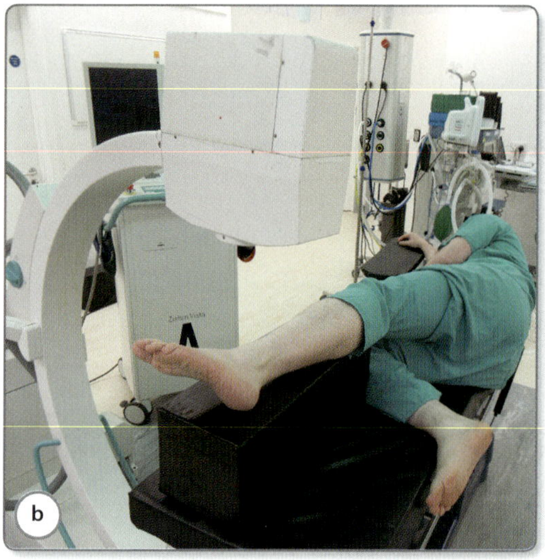

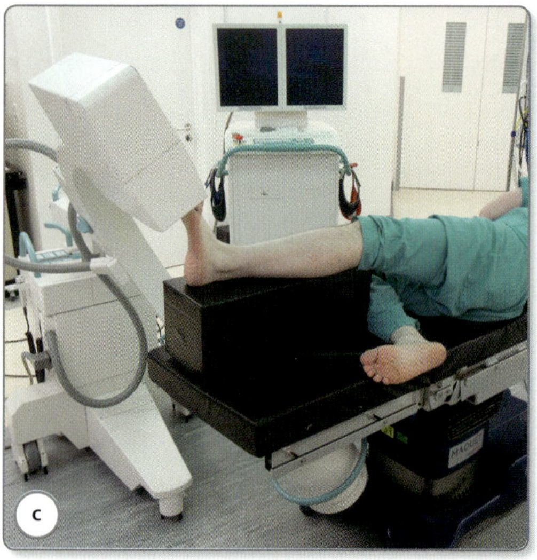

Figure 20.5 (a) Operating room setup and patient positioning. The patient is placed in the lateral decubitus position with the operative extremity on top allowing access for lateral X-ray. (b) Externally rotating leg allows Broden view to be obtained. (c) Harris view obtained by externally rotating the leg and angling the image intensifier by 45°.

Minimally invasive reduction using a lateral approach

- A small straight oblique incision is planned on the lateral aspect of the foot at the fracture site using fluoroscopy, which is typically inferior and posterior to the angle of Gissane
- After the skin and subcutaneous tissues are incised, metzenbaum scissors are used to avoid injuring the sural nerve and peroneal tendons
- The dissection is then carried directly down to bone
- The fracture site is identified and mobilized using a Howarth or periosteal elevator (**Figure 20.3a**)
- A laminar spreader is placed in the fracture site for fracture reduction (**Figure 20.3b**)

Extensile lateral approach

- An L-shaped incision is planned on the lateral aspect of the hindfoot. The horizontal limb is made in line with the 5th metatarsal and the vertical limb is formed between the posterior border of the fibula and the Achilles tendon (**Figure 20.6a**)
- The incision is kept superficial at the most distal and proximal portions of the incision to protect the sural nerve with metzenbaum scissors used for the deeper layers
- The incision in the corner is made directly down to bone to ensure a large full-thickness soft tissue flap
- The scalpel is then used to dissect the flap directly off the lateral calcaneus from distal to proximal until the subtalar joint is adequately visualized. Care must be taken to avoid injuring the peroneal tendons, which should remain in the full-thickness flap with the sural nerve near the subtalar joint
- The fibulocalcaneal and talocalcaneal ligaments are released which then exposes the subtalar joint and sinus tarsi. The subtalar joint capsule is also opened
- Once dissection is complete, 2–3 Kirschner wires are placed in the talus to maintain soft tissue-friendly retraction on the flap
- The lateral wall can now be completely seen and reflected to gain access to the primary and secondary fracture lines and allow for fracture reduction and fixation (**Figure 20.6b**)

Medial approach

The medial approach is typically performed for displaced fractures of the sustentaculum tali.

- A 5-cm incision is made just distal to the medial malleolus toward the navicular that essentially follows the neurovascular structures (**Figure 20.7a**)
- Once through the skin and subcutaneous tissue, the flexor retinaculum is incised which exposes the posterior tibialis tendon along with the posterior tibial artery, tibial nerve and flexor hallucis longus (FHL) tendon. A plane is then created between the neurovascular

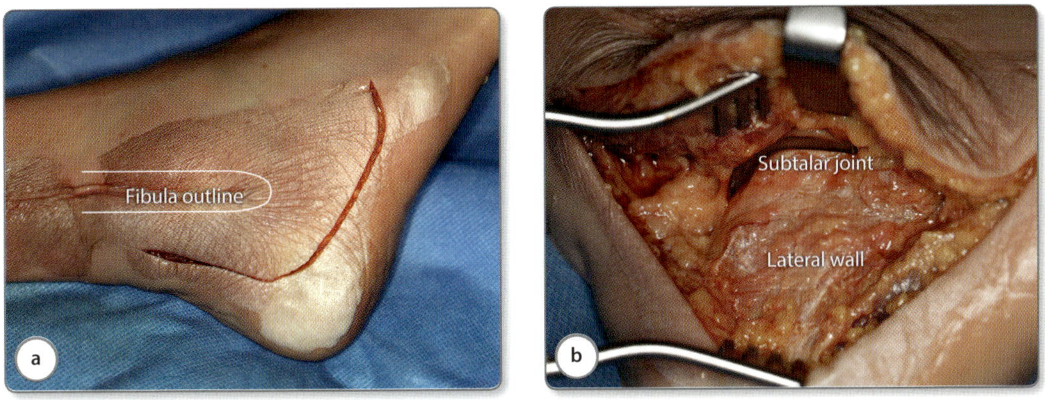

Figure 20.6 (a) Extensile lateral approach skin incision. (b) Full thickness flaps are raised care being taken to elevate the peroneal tendons, allowing access to the lateral wall.

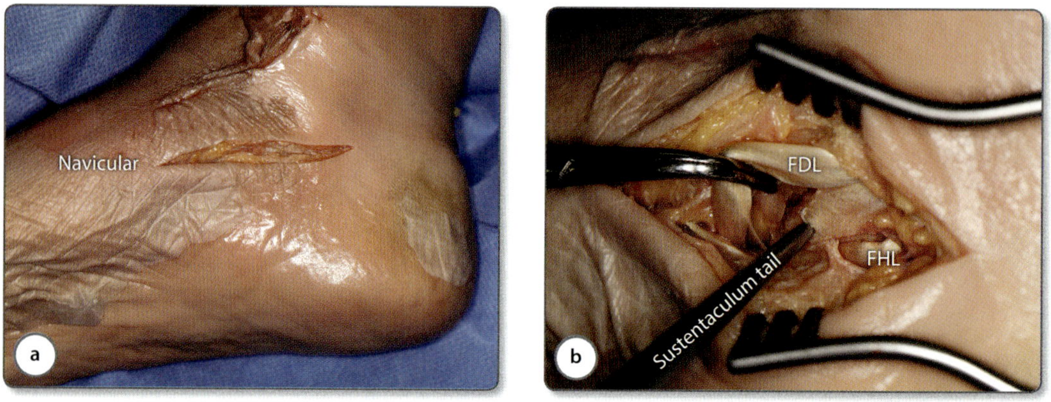

Figure 20.7 (a) Skin incision for medial approach. (b) Following incision of the flexor retinaculum, the tendons are retracted with protection of the neurovascular structures giving access to the sustentaculum tali.

structures and the FHL tendon by retracting the tibial nerve and artery anteriorly and the FHL tendon posteriorly
- The sustentaculum tali is a bony prominence that is immediately identifiable deep to the neurovascular structures (**Figure 20.7b**). Fixation can then be placed directly in to the calcaneus

Foot fasciotomies

- The three-incision technique is most commonly performed for compartment syndrome of the foot with one medial incision and two dorsal incisions (**Figure 20.8**)
- The patient is placed supine on an operating table
- The medial incision is typically 6 cm that runs distally starting at a point that is approximately 4 cm anterior to the posterior aspect of the heel and 3 cm superior to the sole of the foot. This medial incision allows for decompression of the medial and lateral compartments of the foot as well as the superficial and deep central compartments
- The two dorsal incisions are used to decompress the interosseous and adductor compartments. One incision is placed just medial to the 2nd metatarsal and the 2nd incision is formed just lateral to the 4th metatarsal

Equipment requirements

The type of equipment required will depend on the planned surgical procedure and surgeon preference. For a minimally invasive technique, available equipment should include:

- Scalpel and metzenbaum scissors
- Small and large laminar spreaders
- Threaded Kirschner wires
- Grafting material
- Power drill

Additional equipment needed for more extensile medial and lateral approaches:

- Schanz pins
- Nonthreaded Kirschner wires
- Small fragment set
- Foot modular set
- +/– Dedicated lateral calcaneus plates
- Cannulated screws

Reduction and stabilization methods

For a minimally invasive reduction with percutaneous fixation technique:

- Fully threaded Kirschner wires are used to stabilize the reduced posterior facet and tuberosity (**Figure 20.4**)

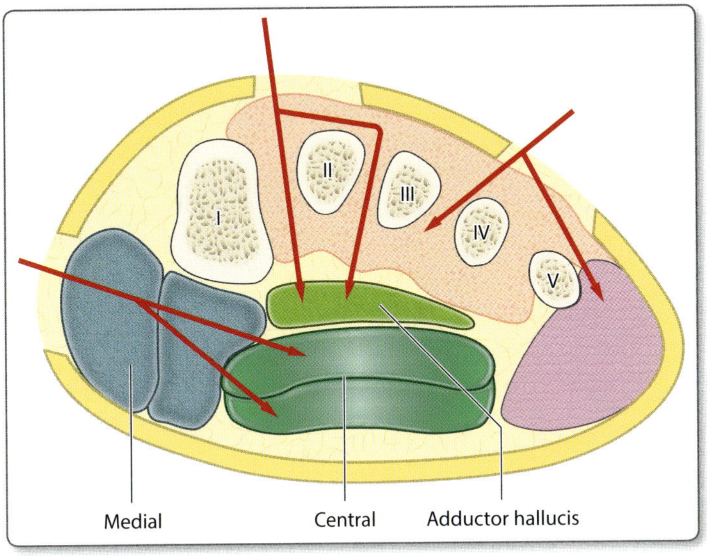

Figure 20.8 Cross-sectional anatomy and proposed skin incisions for foot fasciotomies.

- Place several Kirschner wires (4–6) percutaneously from the posterior aspect of the plantar surface of the foot toward the subchondral bone just under the mid portion of the posterior facet under fluoroscopic guidance
- If further fixation is required, place 2–3 threaded Kirschner wires starting at the mid portion of the calcaneus on the plantar side of the foot heading superior and posterior to the subchondral bone of the posterior facet under fluoroscopic guidance
- Place bone grafting material in to the bone void for further support for the posterior facet and to promote bone healing (**Figure 20.4**)
- Close the small lateral wound
- Cut the Kirschner wires so that a small portion of each wire is sticking outside the skin
- Place a bulky dressing over the wound and Kirschner wires
- Encourage leg elevation and motion to diminish soft tissue swelling

Grafting materials

Several different grafting materials can be used to help treat the large bone void that is typically present after open reduction and internal fixation of calcaneus fractures.

To avoid donor site morbidity, cancellous allograft, tricalcium phosphate or calcium sulfate can be used as a bone void filler (**Figure 20.4**).

Rehabilitation

- The patient remains nonweight bearing for 12 weeks followed by progressive weight bearing
- Range-of-motion exercises can be encouraged 1–2 days postoperatively
- For an extensile lateral approach, close wound monitoring is necessary due to the high complication rate
- Threaded Kirschner wires are removed at 12 weeks postoperatively and full weight bearing is initiated
- Further follow-up is continued to observe for post-traumatic subtalar arthritis.

Avoiding postoperative complications

Wound dehiscence or infection

- Use of minimally invasive techniques
- Wait at least 1–2 weeks for soft tissue stabilization before extensile approaches

- Careful soft tissue handling during the extensile lateral approach
- Adequate wound closure
- Factors that increase wound complications include:
  - Smoking history
  - Diabetics
  - Open injuries

Malunion

- Adequate restoration of calcaneal shape including length, height, width and valgus alignment
- Stable fixation and use of grafting material in large bone voids
- Plantar threaded Kirschner wires to avoid patient noncompliance with non-weight-bearing instructions

Post-traumatic subtalar arthritis

- Accurate posterior facet reduction and stable fixation
- Protected weight bearing and early range of motion
- Often difficult to prevent with displaced fractures with severe comminution of the posterior facet, in which case a primary subtalar fusion is sometimes necessary for Sanders IV fractures

Flexor hallucis longus tendon damage

- Avoid excessively long lateral to medial screws as the tendon travels under the sustentaculum tali

Salvage options after failed fracture fixation

Options are reserved for the treatment of post-traumatic subtalar arthritis.

In situ subtalar arthrodesis (Figure 20.9)

- For patients with subtalar arthritis and normal calcaneal shape

Distraction bone block subtalar arthrodesis (Figure 20.10)

- For patients with subtalar arthritis and calcaneal malunion: patients typically have symptoms and signs of anterior ankle impingement such as anterior ankle pain and limited ankle dorsiflexion

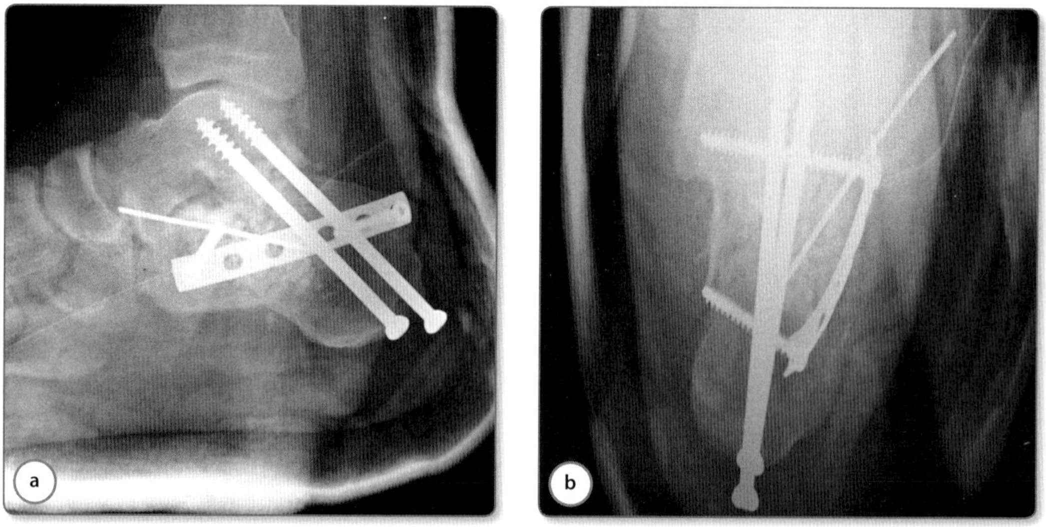

Figure 20.9 (a) Lateral and (b) Harris X-ray views of an in situ subtalar arthrodesis using cannulated partially threaded cancellous screws in a patient who developed subtalar arthritis with a normal calcaneus shape.

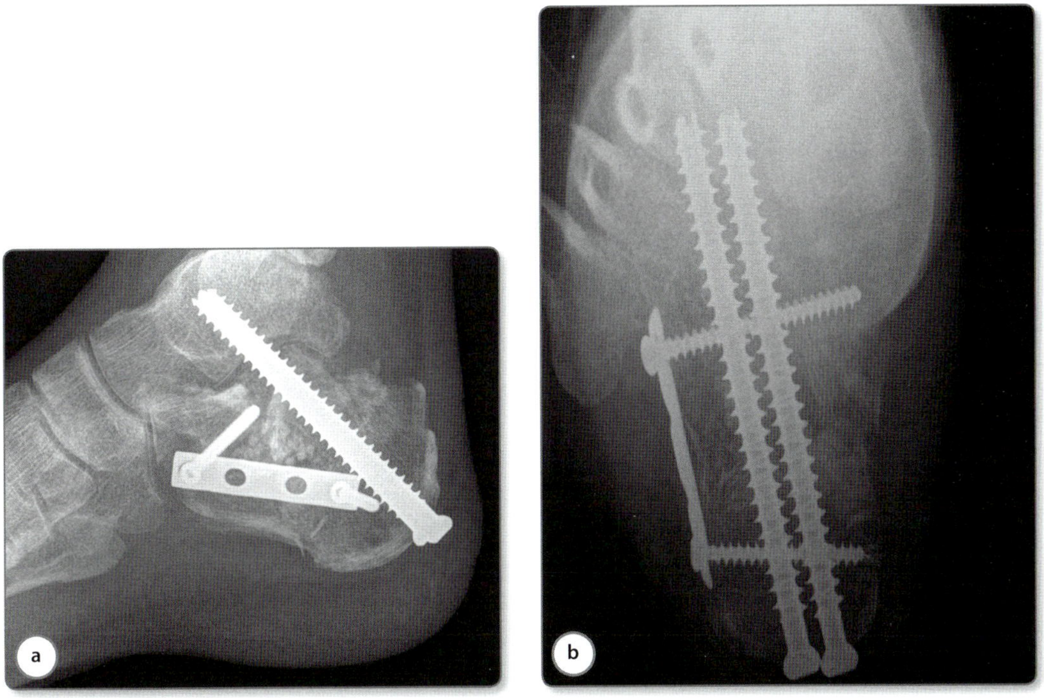

Figure 20.10 (a) Lateral and (b) Harris X-ray views of a distraction bone block subtalar arthrodesis in a patient who developed subtalar arthritis and symptoms of ankle impingement due to abnormal calcaneus shape.

Summary of learning points

- The ideal treatment of displaced, intra-articular calcaneus fractures remains controversial
- Percutaneous operations are becoming increasingly utilized for extra-articular and minimally comminuted intra-articular fractures
- Contrary to extensile exposures, percutaneous procedures should be done early after the injury while the bony fragments remain mobile for ease of reduction
- Restoration of calcaneal shape (length, height, width and valgus alignment) should be the primary goal with accurate posterior facet reduction as a secondary goal
- Grafting materials can be used safely for large bone voids to aid in the maintenance of fracture reduction and stabilization

Further reading

Ågren P-H, Mukka S, Tullberg T, et al. Factors affecting long-term treatment results of displaced intraarticular calcaneal fractures: a post hoc analysis of a prospective, randomized, controlled multicenter trial. J Orthop Trauma 2014; 28:564–568.

Buch BD, Myerson MS, Miller SD. Primary subtaler arthrodesis for the treatment of comminuted calcaneal fractures. Foot Ankle Int 1996; 17:61–70.

Buckley R, Leighton R, Sanders D, et al. Open reduction and internal fixation compared with ORIF and primary subtalar arthrodesis for treatment of Sanders type IV calcaneal fractures: a randomized multicenter trial. J Orthop Trauma 2014; 28:577–583.

Buckley R, Tough S, McCormack R, et al. Operative compared with nonoperative treatment of displaced intra-articular calcaneal fractures: a prospective, randomized, controlled multicenter trial. J Bone Joint Surg Am 2002; 84:1733–1744.

Carr JB. Surgical Treatment of intra-articular calcaneal fractures: a review of small incision approaches. J Orthop Trauma 2005; 19:109–117.

Griffin D, Parsons N, Shaw E, et al. Operative versus non-operative treatment for closed, displaced, intra-articular fractures of the calcaneus: randomised controlled trial. BMJ 2014; 349:g4483.

Sanders R, Fortin P, Dipasquale T, Walling A. Operative treatment in 120 displaced intra-articular calcaneal fractures: results using a prognostic computed tomography scan classification. Clin Orthop Relat Res 1993; 290:87–95.

Sanders R, Vaupel ZM, Erdogan M, Downes K. Operative treatment of displaced intraarticular calcaneal fractures: long-term (10-20 years) results in 108 fractures using a prognostic CT classification. J Orthop Trauma 2014; 28:551–563.

Sivakumar BS, Wong P, Dick CG, et al. Arthroscopic reduction and percutaneous fixation of selected calcaneus fractures: surgical technique and early results. J Orthop Trauma 2014; 28:569–576.

Wallin KJ, Cozzetto D, Russell L, et al. Evidence-based rational for percutaneous fixation technique of displaced intra-articular calcaneal fractures: a systematic review of clinical outcomes. J Foot Ankle Surg 2014; 53:740–743.

21 Complex foot fractures

Faiz Shivji, Ben J Ollivere

Introduction

Amongst the injuries sustained in the foot fractures of the talar neck or body, navicular, and tarsometatarsal (TMT) (Lisfranc) joint are the most difficult to treat. The uncommon nature of such injuries can make decision making challenging. It is essential to maintain the normal load transfer mechanisms within the foot, and these injuries can carry with them significant morbidity. The talus has no tendon attachments, and is responsible for transfering loads from the foot to the rest of the apendicular skelton, whilst the navicular and Lisfranc joints are essential in maintaining the arches.

Incidence

Fractures of the talus and navicular are rare, accounting for less than 1% of all fractures. Whilst the spectrum of Lisfranc injuries accounts for only 0.2% of fractures. These injuries are commonly seen in the multiply injured trauma patient and occur with high energy.

Mechanism of injury

Talar neck fractures result from forced hyperdorsiflexion of the ankle at high energy causing impaction of the talar neck on the tibial plafond. Navicular fractures are often caused by significant axial loading of the foot. Hence, these injuries are associated with road traffic accidents or falls from height. A fall into a plantar flexed foot will tend to result in a midfoot or talus fracture where a fall onto neutral or dorsiflexed foot will result in a calcaneal or pilon fracture.

TMT injuries may be caused by a direct crush flattening the arch; usually seen in industrial workplaces, twisting with axial load during sporting activities leading to forced abduction of the forefoot on the tarsus, or axial loading of a fixed foot during high energy trauma.

Initial management/ prioritization

Advanced Trauma Life Support assessment must be conducted for those involved in high energy trauma. Soft tissue condition must be noted and open fractures managed accordingly. Splintage in a below knee backslab with a foot pump may expedite the reduction of swelling, and prevent equinus contractures. Compartment syndrome is common in fracture dislocations of the forefoot although management is controversial it undoubtedly compromises outcome and rapid reduction and elevation will reduce the incidence.

Considerations for surgery

For all complex foot fractures, the soft tissue envelope requires careful assessment, and definitive fixation should be delayed until swelling has decreased, even though this may take up to 2 weeks. However, fracture dislocations of the talus or navicular require urgent reduction and fixation. In the face of compromised soft tissues, closed reduction and temporary stabilization with buried K-wires or external fixator may effect and maintain reduction allowing swelling to subside. CT imaging is essential for surgical planning. The aims of surgery are to prevent progressive deformity, instability, and arthritis. Where there is diagnostic difficulty (such as in a Lisfranc ligament injury) a weight-bearing axial and lateral film of the foot will yield valuable information about the integrity of the ligamental structures. This may be supplemented by examination under anesthesia with radiographic control.

Theater layout and patient positioning

- The patient is best positioned supine with a thigh or calf tourniquet

Case example: Displaced talar neck fracture

A young man crashed his bicycle into a tree sustaining an ankle injury. A lateral X-ray (**Figure 21.1**) demonstrates an isolated talar neck fracture. In order to gain better access to reduce the medial fracture component, a medial malleolar osteotomy was undertaken, in addition to a standard lateral approach. Working through both approaches simultaneously allowed rotation and alignment to be corrected before the talus was stabilized with lateral plating and a medial partially threaded cancellous screw (**Figure 21.2**).

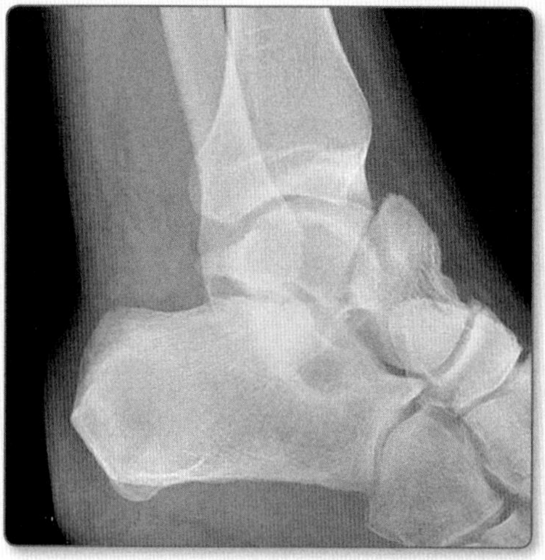

Figure 21.1 Lateral X-ray of talar neck fracture.

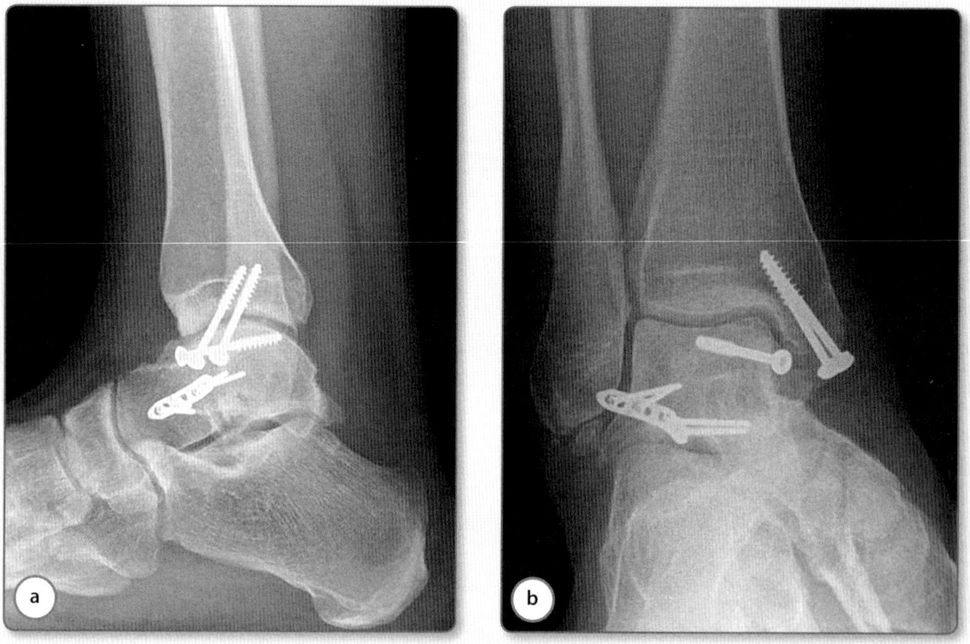

Figure 21.2 (a) Lateral postoperative X-ray. (b) AP postoperative X-ray of medial malleolus osteotomy stabilised with two partially threaded cancellous screws. Lateral 2.7 mm plate and small fragment screw medially.

- A radiolucent table should be used
- Use of a sandbag under the ipsilateral buttock can be useful to hold the foot in neutral, and positioning the patient with the ankles at the end of the table can aid surgical access
- Radiographs are best taken in a 'simulated standing view' with hips and knees flexed (over a supportive triangle as demonstrated) allowing for a weight-bearing anteroposterior (AP) to be taken with the foot flat against an operating table support (**Figure 21.3**)

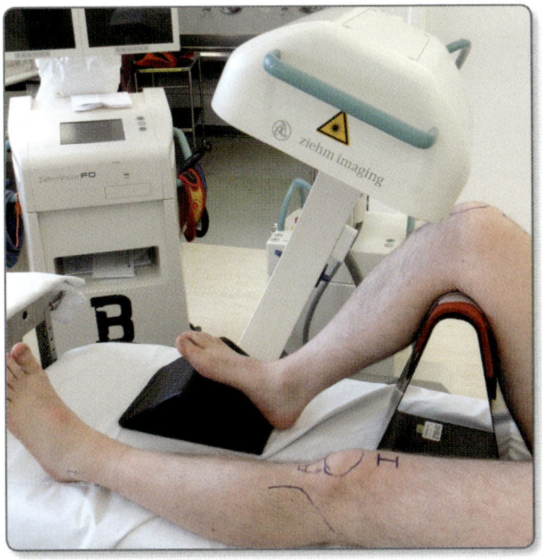

Figure 21.3 Proposed surgical set-up on a radiolucent table.

Review of surgical approaches

Approaches to the talus

The anterior approach to the talus risks disrupting the mains sources of blood supply to the head of the talus, and therefore should be avoided at all costs. Most talus fractures require a dual approach to reduce and fix the fracture. We would recommend anteromedial and anterolateral approaches. A medial malleolus osteotomy is often required to gain access to the talar body.

Anteromedial approach to the talus

- A 5–10 cm longitudinal incision starting anterior to the tip of the medial malleolus and extending distally between the tendons of tibialis anterior and tibialis posterior can be utilized (**Figure 21.4a**). Protect the long saphenous vein and nerve
- Incise the anterior joint capsule to expose the medial side of the talus
- This approach can be extended to include a medial malleolus osteotomy
- A chevron osteotomy can be carefully performed entering the joint at the crural angle (**Figure 21.4b**). Pre-drilling is described; however, we have never found it to be necessary, and a hindrance to obtaining adequate compression following fracture
- The osteotomy should be achieved with small hand osteotomes (Lambottes are ideal) taking care not to injury the tibialis posterior tendon
- The final portion of the osteotomy should be fractured by levering on the subchondral osteotomes to avoid loss of cartilage
- The talus can be exposed by rotating the medial malleolus on the deltoid ligament maintaining the blood supply (**Figure 21.4c**)

Anterolateral approach to the talus

- A 5–10 cm incision starting at the level of the ankle joint, 2 cm anterior to fibula. Curve the incision anteriorly, aiming for the base of the 4th metatarsal (**Figure 21.5a**). Protect the superficial peroneal nerve
- Retract the peroneus tertius tendon laterally, and extensor digitorum tendons medially. The fat in the sinus tarsi will need excising. Incise the joint capsule overlying the talus to expose the lateral aspect (**Figure 21.5b**)

Approaches for tarsometatarsal injuries

- Depending on the exact fracture configuration, a combination of dorsomedial and dorsal approaches will be required for TMT injuries
- For base of 2nd and 3rd metatarsal fracture dislocations, a longitudinal dorsal incision between the 2nd and 3rd metatarsal should be used. These can be located radiographically or via the common extensor tendons. This places the incision lateral to the dorsalis pedis artery and deep peroneal nerve, however when the joint is dislocated the artery can be drawn into the wound and care is required

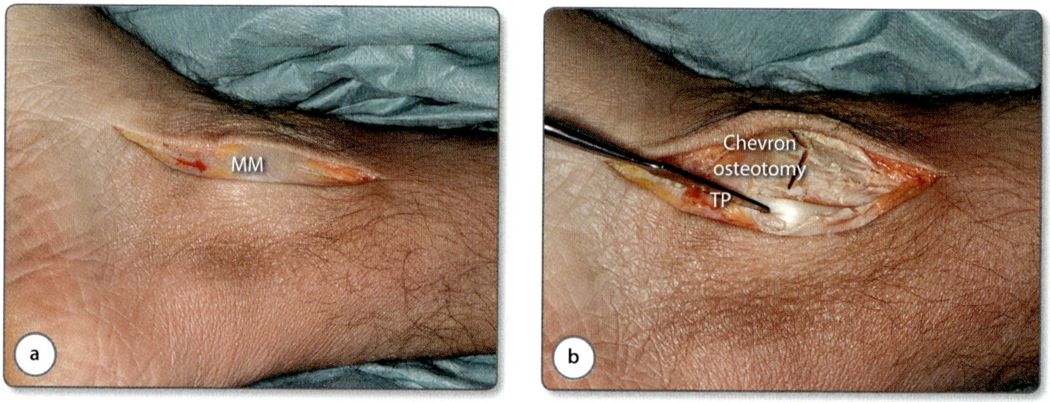

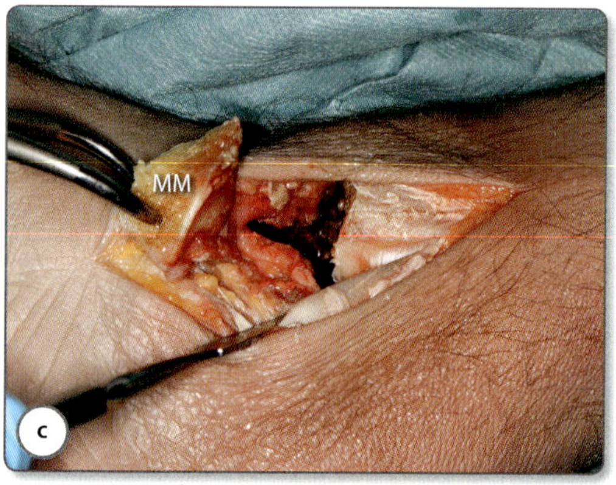

Figure 21.4 (a) Medial based incision over medial malleolus. (b) Inverted chevron osteotomy created with protection of tibialis posterior (TP). (c) Rotating medial malleolus on deltoid ligament gives access to medial surface of talus.

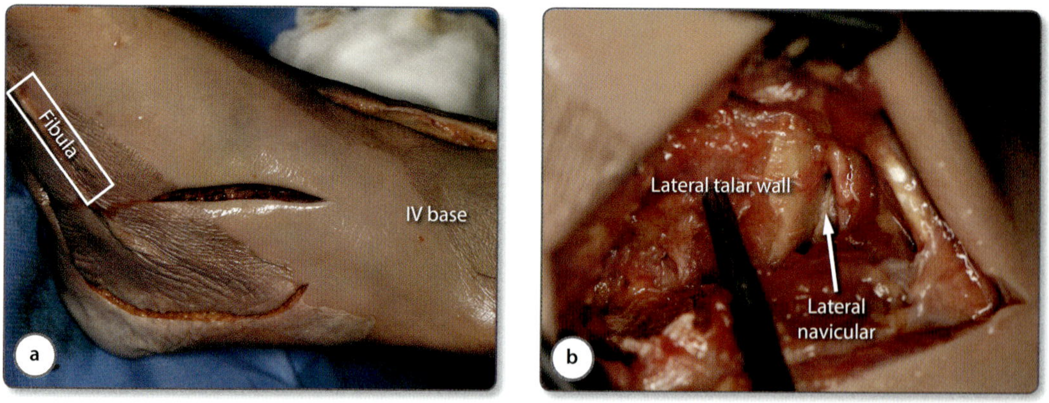

Figure 21.5 (a) Skin incision for the lateral approach to talus. (b) Retraction of peroneus tertius tendon laterally, and extensor digitorum tendons medially exposes the lateral aspect of the talus.

Dorsomedial approach to the first tarsometatarsal joint

- Dorsomedial incision over the first TMTJ can be extended proximally to the talar neck and distally to the metatarsal. The incision is centered over extensor hallucis longus (EHL) (**Figure 21.6a**). The insertion of tibialis anterior lies within the wound and must be preserved

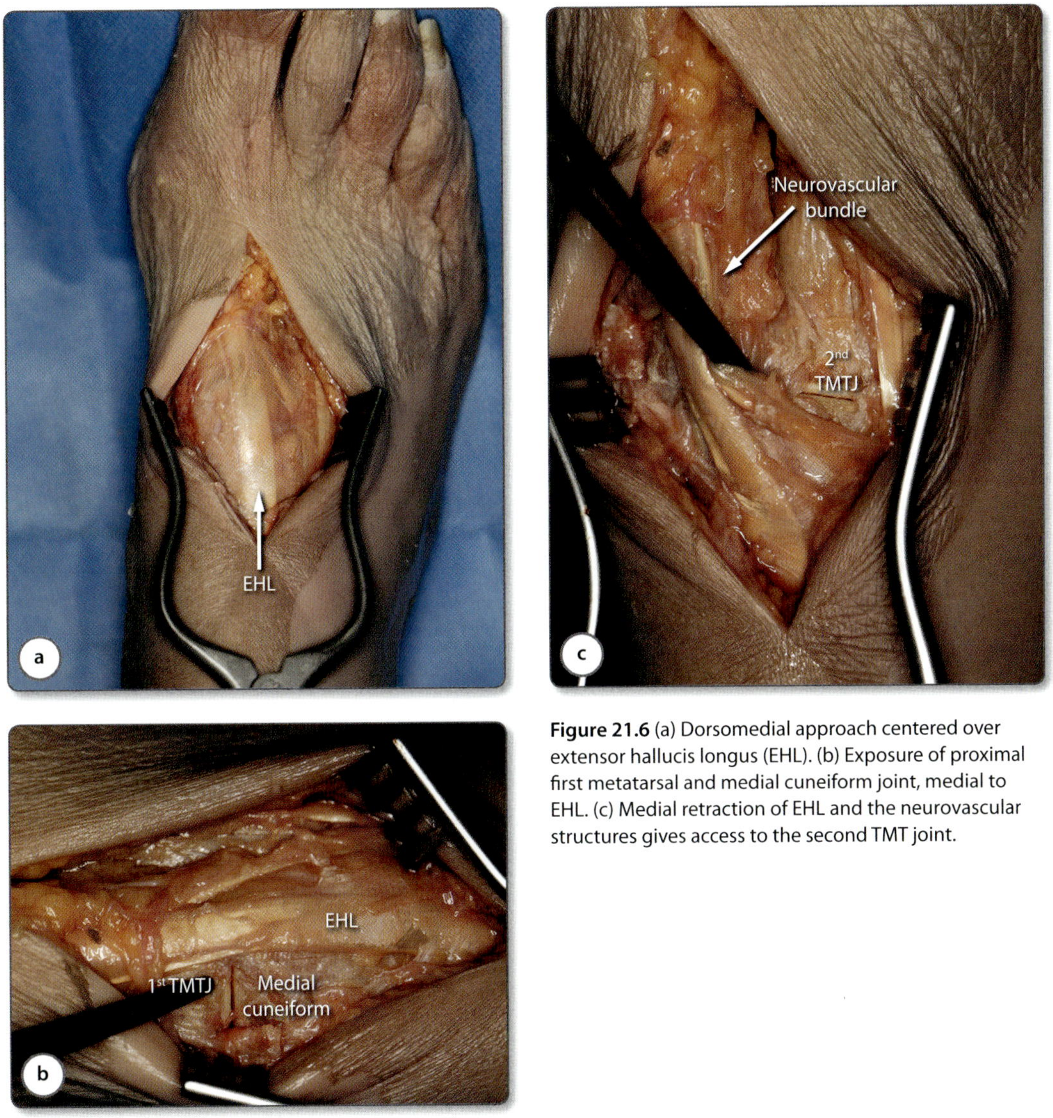

Figure 21.6 (a) Dorsomedial approach centered over extensor hallucis longus (EHL). (b) Exposure of proximal first metatarsal and medial cuneiform joint, medial to EHL. (c) Medial retraction of EHL and the neurovascular structures gives access to the second TMT joint.

- Incise straight to bone, medial to EHL to expose the proximal first metatarsal and medial cuneiform (**Figure 21.6b**). Visualize first TMTJ to enable adequate reduction. The EHL tendon including the neurovascular structures can be retracted medially allowing access to the second TMT joint (**Figure 21.6c**)

Dorsal approach to the second – fourth tarsometatarsal joints

- Dorsal incision between the bases of the 2nd and 3rd metatarsals or the 3rd and 4th
- Sharp dissection through extensor digitorum brevis. Whilst sharp dissection of joint capsule may be required usually in the case of fracture the disruption of the soft tissues is significant and it is easy to expose the fracture without formal dissection

Equipment requirements

- Mini fragment sets with 2–2.7 mm plates and screws for TMTJ fixation. Locking options preferable

- Small fragment set (3.5 mm screws) for talus fixation
- 1.6 mm Kirschner wires
- Reduction clamps
- Saw for medial malleolus osteotomy
- Image intensifier
- Laminar spreader to aid reduction and exposure

Reduction and stabilization methods

Talar fractures

Anteromedial and anterolateral approaches provide good exposure for talar neck fractures, and may be used in combination to check anatomical reduction on both sides. The anteromedial approach also allows the anterior subtalar joint to be checked for adequate reduction via an incision through the deltoid ligament, whilst the anterolateral approach allows the posterior subtalar joint to be checked.

A femoral distractor with pins inserted into the tibia and calcaneus may be useful to improve visibility and aid reduction. K-wires can be used to temporarily hold reduction or joystick fragments into position. Talus fractures are commonly fixed with positional or lag screws. Neck and anterior body fractures can be fixed using one screw from the anteromedial and anterolateral side which converge. Countersink all screws to prevent impingement, or use headless screws. In the more severe injuries plating may be preferable and achieved with either a locking plate or angle blade plate (**Figure 21.2**).

Non-weight-bearing is recommended for 6 weeks, followed by partial weight-bearing for 6 weeks.

The Hawkins sign (subchondral lucency on the mortise ankle radiograph) at 6 weeks postoperative can indicate continued vascularity of the talus.

Tarsometatarsal injuries

If the first TMTJ is subluxed and requires stabilization, a dorsomedial approach with medial plate fixation should be used. The reduction can be maintained temporarily using a 1.6 mm K-wire and maintained with a 2.7 mm LCP plate. The second TMTJ reduction can be achieved using a reduction clamp with one limb placed in the screw hole of the first TMTJ plate, and the other around the base of the 2nd metatarsal. This can be held using a K-wire. For plantar displaced fractures traction is often required and a Howarth distractor can be used to reduce the fracture from the plantar aspect of the foot.

Fixation will vary by fracture type, but the use of dorsal low profile plates has become more common place and primary fusion of the second MTP joint has been shown in some studies to improve postoperative outcomes (**Figure 21.7**). Due to the mobile nature of the 4th and 5th metatarsals rigid fixation is best avoided and Kirshner wire stabilisation is satisfactory.

Rehabilitation

- Advise strict elevation of the limb for 10–14 days postoperatively
- Check that the wounds are healing satisfactorily after 2 weeks
- Serial X-rays should be taken at 2, 6, and 12 weeks to confirm union
- Supervised physiotherapy and progression of weight-bearing with clinical union

Avoiding postoperative complications

- Ensure soft tissue swelling has settled before fixation
- Take CT scans to plan the approach and fixation method
- Avoid developing large skin flaps
- Judicious tissue handling is essential
- Anatomic reduction
- Consider primary fusion in significantly comminuted or purely ligamentous TMT injuries.
- Apply venous thromboprophylaxis
- Prescribe postoperative antibiotics
- Ensure patient compliance with protected weight-bearing

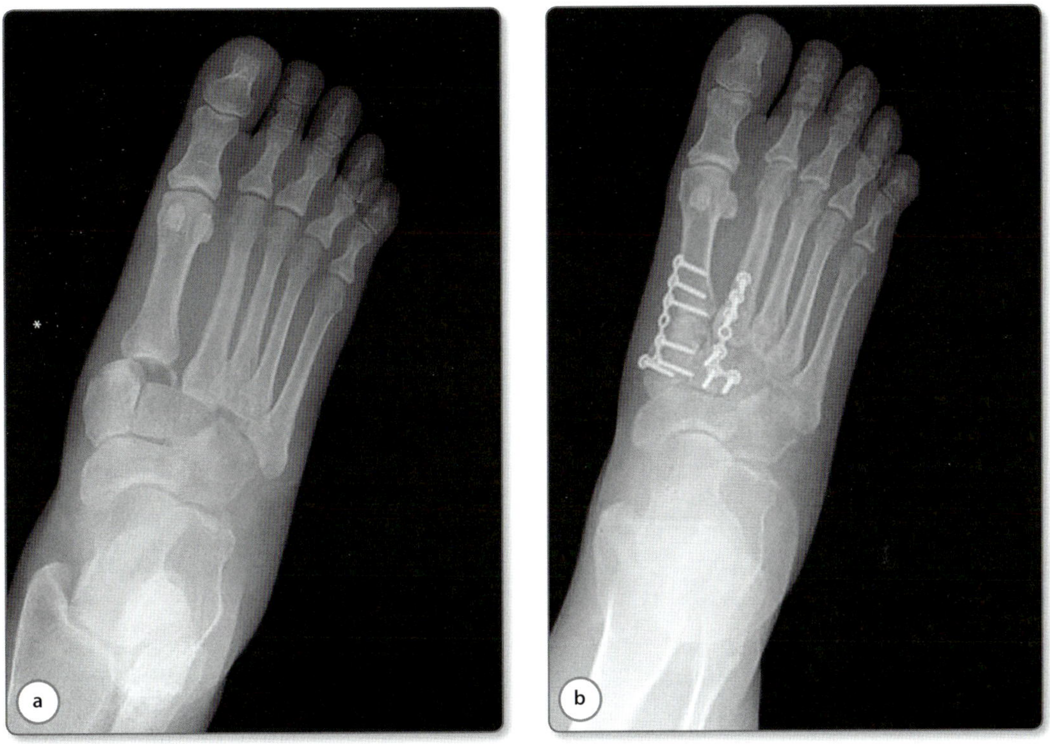

Figure 21.7 (a) Anteroposterior (AP) X-ray of Lisfranc injury. (b) Postoperative AP X-ray of a case treated by low profile dorsal plating with screws avoiding the articular surfaces.

Salvage options after failed fracture fixation

- If there is suspicion of avascular necrosis (AVN) of the talus, MRI is useful for diagnosis
- Significant talar AVN or post-traumatic ankle/hindfoot/midfoot arthritis is treated with arthrodesis procedures
- AVN of the talus may be asymptomatic: conservative management may on occasion be appropriate

Summary of learning points

- Careful history and clinical examination necessary to avoid missing these often subtle injuries
- High index of suspicion for ligamentous mid foot injuries – look for plantar bruising
- Careful review of CT and MRI scans to avoid missing these injuries
- Understanding the 3D anatomy of the mid foot for surgical planning
- Refer to appropriate specialist colleague if not familiar with clinical case management

Further reading

Cronier P, Talha A, Massin P. Central talar fractures--therapeutic considerations. Injury 2004; 35:SB10–22.

Hawkins LG. Fractures of the neck of the talus. J Bone Joint Surg Am 1970; 52:991–1002.

Ly TV, Coetzee JC. Treatment of primarily ligamentous Lisfranc joint injuries: primary arthrodesis compared with open reduction and internal fixation. A prospective, randomized study. J Bone Joint Surg Am 2006; 88:514–520.

Mulfinger GL, Trueta J. The blood supply of the talus. J Bone Joint Surg Br 1970; 52:160–167.

Myerson MS, Fisher RT, Burgess AR, Kenzora JE. Fracture dislocations of the tarsometatarsal joints: end results correlated with pathology and treatment. Foot Ankle 1986; 6:225–242.

Stavlas P, Roberts CS, Xypnitos FN, Giannoudis PV. The role of reduction and internal fixation of Lisfranc fracture-dislocations: a systematic review of the literature. Int Orthop 2010; 34:1083–1091.

22 The physiological response and early appropriate care of the polytraumatized patient

Andrew Gray

Initial patient management

The initial management of seriously injured patients should be focused and streamlined. Optimal physiological stabilization involves the application of basic and well documented Advanced Trauma Life Support principles.

In 2007 the National Confidential Enquiry into Patient Outcome and Death (NCEPOD) report for trauma identified a number of problems with the management of seriously injured patients within England. This retrospective peer review of 795 patients from a range of emergency departments highlighted a number of concerns.

These ranged from:

- Inadequate initial airway management
- Poor initial patient care with a lack of early consultant involvement with a resultant undertriage and treatment delay
- Limited access to CT scanning and initial key diagnostic imaging
- Inadequate distribution of neurosurgical services with less than 10% of receiving hospitals having neurosurgery 'on site'
- Variable resident anesthetic cover with compromised initial patient care

Since 1st April 2012 a structured trauma network within England that involves major trauma centers (MTCs) and trauma units has produced a 20% reduction in mortality for our most seriously injured patients.

Key improvements have included:

- Minimization of delays in delivering the appropriate personnel to the accident scene
- Facilitation of early transfer to and accurate triage of patients in an emergency department having appropriate facilities and personnel to optimally manage the spectrum of presenting injuries
- Early initiation of resuscitation protocols with engrained major hemorrhage and coagulation treatment pathways
- Improved efficiency and effectiveness of MTC emergency departments resulting from the regular handling of high numbers of seriously injured patients complemented by continuous performance review and outcome audit
- Immediate access to total body CT scanning (with contrast) to ensure rapid spinal clearance and the early diagnosis of time dependent injuries
- On-site availability of specialist surgical services ensuring immediately available optimal multidisplinary surgical care supported by specialist intensive care physicians and anesthetists

The triage of our most seriously injured patients to MTCs has ensured an earlier diagnostic workup and a reduced time to surgical intervention. The role of the orthopaedic surgeon within the trauma team initially assessing a polytraumatized patient in the emergency department includes:

- Early identification of muscuoskeletal injuries that are life- or limb-threatening
- Interpretation of total body CT scan (with contrast). This enables early spinal clearance and can define fracture patterns and bleeding sources from pelvic injuries
- The appropriate and correct positioning of a pelvic binder (centered on the hip trochanters and not the iliac crests)
- Ensuring an adequate secondary survey
- Being present for the patient log roll to identify clinical signs of spinal injury
- Identifying open fractures with the application of a sterile dressing and checking administration of antibiotic and tetanus prophylaxis

- Reducing and splinting obvious skeletal deformity to minimize skin pressure and restore neurovascular function (e.g. dislocated ankle or elbow; deformed femur or tibia)
- Appropriate and timely ordering of plain X-rays during the initial emergency department patient management to properly define extremity injuries but without delaying or impeding patient care
- Early communication with other allied surgical specialties in order to prioritize injuries and formulate a treatment plan and order is vital. Intensive care and anesthetic specialists should be involved early to optimize oxygenation, with fluid and blood administration and early use of fresh frozen plasma (FFP) and platelets to help prevent coagulopathy in the bleeding patient
- The availability of theater and adequately trained orthopaedic staff should be ascertained. Good communication with the trauma theater coordinator is needed to ensure theater efficiency. The use of a radiolucent table, describing the surgical sequence, ordering the correct kit and instrumentation, ordering X-ray screening imaging and setting up the theater in terms of trays, X-ray and patient positioning are all factors that will optimize and reduce surgical time

Pathophysiology and injury severity

Injury severity

Higher injury severity is linked directly to poorer outcome. In a large prospective study of over 7,000 injured patients White et al. demonstrated patterns of injury that had a higher incidence of poor outcome and systemic complications. These included a high Injury Severity Score (ISS); the presence of a femoral fracture and hemodynamic compromise on admission. A higher ISS increases the likelihood of developing a systemic inflammatory response to trauma and the occurrence of acute respiratory distress and multiple organ dysfunction.

Hypovolemia

The correction of hypovolemic shock is paramount to any resuscitation protocol and there has been the development for transfusion protocols that replace blood earlier and have a lower threshold for the early use of platelets and FFP in order to maintain clotting. Massive transfusion protocols are now standard throughout most major trauma centers.

Elevated lactate levels indicate inadequate resuscitation with prolonged and persistent metabolic acidosis proven to increase mortality after serious injury. Patients who have lactate levels greater than 2.5 mmol/L have a higher incidence of respiratory problems after early intramedullary femoral stabilization.

Vallier et al. examined over 1400 injured patients with a severity score that ranged from 9–57 (mean 24.7). 22% had a complication during their initial treatment phase with the most frequent cause being either a pneumonia (8%) or a thrombosis (6%). Respiratory complications had a direct correlation to higher lactate values and base excess. Those patients who were slower to respond to resuscitation and who still had uncorrected metabolic acidosis 24 hours after admission had a greater complication risk and higher mortality rate. The presence of a chest injury and delayed fracture stabilization were also linked to higher levels of morbidity.

Fat embolus

Fat emboli are produced after long bone fractures and subsequent surgical stabilisation. Transient arterial hypoxemia can commonly be detected after such events but the incidence of a true 'fat embolus syndrome' after injury is low and incidence linked to the severity of injury.

Fat embolism syndrome is defined by the production of specific symptoms and signs associated with fat embolus. Major clinical criteria included: axillary and/or subconjuctival petichiae; hypoxemia ($PaO_2 < 60$ mmHg) and neurological symptoms (confusion) out of proportion to the degree of hypoxaemia. Minor criteria included a tachycardia (> 110 per minute), pyrexia (> 38.5) and fat macroglobulinemia.

The 'iceberg' phenomenon of fat embolus syndrome has been suggested and describes more frequent but less severe and sub-clinical forms of the condition.

The pathogenesis of fat embolus syndrome is linked to mechanical and biochemical effects. Fat emboli produced at a fracture site by trauma or surgery. These can cause mechanical blockage of pulmonary capillaries and microvasculature. Pulmonary arteriovenous shunts or a patent foramen ovale (present in 20% of patients) are methods by which emboli can enter the systemic circulation and affect other end organs such as the brain and kidneys. The biochemical theory is based upon the conversion of benign fat being to more toxic free fatty acids by enzymes produced by end organ endothelium after trauma. Symptoms are similar to the systemic inflammatory response seen after injury.

Instrumentation of the medullary canal can generate embolic material and can produce secondary pulmonary injury. Such emboli are detectable on transesophageal echocardiography of the pulmonary trunk. Instrument design and surgical technique aim to reduce this embolic 'hit.' Unreamed nails, fluted reamers, reamer irrigation aspiration systems and medullary canal venting are methods available to reduce the embolic load.

Coagulation

The presence of fat and marrow emboli in the pulmonary and systemic circulation after long bone fracture activates the coagulation and fibrinolytic pathways. Surgery further stimulates this thrombogenic process.

Activation and loss of coagulation control after serious injury has been linked to the development of acute lung injury and other systemic complications. Intramedullary reaming and nailing stimulates the coagulation mechanism and may contribute toward complications seen.

Reamed nailing was seen to activate the coagulative systems with a prolonged activated partial thromboplastin and prothrombin times as well as a consumption of fibrinogen and platelets with elevated levels of D-dimer and thrombin degradation products. The pulmonary embolic load measured by transesophageal echocardiography at the pulmonary trunk during surgery has been shown to closely correlate to the degree of activation. A larger embolic load is associated with a more pronounced coagulative response, with greater hypoxemia, raised pulmonary arterial pressure and respiratory compromise after surgery.

Inflammation

The systemic inflammatory response syndrome (SIRS) has been applied to the generalized inflammatory response that occurs after injury. This initial proinflammatory stress response is produced predominantly from macrophages and is primarily involved in removing damaged tissue and beginning the repair processes. The initial stress response is short lived and monocytes become deactivated and unable to respond to fresh stimuli.

A compensatory anti-inflammatory response (CARS) is activated with mediators directly linked to the development of immunosuppression after trauma.

An immune imbalance can result with the patient having a period of increased immune susceptibility. A more pronounced immunodepression is seen with increasing levels of injury, with hemorrhage and tissue damage acting in synergy. The effects of this immune imbalance can be to exacerbate shock, coagulation defects and predispose to future infection.

This occurs in the early days after injury and corresponds to the scheduling time for many surgical procedures, which involve further tissue trauma.

A recent development has been the use of pro- and anti-inflammatory markers in the prediction of patient outcome after serious injury. Both may play a role in the determination of which patients may benefit from damage control surgical techniques.

Interleukin 6 (IL-6) is a pro-inflammatory cytokine with a half-life of 6 hours. IL-6 levels correlate to the level of blunt injury and are one potential marker of injury severity and also the patient response to subsequent treatment and surgery. A correlation between serum IL-6 levels and the development of multiple organ failure and acute respiratory distress in patients following polytrauma has been demonstrated.

In a prospective study, Pape et al. demonstrated a comparable increase in IL-6 levels in patients undergoing elective hip arthroplasty with those having intramedullary fixation of an isolated femoral diaphyseal fracture. This study also included polytrauma patients and a 'control' group undergoing ankle fixation. The latter group showed no increase in IL-6 postoperative levels whereas the polytrauma group showed the highest preoperative IL-6 levels with substantial further increases after intramedullary femoral fracture fixation. The effects of intramedullary fracture fixation surgery have been clearly shown not to be inconsequential after major injury.

During the early phase after injury it has been suggested that the cytokine proinflammatory cascade is significantly up regulated within the pulmonary parenchyma to produce a different pattern in concentrations of pulmonary and systemic inflammatory mediators. Keel studied 16 patients with a severe injury (average ISS = 34). Amplified levels of pro-inflammatory cytokines IL-1β and IL-8 were demonstrated from bronchoalveolar lavage samples. However, there was no corresponding rise in systemic (serum) concentrations. Measurements of pro-inflammatory cytokines within the lung, but not in the systemic circulation may indicate an amplified local inflammatory response early after injury. This may account for the apparent susceptibility of the pulmonary parenchyma to inflammatory damage after trauma.

In summary, immunological evaluation may offer an accurate method to categorise patients and quantify the degree of initial injury in order to determine the optimal surgical strategy. In addition it could help identify at an early stage which patients are developing acute respiratory and systemic complications unexpectedly after less severe and isolated injuries.

Early total care, damage control and early adequate surgery

It is now recognized that trauma to the patient results in an immediate systemic stress response related to the degree of initial injury. The clinical outcome is determined by the magnitude of the initial insult and by an individual's systemic response both to the initial injury and subsequent treatment. The term 'second hit' has been applied to the process whereby an injured and physiologically vulnerable patient is exposed to further trauma as a result of the surgical management of their injuries.

Peripheral limb injuries involving femoral and tibial diaphyseal fractures constitute a leading cause of hospitalization related to nonfatal injury. It became apparent that early skeletal stabilization did reduce the incidence of injury related systemic and respiratory complications and improve outcome by minimizing further tissue trauma and reducing hemorrhage and fat embolus release.

Early total care

The term 'early total care' (ETC) refers to the definitive and early (< 24 hours from injury) stabilization of long bone fractures. This involves reamed intramedullary fixation of femoral and tibia diaphyseal fractures.

Bone et al. demonstrated a reduction in morbidity and mortality using ETC in seriously injured patients with long bone fractures in two separate studies. The key factor was that these were patients that were adequately resuscitated.

The first paper (1989) was a prospective study involving patients with acute femoral fractures. A delay of more than 48 hours before intramedullary fracture stabilization resulted in an increased incidence of respiratory complications in those patients who had significant associated injuries.

A subsequent multicenter trial that involved over 600 patients demonstrated that early (< 24 hours) intramedullary femoral fracture stabilization was responsible for marked reductions in mortality in patients with severe musculoskeletal injuries. By the early stabilization of peripheral limb fractures, patient mobilization was encouraged and the length of time spent in both intensive care and hospital subsequently fell. The morbidity associated with prolonged immobilization was reduced and a fall in healthcare costs clearly demonstrated. However, concerns were raised regarding secondary pulmonary and systemic fat embolic events thought to be linked to reamed intramedullary techniques in the seriously injured patients. Reynolds retrospectively reviewed 424 patients who had acute femoral fractures treated by reamed intramedullary stabilization. Patients with a low severity of injury benefitted from early stabilization with fewer respiratory complications. However, this benefit was not seen in patients with a higher ISS (> 18). It was concluded that modest delays in definitive fracture stabilization in the more seriously injured cohort did not adversely affect prognosis.

Damage control

Pape and the Hannover group investigated the above concerns extensively.

In the early 1990s a retrospective study investigated an apparently high incidence of respiratory complications in patients who had primary reamed intramedullary femoral fixation with an associated blunt chest injury. At that time the Hannover unit was following the policy of 'early total care'. This review revealed a higher rate of acute respiratory distress in those patients who had a thoracic injury and early reamed intramedullary stabilization compared to patients who had an isolated chest injury.

A subsequent change in the management of acute femoral fractures in the most seriously injured patients from definitive intramedullary stabilization to initial external fixation was implemented in this major trauma center. A retrospective review indicated that this change in surgical protocol was at least partially responsible for improvements in the rates of multiple organ failure and acute respiratory distress subsequently seen.

'Limited' surgical techniques with reduced operative time and tissue insult have been proposed in seriously injured patients to minimize the 'second hit' and possibly improve outcome. The term 'damage control' has been applied to these surgical techniques. With regards to femoral fractures this involves the initial application of an external fixator with delayed conversion to definitive intramedullary stabilization once the patient's condition has been optimized (usually in an intensive care or high dependency environment).

The Hanover group proposed a practical use for damage control orthopaedics. They recommended its use in certain groups of patients:

- ISS > 20 with an associated chest injury
- ISS > 40 with no associated chest injury
- Combined pelvic and abdominal trauma with hypovolemic (Systolic BP < 90 mmHg)
- Pulmonary arterial pressure measurement of > 24 mmHg
- Bilateral lung contusions on chest radiographs

Nowotarski demonstrated successful delayed conversion of external fixation to intramedullary stabilization of femoral diaphyseal fractures in the multiply injured. This retrospective review of 1500 femoral fractures documented that primary external fixation was used in 4% of admissions. This procedure was again reserved for the more seriously injured patients with a mean ISS of 29. Conversion to intramedullary fixation was performed at an average of seven days after initial surgery with low infection rates (1.7%).

Although there is much debate about the optimal method of initial fracture fixation there is general agreement that initial skeletal stabilization should not be delayed and that the degree of initial trauma has a more direct correlation with the development of subsequent systemic complications than the method or timing of any peripheral extremity fracture stabilization. The main debate has centerd upon quantifying the relative physiological effects of fracture treatment compared to the consequences of injury alone.

Early adequate care

In 2013 Vallier et al. published an article that should change clinical practise. This retrospective review of over 1400 seriously injured patients helped clarify injury patterns and physiological parameters that warrant definitive fracture management being delayed.

Chest injury was the strongest predictor of subsequent pulmonary complication.

The patient's physiological status measured by acidosis is predictive of complications regardless of injury sustained to another body system (e.g. head or abdomen).

The degree of acidosis on admission and inability to respond to resuscitation were directly linked to poor outcome. Uncorrected acidosis at 24 hours was directly linked to pneumonia and respiratory morbidity.

Their protocol for early appropriate care recommends definitive management of mechanically unstable fractures of the pelvis, acetabulum, proximal femur, femoral shaft, and spine within 36 hours of injury as long as the patient has demonstrated response to resuscitation as based on improvement of acidosis with lactate, 4.0 mmol/L, pH .7.25, or BE < 25.5 mmol/L.

Therefore, during persistent acidosis, a DCO strategy is used, and the patient is continually reassessed to determine the timing of definitive care.

Case example: Appropriate early total care

A 68-year-old man suffered a high energy motorbike accident. His airway and breathing were normal, but he had mild tachycardia (100 bpm). Blood pressure was stable. Intravenous access was obtained and intravenous crystalloids commenced. His Glasgow coma score (GCS) was 15. A whole body trauma pan scan CT was undertaken within 30 minutes of admission to the emergency department. There was no evidence of intracranial, thoracic, abdominal or pelvic injury. Cervical and thoracolumbar spines were cleared. On secondary survey, there was evidence of gross lower limb deformity. These were closed injuries with no neurovascular defects. The patient was sent for X-rays. Bilateral segmental femurs with a right basocervical proximal femoral fracture were seen (**Figure 22.1**).

A decision was made to proceed with definitive fracture stabilization. Arterial base excess was 3.5 mmol/L. Cross-matched blood, FFP and platelets were ordered. The patient was consented for bilateral retrograde nailing and right four-hole sliding hip screw fixation of the proximal femoral neck fracture. Retrograde nailing is a good option for bilateral femoral fractures due to speed of surgery and ease of patient set up, with use of a radiolucent table and the avoidance of a traction table. Combined femoral shaft and neck fractures are often easier to stabilize with two devices rather than a single-antegrade reconstruction type nail (cephalomedullary)

The surgical plan was to allow the retrograde nail to bypass the most distal aspect of the sliding hip screw in order to prevent a potential stress riser. The plan was to only use the two most proximal screws holes of the four-hole SHS (this leaves the potential to lock the proximal aspect of the nail through one of the two most distal holes).

The patient was informed that if he was to deteriorate physiologically during the procedure, then the femurs would be temporarily stabilized with spanning external fixators. A high-dependency bed was booked following team discussion between the trauma anesthetist and the intensive care physician.

The patient's physiological compromise had been underestimated, with only 500 mL of normal saline given over a 3-hour period in the emergency department. He was also quite hypothermic (34.5°C) by the time he arrived in theater reception. Each closed femoral shaft fracture has the potential to lose >1.5 L of blood. The patient was a well 68-year-old male but his age means that his physiological reserve is lower than that of a younger patient.

Blood, warm fluids, fresh frozen plasma (FFP) and platelets were given throughout the procedure as well as the application of a warming device. The patient's physiological status improved throughout the duration of surgery.

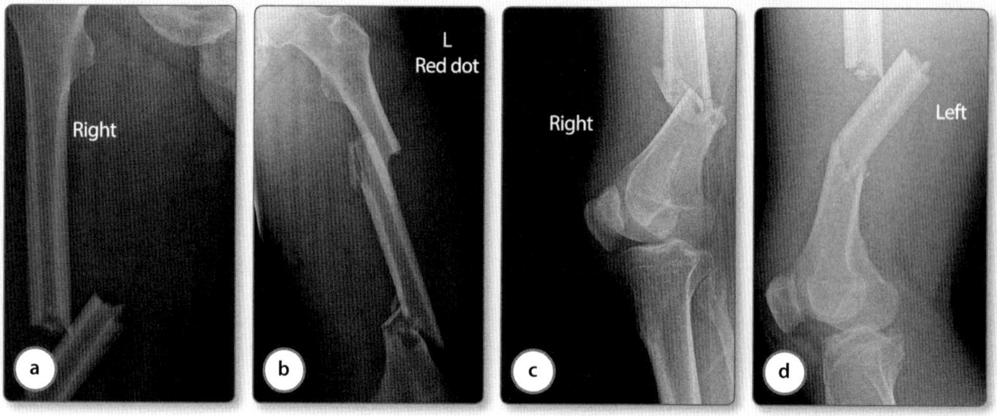

Figure 22.1 (a-d) Bilateral segmental femurs with a right basicervical proximal femoral fracture (not shown in Figure 22.1a).

Case example: *continued.*

Definitive fracture stabilization is demonstrated in **Figure 22.2**. Radiolucent table and triangles were used for freehand retrograde nailing and hip screw insertion (**Figure 22.3**)

The patient was admitted overnight to the high-dependency unit and made a rapid recovery after extubation, being able to be transferred back to the standard orthopaedic trauma ward within 24 hours of surgery.

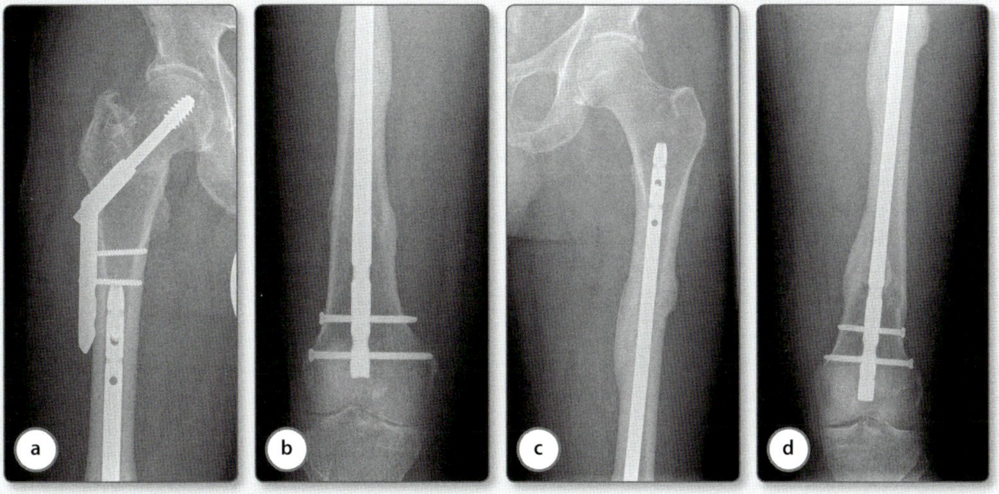

Figure 22.2 (a-d) Management of case example. Bilateral retrograde nailing with SHS stabilisation of proximal right femoral fracture. The four-hole plate (a) has been chosen to avoid the potential stress riser caused by the retrograde nail. The retrograde nail should finish proximally above the level of the lesser trochanter.

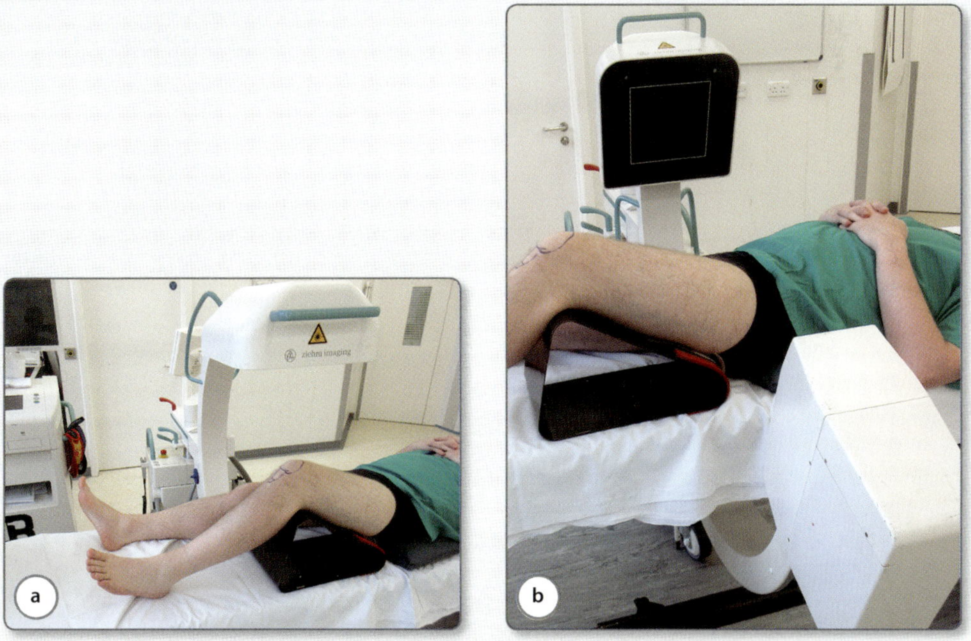

Figure 22.3 (a, b) Proposed setup for bilateral retrograde nailing and insertion of hip screw. An oblique lateral is required at the proximal aspect to assess proximal locking and guide wire placement in the head and neck for SHS insertion.

Further reading

White TO, Jenkins PJ, Smith RD, et al. The epidemiology of posttraumatic adult respiratory distress syndrome. J Bone Joint Surg Am 2004; 86-A:2366–2376.

Crowl AC, Young JS, Kahler DM, et al. Occult hypoperfusion is associated with increased morbidity in patients undergoing early femur fracture fixation. J Trauma 2000; 48:260–267.

Vallier HA, Wang X, Moore TA, et al. Timing of orthopaedic surgery in multiple trauma patients; development of a protocol for early appropriate care. J Orthop Trauma 2013; 27:543–551.

Pape HC, Schmidt RE, Rice J, et al. Biochemical changes after trauma and skeletal surgery of the lower extremity: quantification of the operative burden. Crit Care Med 2000; 28:3441–3448.

Keel M, Ecknauer E, Stocker R, et al Different pattern of local and systemic release of proinflammatory and anti-inflammatory mediators in severely injured patients with chest trauma. J Trauma 1996; 40:907–912.

Bone LB, Johnson KD, Weigelt J, Scheinberg R. Early versus delayed stabilization of femoral fractures. A prospective randomized study. J Bone Joint Surg Am 1989; 71:336–340.

Bone LB, McNamara K, Shine B, Border J. Mortality in multiple trauma patients with fractures. J Trauma 1994; 37:262–264.

Reynolds MA, Richardson JD, Spain DA, et al. Is the timing of fracture fixation important for the patient with multiple trauma? Ann Surg 1995; 222:470–481.

Pape HC, Auf'm'Kolk M, Paffrath T, et al. Primary intramedullary femur fixation in multiple trauma patients with associated lung contusion – a cause of posttraumatic ARDS? J Trauma 1993; 34:540–547.

Pape HC, Hildebrand F, Pertschy S, et al. Changes in the management of femoral shaft fractures in polytrauma patients: from early total care to damage control orthopedic surgery. J. Trauma 2002; 53:452–461.

Nowotarski PJ, Turen CH, Brumback RJ, Scarboro JM. Conversion of external fixation to intramedullary nailing for fractures of the shaft of the femur in multiply injured patients. J. Bone Joint Surg Am 2000; 82:781–788.

23 Pediatric case examples

Antoine de Gheldere, Philip Henman

SUPRACONDYLAR ELBOW FRACTURES

Introduction

Supracondylar fractures (SCF) of the elbow are metaphyseal fractures of the distal humerus. They can be challenging to treat, even in experienced hands. Unsatisfactory results after surgery have been reported in 3–16% of cases. As remodeling at the elbow is limited, residual rotational deformity will remain. Any such malunion will have a cosmetic – and sometimes functional – consequence.

Incidence

SCF represent 18% of all pediatric fractures and are the most frequent fractures of the elbow in children (60%). The extension-type SCF is much

Case example: Supracondylar elbow fracture-extension type

A 5-year-old girl was playing outside when she fell over a low wall, injuring her left elbow. Initial X-rays are show in **Figure 23.1**. A full neurovascular examination was undertaken before and after limb splintage. She was admitted for reduction and stabilization (**Figure 23.2**).

Flexion supracondylar fractures, although much less common and often with only moderate displacement, often have a poorer functional outcome (**Figure 23.3**).

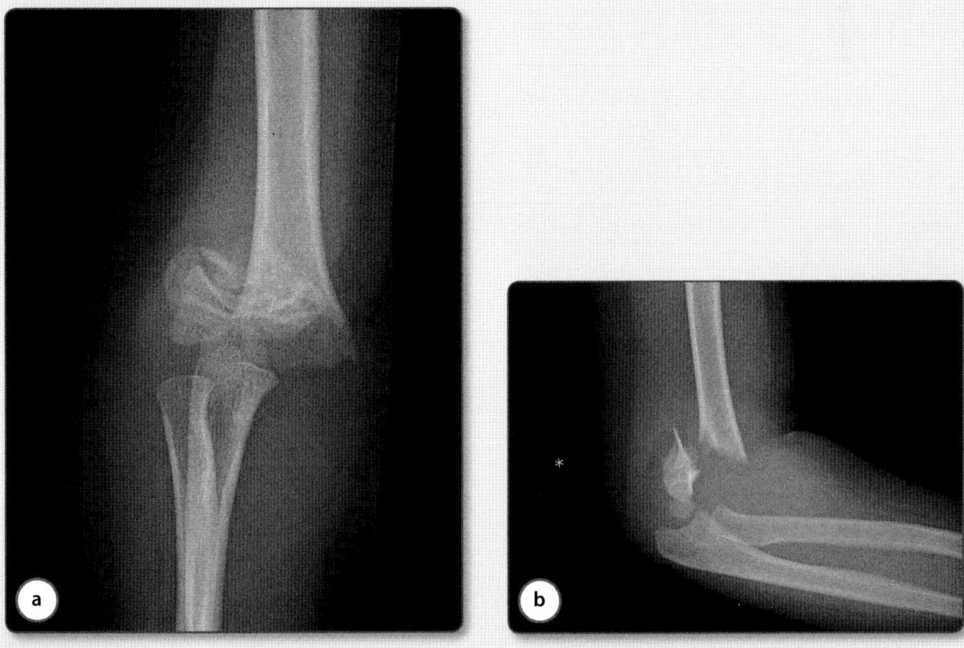

Figure 23.1 (a, b) Radiographic images of unsupported supracondylar fracture: extension fracture pattern (Garland 3 or AO 4 are the most common types).

Case example: *continued.*

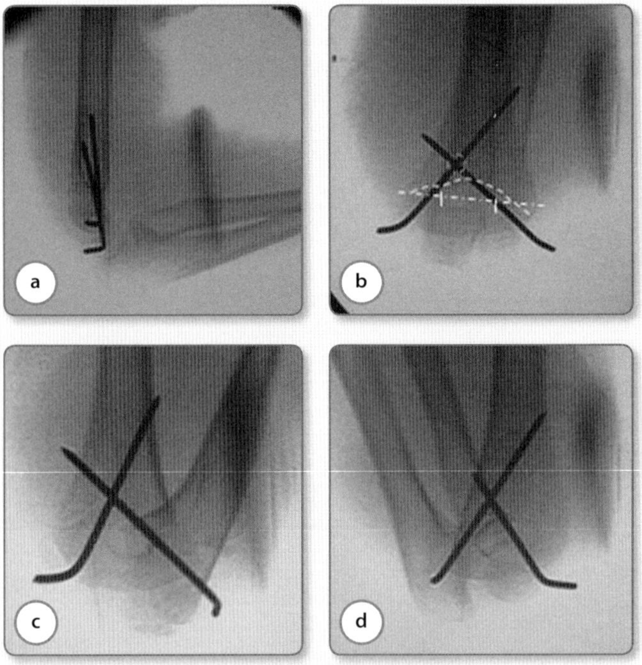

Figure 23.2 Intra-operative X-rays of the fracture shown in Figure 23.1. (a) Lateral view confirms anatomic reduction. (b) AP view shows the stability criteria. (c, d) Oblique views confirm the anatomic reduction of both columns.

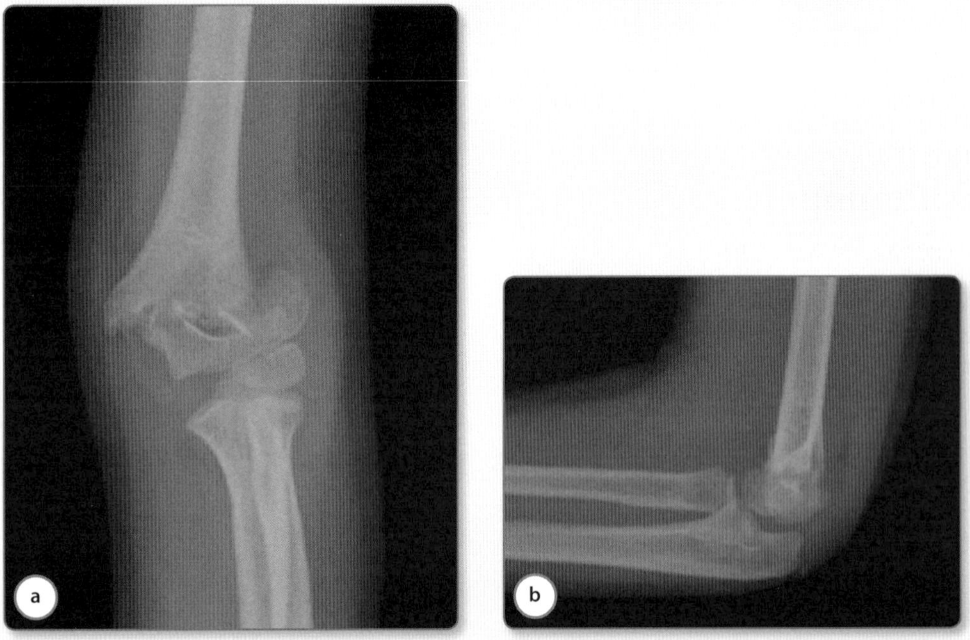

Figure 23.3 (a, b) AP and lateral X-rays of flexion pattern.

more frequently seen (95%) than the flexion-type SCF (5%).

Mechanism of injury

Falling onto an outstretched hand (e.g. when running, trampolining, falling from a swing, etc.)

Initial management/ prioritization

Appropriate pain management and splintage allows for a more reliable neurovascular examination. Vascular compromise is rare, but requires an urgent reduction. Nerve injuries are more frequent (especially the anterior interosseous branch). It is not necessary to explore the nerve when the reduction of the fracture is anatomical, but the recovery can take several months.

X-rays (lateral and AP views of the elbow) help to classify the fracture according the widespread Gartland classification or the more recent AO classification.

Considerations for surgery

Unstable fractures (Gartland 2 and higher or AO type 2 and higher) are indications for surgical management.

Theater layout and patient positioning

Under general anesthesia, the patient is positioned supine with an arm table. The image intensifier is parallel to the patient to be able to perform an anterior and lateral view without moving the arm (**Figure 23.4**). The surgeon stands at the edge of the hand table and the assistant is positioned on the opposite side, ready for contratraction.

Review of surgical management

Stages in reduction

- Gentle, continuous and progressive axial traction his performed under image intensifier screening (**Figure 23.5a**)
- Medial – lateral translation is corrected with direct pressure, but rotation is corrected with a pronation-supination motion at the wrist (**Figure 23.5b**)
- When the reduction is good on the anteroposterior (AP) and lateral views; the elbow is flexed with pressure on the distal humeral epiphysis and olecranon (**Figure 23.5c**). This controls the reduction and allows further imaging and subsequent stabilization

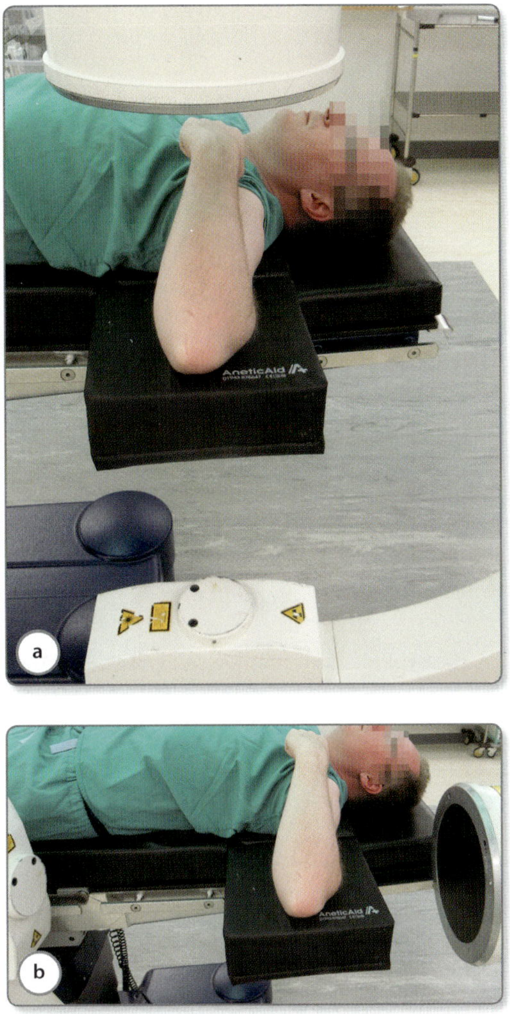

Figure 23.4 (a, b) Clinical positioning of patient and C-arm for surgical procedures: allows maintenance of fracture reduction and orthogonal images obtained by moving the C-arm.

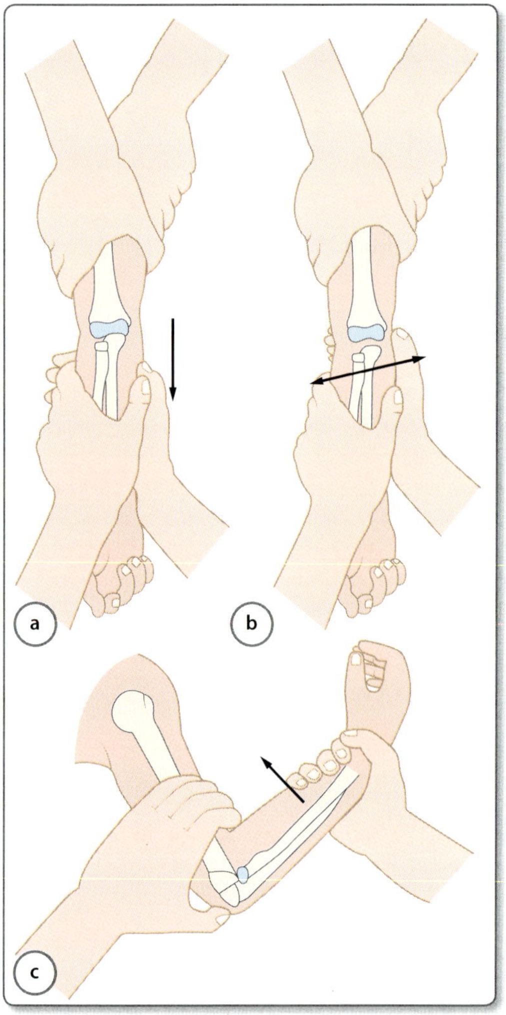

Figure 23.5 Reduction manoeuvers for supracondylar fractures. (a) Traction. (b) Translation correction. (c) Forearm flexion with thumb pressure on elbow.

Equipment requirements

- Tourniquet (optional; becomes useful when open reduction is required)
- 1.6 mm or preferably 1.8 mm K-wires (BOAST 11 recommends the two lateral K-wire technique which requires wider 2 mm K-wires to confer necessary stability to the fixation, but often in the small child these are too robust)
- Wire driver
- Wire cutter

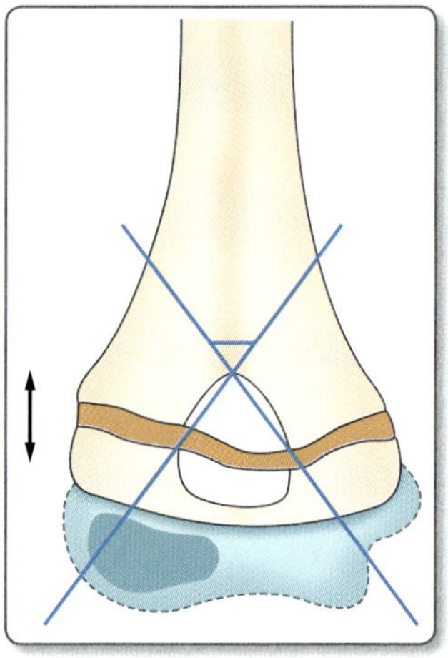

Figure 23.6 The K-wires should cross each other proximal to the fracture.

- Orthopedic pliers
- Basic instrument (if open reduction is required)

Reduction and stabilization methods

As often in trauma, the key is to reduce the fracture. With patience and good technique, most supracondylar fractures can be managed with closed reduction and percutaneous fixation on the lateral side (with one or two wires) and a mini-incision on the medial side in order to identify and protect the ulnar nerve. In some rare cases, the fracture is irreducible because of soft tissues impingement. An open reduction through a medial approach is then indicated. In all cases, leaving the wires outside the skin enables removal without general anesthesia.

Principle of stability after pinning

On an AP view, both K-wires should cross the fracture line at its lateral and medial one-third. The K-wires should cross each other proximal to the fracture and not at the fracture site (**Figure 23.6**).

Rehabilitation

- Elbow stiffness is common for 2–3 months following removal of cast (and K-wires)
- Patients who had physiotherapy did not show better elbow function compared to patients without physiotherapy at 6 months of follow-up

- The patient and their family should be informed from the outset that recovery of full range of motion (ROM) can take up to 12 months
- Patients can return to sports safely when they have recovered a functional range of elbow motion: 30° flexion to 130° flexion

Avoiding postoperative complications

The common complications are:

- Reoperation (2%)
  - Accurate fracture reduction
  - Bicortical wire placement
  - Appropriately sized wires for patient body habitus
  - Wires not crossing at fracture site
- Malunion
  - Attention to surgical detail – appropriate reduction and fixation
  - Appropriate clinical experience
- Volkmann's ischemic contracture
  - Often determined by seriousness of injury
  - Avoidance of undue delays to surgery
  - Constrictive splints
  - Missed vascular compromise
- Cellulitis or osteomyelitis
  - Antibiotics
  - Efficient surgical techniques
  - Nerve palsy

Salvage options after failed fracture fixation

Secondary displacement can be re-operated on within 10 days of the initial procedure. After 10 days of the initial trauma, it is very difficult to move the fragments to achieve an anatomical reduction. The best option in this case is to let the fracture heal and to refer the patient to a pediatric orthopaedic surgeon to discuss further treatment options.

FOREARM FRACTURES

Introduction

Forearm fractures are a large group of fracture with different patterns according to the velocity of the trauma, the age of the patient and the position of the forearm at the time of impact.

- Bowing deformity (toddlers and young children)
- Greenstick fracture (incomplete fracture)
- Complete fracture (older children, teenagers)
- Monteggia injury (when a fracture of the ulna is associated with a dislocation of the radial head)
- Galeazzi injury (when a fracture of the radius is associated with a dislocation of the distal radioulnar joint)

Incidence

The incidence of forearm fractures is 5% of all fractures in children.

Mechanism of injury

These fractures are often the result of an indirect blow, usually cased by falling on an outstretched hand. A direct blow can be suspected in a one-bone fracture of the forearm.

Initial management/ prioritization

- Pain management and splintage
- Neurovascular examination and assessment of compartments
- X-rays of the entire forearm with the elbow and wrist joints to exclude Monteggia or Galeazzi fractures

Considerations for surgery

If the forearm is grossly deformed and/or the X-rays show more than 10° of angulation (any views) or overlapping of the bone fragments, a closed reduction of the fracture under general anesthesia is indicated. Occasionally, when a closed reduction cannot be achieved, an open reduction is indicated. The stability of the fracture depends on the integrity of the periosteum. Therefore, stabilization of the fracture is achieved with a long-arm cast in supination (periosteum partially intact) or the use of elastic nailing technique (complete periosteum rupture). When surgeons are experienced in the technique of elastic nail fixation of forearm fractures there are almost no indications for plate fixation of diaphyseal forearm fractures in children.

The goal of the technique is to restore the tension – and therefore stability – of the

Case example: Both bone forearm fractures

a 8-year-old girl fell in the school playground while running, sustaining a clinically deformed forearm. She was assessed, the arm splinted, and re-examined before X-rays were obtained (**Figure 23.7a, b**). She subsequently underwent closed reduction and intermedullary wire stabilization of both forearm bones (**Figure 23.7e, f**).

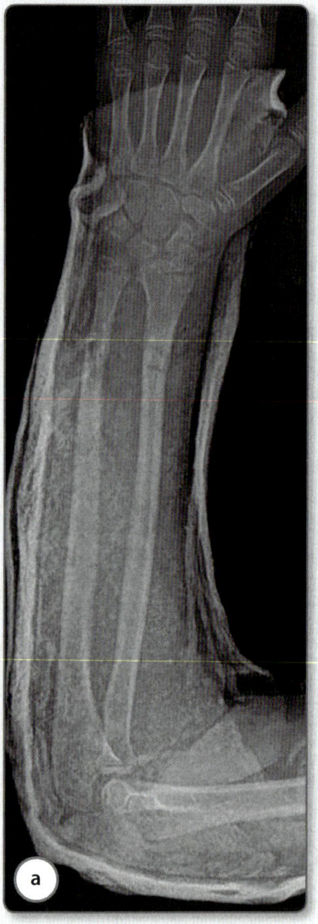

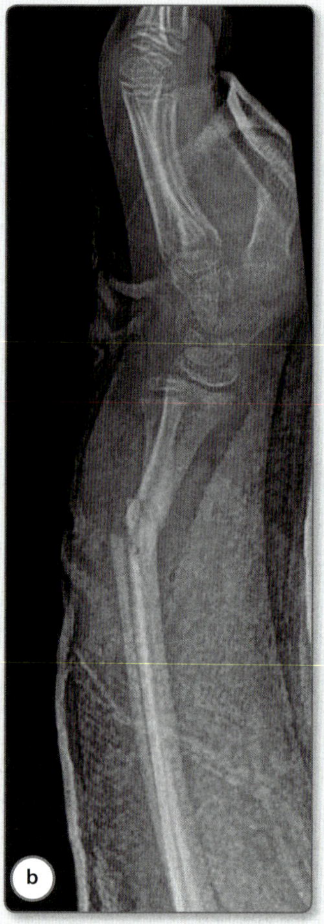

Figure 23.7 (a, b) Preoperative AP and lateral radiographs of a both-bone forearm fracture. (c) Proposed radial-based entry point (other options include Lister's tubercle dorsally). (d) Proposed safe proximal ulnar entry point. (e, f) Postoperative radiographs of the same case, showing solid healing with remodeling. *Continues overleaf*

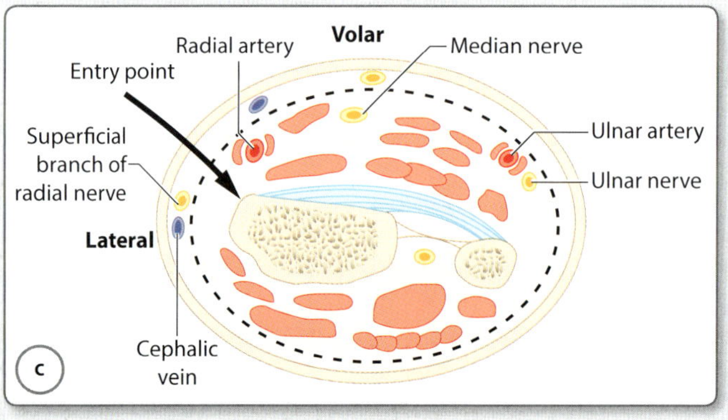

Case example: *continued.*

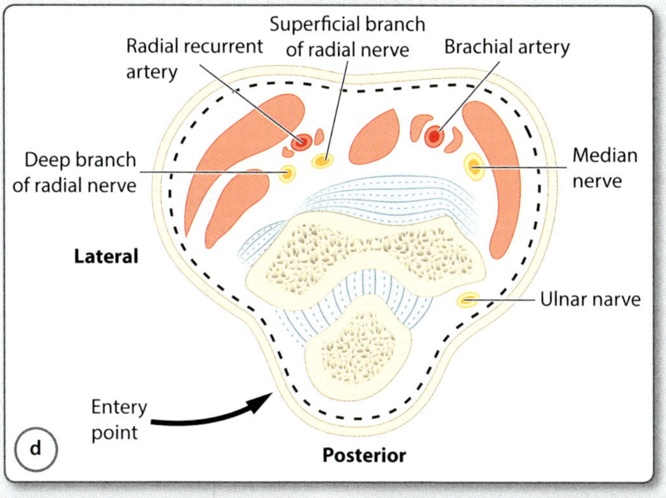

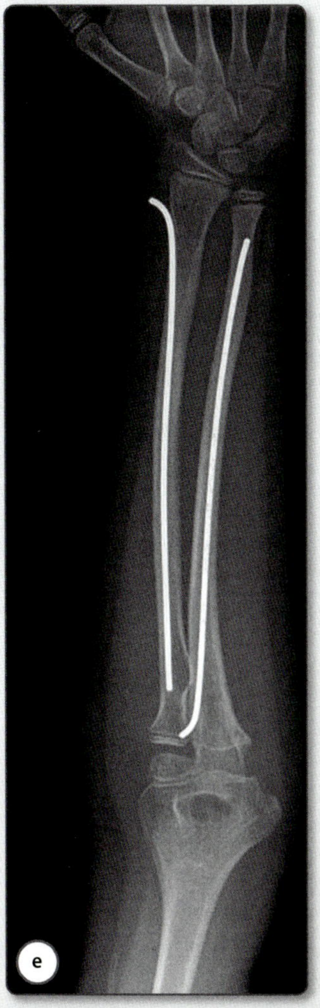

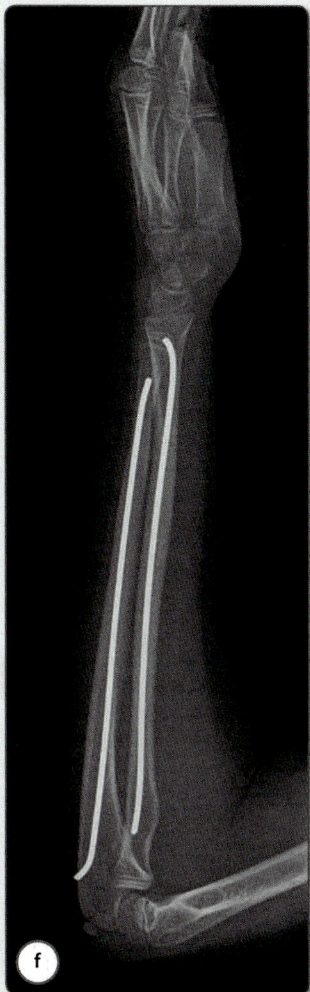

interosseous membrane. Most of the time, the elastic stability is enough and a postoperative cast is not required. Full ROM is often recovered after 2–6 weeks. It is unsafe to remove the nails before 6 months. Any removal of nails before 6 months increases the risk of re-fracture.

Theater layout and patient positioning

Under general anesthesia, the patient is positioned supine with an arm table at the injured side. The image intensifier is perpendicular to the patient and the surgeon sits on the radial side of the upper limb. The assistant is on the opposite side of the arm table.

Equipment requirements

- Closed reduction and cast:
  - Double layer of stockinet (no soft band)
  - Plaster of Paris (soft cast or fiber glass)
- Elastic nailing technique:
  - Tourniquet (to avoid the nerve during the approach)
  - Basic instrument for mini-incision
  - Elastic nailing set (stainless steel); use pre-bent nails or bend it manually
  - If not available: smooth K-wire with T-handle and wire cutter
  - Appropriately sized wires for body habitus
  - Nail sizes used: 1.5 mm (6–8 years); 2.0 mm (8–10 years); 2.5 mm (> 11 years)

Reduction and stabilization methods

Closed reduction and cast

- Gently align the two bones to < 10°
- Use the three point molding technique
- Cast position in supination

Elastic nailing technique

- Entry points identified and created with awl or small drill and tissue protector (**Figure 23.7c, d**; be aware of the nerves)
- Start with the radial bone
- Push the wire by hand to the fracture site
- Perform the same procedure with the ulna
- Use a hammer (gently) if necessary to pass the wire through the fracture site
- Continue pushing by hand
- Turn both nails to restore tension to the interosseous membrane
- Assess for passive forearm ROM and fracture stability

Postoperative X-rays of the illustrated case example after treatment with flexible intramedullary nails are shown in **Figure 23.7e, f**.

Rehabilitation

- No rehabilitation is required

Avoiding postoperative complications

Compartment syndrome

It seems to have a higher incidence when the surgical management has been delayed. The authors recommend early splintage and elevation. After final treatment (closed reduction and/or nailing); elevation of the arm should be continued until the patient can move freely and without pain in the fingers.

Nonunion/delayed union

Nonunions are extremely rare. Delayed union is more frequent in cases of open fractures or open reduction.

Re-fractures

Re-fractures are the most common significant complication of this injury. It is best to avoid an early return to contact sports and early removal of flexible nails. In children over the age of 4 years, the period in a cast can be up to 12 weeks or until the intramedullary canal has re-formed. Children should refrain from contact sports until the medullary canal has recannulated.

Malunion

Malunion is often iatrogenic, resulting from:

- Poor initial fracture reduction
- Poor quality of cast application
- Neglected secondary displacement

Nerve palsy

Nerve palsy can occur with the fracture displacement, but is more often related to a poor nailing technique and multiple attempts of closed reduction (iatrogenic).

SLIPPED UPPER FEMORAL EPIPHYSIS

Introduction

A slipped upper femoral epiphysis (SUFE) is the relative displacement of the proximal epiphysis of the femur on his metaphysis. The epiphysis looks posteriorly displaced, but in fact it stays in the hip joint. Therefore, the metaphysis (and the rest of the lower limb) is anteriorly displaced with external rotation (**Figure 23.8a**).

The clinician normally sees two types of SUFE, the presentation, treatment and prognosis of which are very different:

- *Unstable type:* often acute, with a high risk of avascular necrosis
- *Stable type*: often chronic, but can become acute if diagnosis is delayed

Incidence

The true incidence of SUFE is probably underestimated (2:100,000), but it is the most serious hip condition in teenagers before they reach skeletal maturity. SUFE is more common in boys than girls, with a 3:1 ratio. Bilateral SUFE is present in 20–50% of patients with 0–18 months of initial presentation.

Etiology

The etiology remains unknown and is probably the result of different factors (mechanical, hormonal and metabolic abnormalities). Mechanical factors involve increased shear forces across the growth plate and biological factors seem to weaken the growth plate with a pathophysiology that remains unknown.

Initial management/ prioritization

Patients with an unstable SUFE often present to accident and emergency departments. The presentation is very similar to someone with a femoral neck fracture. The optimal treatment option remains unknown and the patient should be urgently referred to a specialist center. This contrasts with the difficulty in making the diagnosis in patients with a stable SUFE.

Typically, the patient has been limping for a few weeks or months and the changes seen on X-rays can initially be subtle. Clinically, the excess of external rotation should be compared to the other side and a 'frog view' X-ray of the pelvis should always be requested.

Considerations for surgery

A patient with a stable SUFE should be treated as soon as possible, not only to avoid further displacement, but also to avoid the risk of the SUFE becoming unstable. The treatment of an unstable SUFE is often pinning in situ or an appropriate osteotomy (which is outwith the remit of this chapter), and should be referred to a specialist center.

Theater layout and patient positioning

- The patient is supine on a traction table or supine on a radiolucent table with free leg draping
- Confirm orthogonal image intensifier views can be obtaining before commencing the procedure

Equipment requirements

- Traction table (without any traction) or radiolucent table
- Cannulated screw size 6.5 or 7.3 mm

Reduction and stabilization methods

- No reduction is required for stable SUFE
- The patient is positioned supine on a radiolucent table or traction table depending on the surgeon's preference
- The technique is undertaken percutaneously using the image intensifier
- The principle is to enter the proximal femoral growth plate with the screw perpendicular (90°) to the plane of the physis on AP and lateral view, so the degree of slip will influence the position of the guide wire entry point (**Figure 23.8f**)

Case example: Slipped upper femoral epiphysis (acute on chronic)

A 9-year-old boy had acute, sudden and worsening right hip pain, having previously stopped sporting activities 3 months prior due to hip discomfort (**Figure 23.8b, c**). A SUFE such as this is obvious and does not cause diagnostic confusion, but the radiographic features can still be subtle, as shown in **Figures 23.8d** and **23.8e**. The patient was taken to theater and the slip stabilized with a percutaneous cannulated screw.

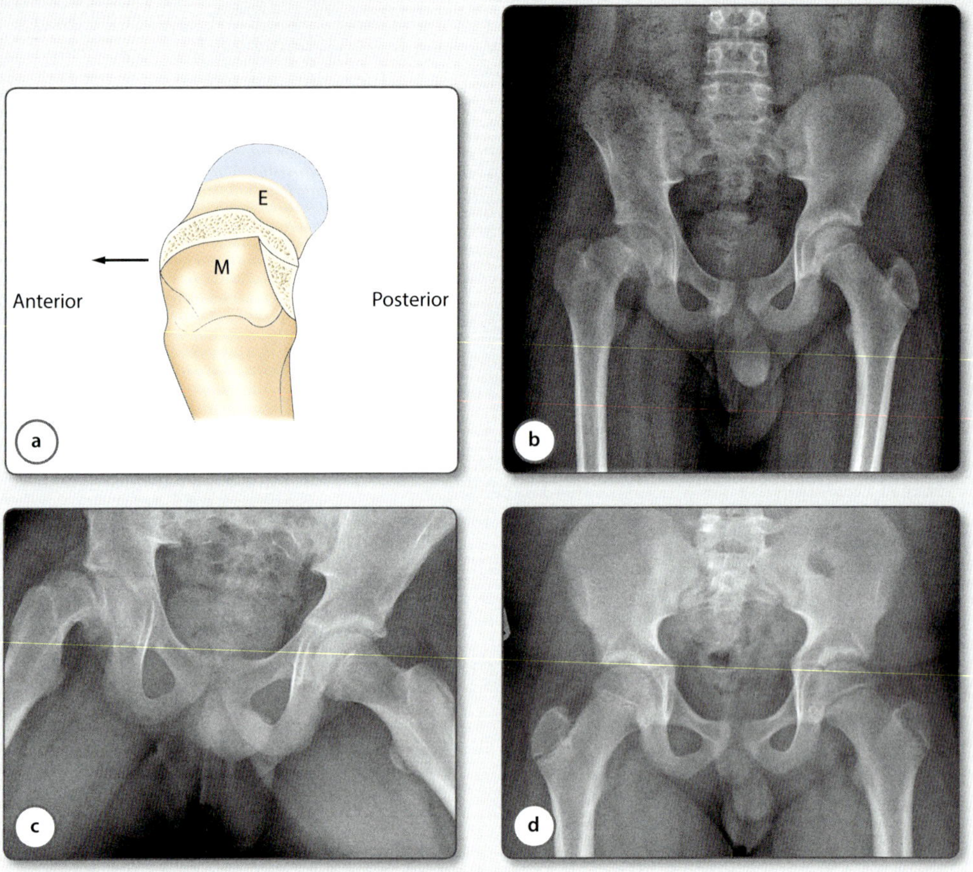

Figure 23.8 (a) Relative displacement of metaphysis anteriorly which is associated with clinical shortening and external rotation of the affected limb. (b, c) AP and lateral X-rays showing acute (or acute on chronic) right-sided SUFE. (d, e) The AP pelvic view looks 'normal', but the 'frog' lateral view confirms a SUFE of the left hip. If the left hip is not stabilized as soon as possible, there is a risk of greater displacement and worsening outcome. (f) Landmark on the skin for the proposed entry point. Line TD follows palpation of the lateral femur from the greater trochanter (T) to the diaphysis (D). H is the center of the femoral head under image intensifier. Line H0 follows the anatomic axis of the femoral neck under image intensifier. The entry point is somewhere on this line between 0 (no slip) and half way along the H0 line (45° slip). The slip angle is calculated on preoperative X-rays.

Case example: *continued.*

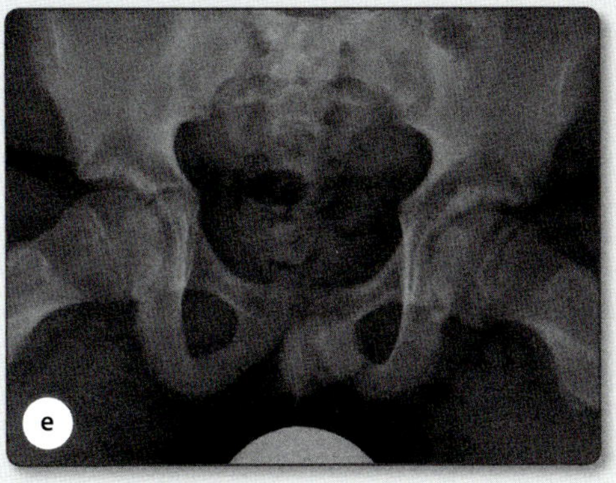

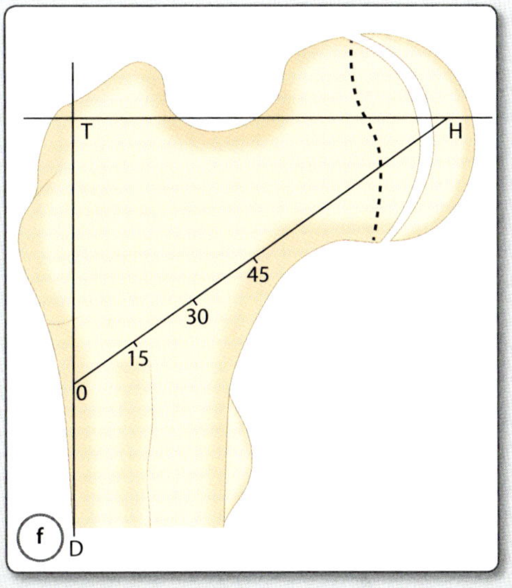

Figure 23.8 *Continued*

Rehabilitation

- Protected weight-bearing under physiotherapy supervision
- Progression of mobility as symptoms allow
- Avoidance of contact sports until the growth plate has fused
- The patient and family should be informed that the affected leg will remain in slight external rotation after the surgery. However, if sufficient growth potential remains, slow remodeling may occur and progressively correct the residual deformity

Avoiding postoperative complications

To avoid the risk of avascular necrosis, no traction or attempt to reduce the SUFE should be attempted. To avoid the risk of iatrogenic chondrolysis, the surgeon should control the screw position under image intensifier with several different angled views. The goal is to make sure that there is no penetration of the screw in the hip joint. Many studies recommend not removing the screw (especially if it is not affecting the patient) as the procedure can be difficult and lead to unnecessary complications.

In case of fixation of a moderate/severe stable SUFE, the patient can develop later groin pain as a result of a femoral acetabular impingement. It remains unclear whether a more aggressive initial treatment is superior to a simple percutaneous fixation of the femoral head. These patients should be referred to a specialist center to discuss further treatment options.

SEPTIC HIP WASHOUT

Introduction

A pediatric hip infection can result in dramatic consequences when the diagnosis is delayed and can become an orthopaedic emergency. Bacteria and leukocytes create proteolytic enzymes, which are then responsible for joint destruction.

Incidence

The true incidence of hip infection is unknown; around 50% of the samples taken from joint aspirate and/or blood come back negative (i.e. normal). The main clinical suspicion signs are:

- Painful hip
- Fever
- Sick child
- Non-weight bearing or antalgic posture

Kocher's criteria are worth considering as they highlight that a limping child with only moderately raised temperature, white cell count and inflammatory markers nevertheless has a high chance of infection, but not necessarily of the joint.

The Kocher algorithm (**Table 23.1**) comprises four parameters:

1. Non-weight bearing
2. Fever > 38°C
3. ESR > 40 mm/hr (CRP > 20)
4. WBC > 12,000/mm^3

Table 23.1 Kocher algorithm – probability of septic arthritis

Parameters present	Probability of septic hip
4 out of 4	99%
3 out of 4	93%
2 out of 4	40%
1 out of 4	3%

Initial management/ prioritization

The main challenge remains to make the initial diagnosis. The presentation in babies and young children can be tricky and the clinical examination difficult in inexperienced hands. A blood test is performed to confirm the WBC, ESR and CRP.

Imaging of the hip is helpful. This can be easily done by a hip ultrasound but this modality is highly operator-dependent. A MRI scan often requires general anesthesia or deep sedation required in young children. Most importantly, time should not be wasted on imaging investigations if drainage is clinically indicated.

Considerations for surgery

Some clinicians use Kocher's algorithm (**Table 23.1**) to differentiate a septic hip and an irritable hip. This can be helpful in the decision-making process, but needs to be weighed carefully with the fact that a mistreated septic hip can permanently alter joint function.

Theater layout and patient positioning

- Supine positioning on a radiolucent table if an image intensifier is to be utilized
- Legs are in abduction or the frog position to be able to palpate the adductor longus tenon/ muscle
- The image intensifier come from the opposite side and the screen is near the head of the patient

Review of surgical approaches

Under general anesthesia and aseptic conditions, the patient is placed in a supine position on the operating table. The surgeon stands on the side of the affected hip.

Hip aspiration: medial approach

- The leg is placed in abduction-flexion-external rotated position (**Figure 23.9c**)
- The surgical site is prepared and draped appropriately
- A 20G spinal needle is introduced at the junction of the skin fold and just under the adductor longus tendon (**Figure 23.9**)
- The needle is kept horizontal and advanced toward the iliac crest. A resistance can be felt when going through the capsule. The position of the needle is controlled under image intensifier guidance
- Injecting 0.5 mL of saline without resistance confirms that the needle is in the joint

Case example: Septic arthritis of the hip joint

A 1-year-old child presented with general malaise, raised temperature and associated limping over 2-day period. Following clinical examination and routine blood tests, an ultrasound scan was undertaken (**Figure 23.9a**).

MRI, when available, can give additional information. In this case, the child refused to weight-bear, and had a fever and an abnormal WBC count. The MRI revealed not only fluid in the joint (septic arthritis of the hip), but also high-intensity signal change in the femoral neck (osteomyelitis) (**Figure 23.9b**).

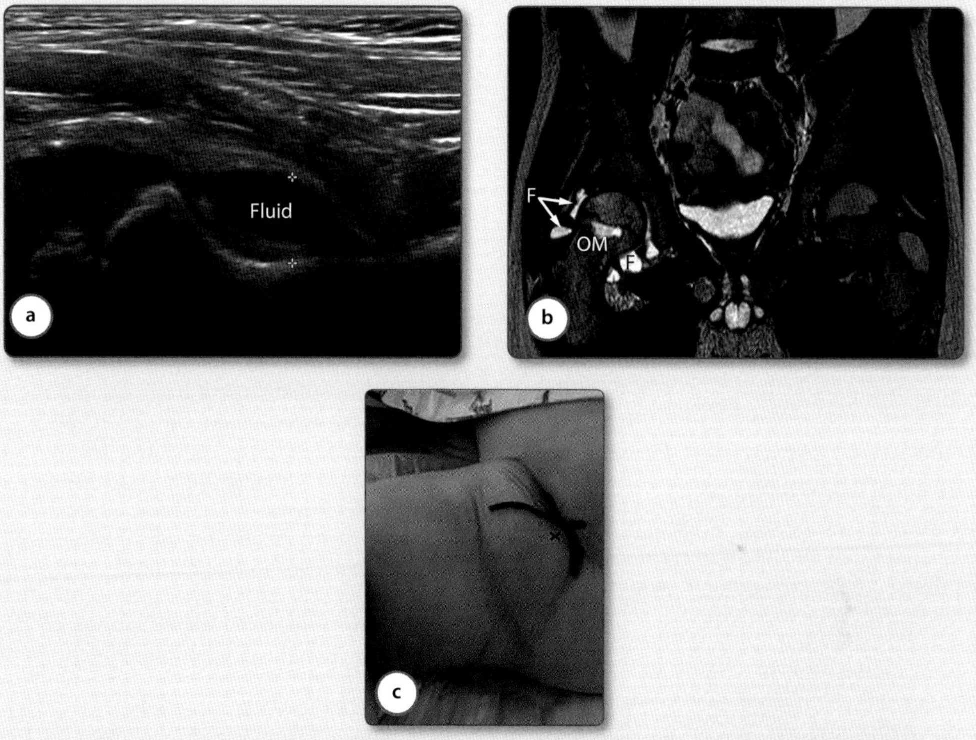

Figure 23.9 (a) Ultrasound of the hip (anterior approach) confirms the presence of fluid in the right hip joint (concave shape of the capsule). The history and clinical examination are suspicious of a septic arthritis and there is a strong indication to at least aspirate the joint. (b) MRI showing fluid in the joint (F, fluid), as well as a high intensity spot in the femoral neck (OM, osteomyelitis). (c) Hip aspiration through a medial approach. The patient is supine at the end of the table: the image intensifier comes from the opposite side. The horizontal line follows the adductor longus tendon. The vertical line follows the skin crease. Enter the needle in the inferior-lateral quadrant (x), horizontal to the floor (or slightly posterior), toward the iliac crest.

- Aspirate the fluid and send it for analysis
- A washout of the joint can be done by injecting and aspirating clear saline through the same needle. This is performed until the aspirated fluid comes back clear

Hip aspiration: anterior approach

- The anterior approach is easier to use for adolescent patients because of the amount of soft tissues in the groin
- The leg is held in a neutral position and preparation of the groin and upper thigh is undertaken
- The spinal needle can be inserted under image intensifier control touching the anterior femoral neck just under the growth plate
- An assistant can then gently flex the hip to loosen the capsule
- Injecting 0.5 mL of saline without resistance confirms that the needle is in the joint. Aspirate the fluid and send it for analysis
- A washout of the joint can be done by injecting and aspirating clear saline through the same needle. This can be performed until the aspirated fluid comes back clear

Hip arthrotomy: Smith-Peterson anterior approach

- An arthrotomy (opening the joint) of the hip is indicated when the fluid (pus) is too thick to be aspirated or when the surgeon wants a more efficient washout of the joint
- The entire lower limb is prepared and draped
- A small Smith-Peterson approach is recommended. Although the interval is the same as that described in Chapter 12 (Figure 12.6a–d), a mini horizontal bikini incision in the skin crease lines can be undertaken
- Sometimes, muscle fibers of the psoas can be attached on the capsule and need to be pushed medially
- A small window (0.5 cm in diameter) of the capsule is made to aspirate specimens and washout the hip joint
- When the joint is clean, leave the window open and close the subcutaneous tissues and skin only

Equipment requirements

Hip aspiration: medial or anterior approach

- G20 spinal needle
- 2 mL syringe of injectable saline
- 5 mL syringe of injectable contrast
- Universal containers for the specimens
- Dressing or spray dressing

Hip arthrotomy: anterior approach

- This will depend on the size of the child, but universal soft tissues set with different sizes Langenbeck retractors (or similar) should be enough to reach the capsule.
- Suction
- 10 mL syringe
- Injectable saline

Rehabilitation and avoiding postoperative complications

The temperature and inflammatory markers are monitored regularly until clinical improvement. Any change of the antibiotic treatment should be undertaken in collaboration with the infectious disease team. Ideally, a protocol for antibiotic treatment should be agreed with the local pediatric team or regional pediatric infectious disease unit. A current tendency is to switch to oral antibiotics as soon as there are signs of efficacy of the treatment. The family should be informed that a few weeks or months may be necessary in order for the patient to recover a normal gait. Protected weight-bearing is recommended in the older population for few weeks.

FEMORAL FRACTURE MANAGEMENT

Introduction

The management of femoral fracture is guided by the site of the fracture, but also by the age of the patient. Fractures of the head and neck of the femur are not discussed in this chapter. They represent less than 1% of all paediatric fractures. Patients with such fractures need to be referred (and/or at least discussed) with specialist centers as an urgent matter. The main complication to avoid is an avascular necrosis of the femoral head. They are also occasionally a predilection site for pathological fractures and require special attention (e.g. MRI scan and/or biopsy).

Types of femoral-shaft fractures:

- Birth injury
- Femoral fracture before school age
- Femoral fracture in older children
- Femoral fracture in teenagers

Incidence

Femoral shaft fractures represent less than 2% of all pediatric fractures. The distribution is bimodal, with a peak incidence at 2 and 12 years of age. The clinician should be aware that femoral fractures in patients under the age of 18 months are a common feature of non-accidental injuries and they should instigate an appropriate pathway for investigation of such injuries within their institution.

Mechanism of injury

The mechanism of injury is often an indirect blow following a fall with moderate velocity (e.g. sport trauma, bicycle fall, etc). The adolescent population requires a higher-energy impact to result in the same injury.

Initial management/ prioritization

Pain management, splintage and traction combined with assessment for associated injuries/fractures are the two priorities.

Definitive treatment

Femoral shaft fractures under the age of 6 months can be treated conservatively in a Pavlik harness for 3–6 weeks.

After 6 months, but before school age (4–5 years), the hip single-leg spica cast is the authors' preferred treatment method. This can be delayed with a few days of traction to reduce the risk of compartment syndrome and avoid the need for a general anesthetic to apply the cast. Definitive traction treatment is also an option. The decision regarding which method should be followed can be made after discussion with the family/carers.

For these two conservative treatments, the aim is not to reduce the fracture, but simply to provide sufficient external stabilization to reduce the discomfort. The remodeling will then correct most of the malunion and shortening.

After school age, the aim is to restore the function of the broken limb as quickly as possible to minimize school non-attendance. Therefore, a minimally invasive technique, such as elastic stable intramedullary nailing (ESIN), is often offered to the family. The limit of this technique is the size of the nails that can be used. Teenagers over 50 kg in weight are better managed with an intramedullary nail, but it is mandatory to lock the distal bolt above the distal femoral growth plate. In older children where the fracture extends to the metaphyseal region or the medullary canal is too narrow for locked intramedullary nailing, submuscular plate fixation using a minimally invasive plate osteosynthesis (MIPO) technique is an alternative strategy.

Theater layout and patient positioning

The patient is positioned supine with free leg draping on a radiolucent table.

Review of surgical approaches

Bilateral distal entry points

Bilateral distal entry points are created in the bone with an awl or drill which is angled proximally to make passage of the nails easier (**Figure 23.11b**). This is the common technique for most of the femoral shaft fractures treated with ESIN. Both medial and lateral entry points can be created with a drill 2–3 cm above the distal femoral growth plate. The nails can then be progressed proximally simultaneously.

Proximal femur entry points

When the fracture is too distal for distal nail insertion to control the fractures, two entry points are made at the proximal femur on the lateral side at the level of the lesser trochanter. As the bone is more solid in this region, the authors recommend two separated drill entry holes with 1–2 cm of gap between both for nail insertion.

Case example: Non-operatively managed femoral fracture

A 3-year-old boy fell off a low wall, landing awkwardly on concrete. He was unable to weight-bear subsequently and brought to the emergency department. Initial X-rays (**Figure 23.10a, b**) confirm a spiral diaphysial femoral fracture. He was initially managed using skin traction followed by hip spica application on the ward after approximately 10-days. X-rays taken after removal of the hip spica confirm union (**Figure 23.10c, d**). The residual deformity will continue too remodel whilst the femur grows.

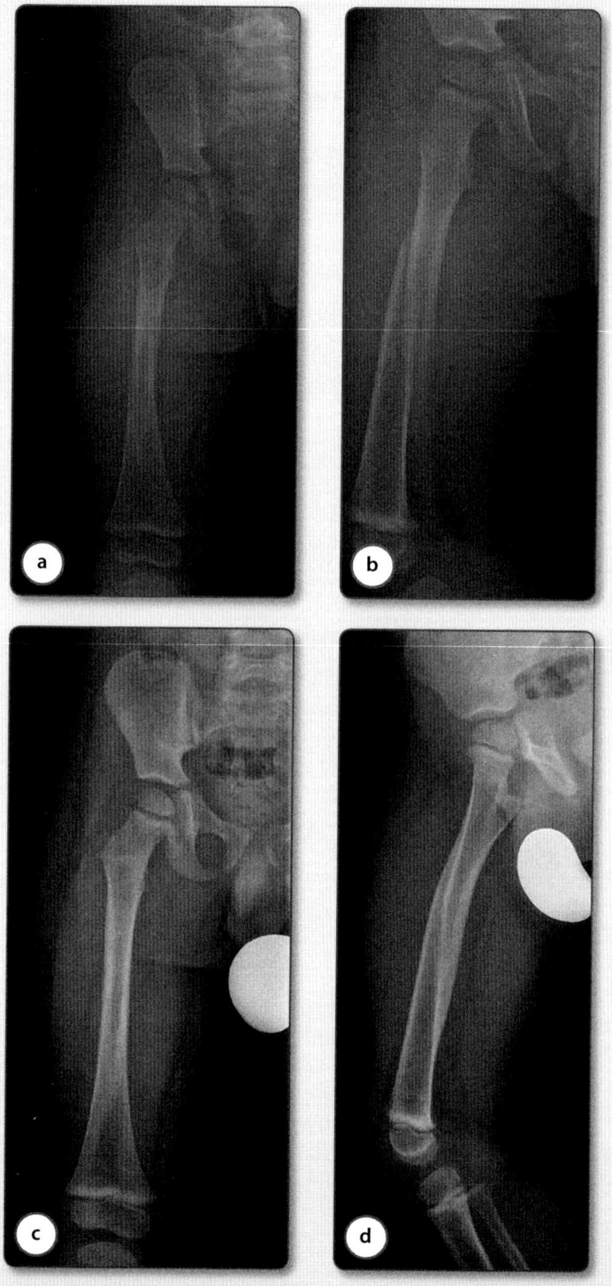

Figure 23.10 (a, b) AP and lateral X-rays of right spiral femoral fracture. (c, d) X-rays following conservative treatment (traction and spica cast) at 7 months post-injury.

Case example: Surgically stabilized femoral fracture

An 8-year-old girl fell out of a tree and injured her left leg. The clinical deformity was corrected with traction in the emergency department and X-rays taken (**Figure 23.11a**).

She was admitted to the pediatric ward for planned theater, in order to reduce her hospital stay and improve fracture alignment and rotation. She underwent fracture stabilization with retrograde flexible nails as per **Figure 23.11c, d**.

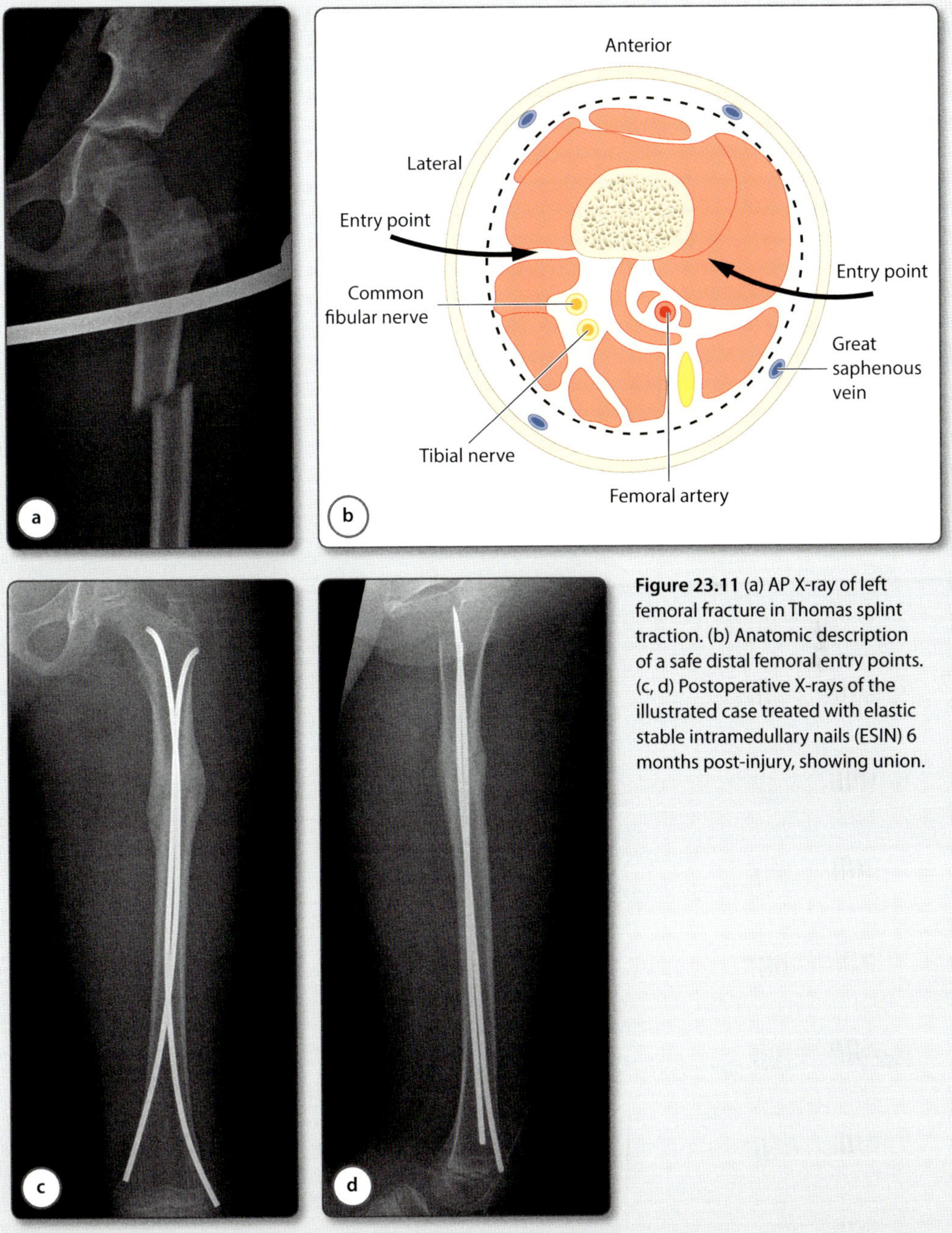

Figure 23.11 (a) AP X-ray of left femoral fracture in Thomas splint traction. (b) Anatomic description of a safe distal femoral entry points. (c, d) Postoperative X-rays of the illustrated case treated with elastic stable intramedullary nails (ESIN) 6 months post-injury, showing union.

Equipment requirements

- Basic instrument for the mini incision
- Elastic nail instruments and implants
- Image intensifier
- Drill to create entry points
- Nail sizes used: 3.0 mm (6–8 years); 3.5 mm (8–10 years); 4.0 mm (>11 years)

Reduction and stabilization methods

It is not difficult to restore the length of the femur when the patient is asleep with muscle relaxant medication. There is therefore no need to use a traction table. However, the pattern of the fracture can make the reduction difficult. Most of the elastic nail instrument sets include a reduction tool that can be useful. Often, both nails are inserted to the level of the fracture and then progressed, while reduction is maintained. Excessive rotation of the nail in the intramedullary canal should be avoided to avoid the 'plait' effect. Other difficulties include maintaining the rotation (transverse fracture) and avoiding residual angulations (oblique/spiral fracture).

Rehabilitation

- Progressive weight bearing under physiotherapy supervision
- Maintenance of knee and hip ROM, as distal aspect of elastic nails can irritate the soft tissues
- Progressive muscle strengthening as rehabilitation increases
- planned elective removal of metal work after 12 months

Index

Note: Page numbers in **bold** or *italic* refer to tables or figures, respectively.